NUTRIENT TIMING

Metabolic Optimization for Health, Performance, and Recovery

NUTRIENT TIMING

Metabolic Optimization for Health, Performance, and Recovery

Edited by

CHAD M. KERKSICK

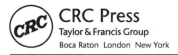

CRC Press
Taylor & Francis Group
Boca Raton London New York

CRC Press is an imprint of the
Taylor & Francis Group, an **informa** business

CRC Press
Taylor & Francis Group
6000 Broken Sound Parkway NW, Suite 300
Boca Raton, FL 33487-2742

First issued in paperback 2019

© 2012 by Taylor & Francis Group, LLC
CRC Press is an imprint of Taylor & Francis Group, an Informa business

No claim to original U.S. Government works

ISBN-13: 978-1-4398-3889-1 (hbk)
ISBN-13: 978-0-367-38223-0 (pbk)

Library of Congress Cataloging-in-Publication Data

Nutrient timing : metabolic optimization for health, performance, and recovery / editor, Chad M. Kerksick.
    p. ; cm.
Includes bibliographical references and index.
ISBN-13: 978-1-4398-3889-1 (hardcover : alk. paper)
ISBN-10: 1-58488-558-0 (hardcover : alk. paper)
    1. Athletes--Nutrition. 2. Energy metabolism. 3. Bioenergetics. I. Kerksick, Chad M.
    [DNLM: 1. Athletic Performance--physiology. 2. Nutrition Processes. 3. Dietary Proteins--metabolism. 4. Energy Metabolism--physiology. 5. Resistance Training. QU 145]

TX361.A8N82 2012
613.2024796--dc23   2011017672

Visit the Taylor & Francis Web site at
http://www.taylorandfrancis.com

and the CRC Press Web site at
http://www.crcpress.com

Dedication

This book and the efforts it represents are first dedicated to my grandparents. Within a year of each other, the family lost my Dad's parents, Grandpa Arvie and Grandma Dixie. Sadly, within the next year we lost my Mom's father, Grandpa Don, as well. All left me too early, and living documents such as this book will document for years the impact they made and the love they left behind. Then there is Grandma Jeanie, my lone living grandparent. In no way can I explain in a few sentences the impact and memories I have of this woman. One day our lives will too part, but I want you and anyone else who reads this book to know that I love you, and I thank you for all the cookies you've baked, hems you've stitched, and the conversations we've shared.

Finally, this book is also dedicated to fellow scientists across the world who study the things they do for reasons that many people likely don't understand or appreciate, but I for one am thankful for all of your efforts.

Contents

Preface

This book is part of the continual efforts of CRC and Taylor & Francis to provide relevant, meaningful titles in areas that relate to exercise, nutrition, and health. Nutrient timing is a concept that has evolved into a practice. While it certainly is considered as an aspect of nutrition, its existence lies particularly in the application of knowledge. Whereas some areas are considered foundational content, the timing of nutrients surrounding exercise or other periods of stress has been and continues to be widely considered as a strategy or method performed by athletes or other active individuals that may confer improved adaptations to the exercise or stressor invoked. Make no mistake about it, this mind-set or concept overall is in its infancy as the number of studies that have particularly been designed to examine timing are limited. Researchers, coaches, and athletes abroad have jumped onboard and fueled its flames, resulting in it growing into something that is discussed on many continents and in many sports nutrition or applied physiology laboratories throughout the world.

The book is separated into three sections. The first section operates as an introduction, with Chapter 1 leading the way as a "placement" of nutrient timing into the world of sports. Concluding this section are chapters focusing on the macronutrients and a general overview of their role in sporting activity and a chapter focusing on vitamins and minerals. The middle section could be considered the "meat" of the book as this section consists of chapters that focus exclusively on the preexercise, during exercise, and postexercise considerations for both resistance and aerobically mediated activity. The final section could be looked upon as "the future" or the "speculative/daring" aspect of the book. Chapters in this section are devoted to concepts themselves inside nutrient timing. Here, the impact of protein source is considered in the context of timing. In addition, nutrient timing is discussed regarding how it can fit in with a comprehensive recovery program. Finally, two chapters are exclusively devoted to discussing the application of these concepts in alternative/unique populations, including the aged, the military, and populations interested in weight loss. Organization of this task began with corralling the single best group of scientists, future scientists, and practitioners that I could to complete the work. I was humbled by the response as the authors represent five countries and three continents, and many of these people are truly the best in the business in not only their respective universities, but also their respective countries. Thus, it was my hope to deliver one of the most authoritative books to date discussing the scientific application of the concept of nutrient timing. I leave it up to its readers to decide whether this goal was achieved.

Chad M. Kerksick, PhD
Health and Exercise Science Department
University of Oklahoma
Chad.Kerksick@gmail.com

Acknowledgments

First to my parents, Gary and Kathy, who taught me so many important things about life: how to work hard, how to love, how to care, and how to have fun: Thank you! Thanks to my sister, Kelly, and for the strength with which our relationship grew during our time together in Memphis; those times will remain as some of the best of my life. Acknowledgment goes to Dr. Jerry Mayhew, Dr. Fontaine Piper, Dr. Chris Lantz, Clint Thompson, and Michelle Boyd, all at Truman State University; thank you for the opportunities, love, and energy you showed a young mind filled with energy and little direction. Dr. Richard Kreider, whom I first met at the University of Memphis and followed to Baylor University, provided me with countless opportunities to grow, write, and present and who I still count on for honest, professional advice. I hope a work such as this gives you great satisfaction knowing you had a major role in its development. Thank you to Darryn Willoughby and Mike Greenwood for the compassion and opportunities you've provided and lessons you gave me. I am grateful to Joel Cramer and Jeff Stout at the Health and Exercise Science Department at the University of Oklahoma who have proved to be true and supportive colleagues. Other professional colleagues such as Lee Brown, Mike Iosia, Mark Faries, the "Trailblazers," and "The Six Pack" made graduate school fun and productive.

Next, the devotion and expertise provided by the contributors of this textbook is, as I said before, humbling. Many of you are so busy, but yet your passion and devotion somehow created time for this project. Without your minds and hearts, this book would not have been possible.

Finally, to Adrien, my newest and the most important member of my family, thank you for saying yes to my proposal a few short years ago. Your devotion, dedication, and understanding of my imperfections early on in our marriage are something I hope to pay forward more than a few hundred times over. I do want you to know that I truly do love you and all that you are. To me, you are and always will be perfect. I continue to remain very excited about what life has in store for us.

Chad

About the Editor

Chad M. Kerksick, PhD, FACSM, FISSN, ATC, CSCS*D, NSCA-CPT*D, is currently an assistant professor of exercise physiology in the Health and Exercise Science Department at the University of Oklahoma. He founded, developed, and directs the Applied Biochemistry and Molecular Physiology Laboratory and holds adjunct positions in the Endocrinology and Diabetes Section with the Department of Pediatrics and Department of Physiology at the University of Oklahoma Health Sciences Center. He received his PhD in exercise, nutrition, and preventive health from Baylor University; his master's degree in exercise and sport science from the University of Memphis; and has a bachelor of science in exercise science with an emphasis in athletic training and exercise physiology from Truman State University. He is recognized as a Fellow of the American College of Sports Medicine and International Society of Sports Nutrition and currently holds national certifications as an athletic trainer (ATC) by the National Athletic Trainers Association (NATA) and strength and conditioning specialist (CSCS*D) and personal trainer (NSCA-CPT*D) with distinction from the National Strength and Conditioning Association. He currently teaches exercise testing and prescription at both the undergraduate and graduate levels in addition to exercise and nutritional biochemistry at the doctoral level. He has worked with numerous athletes in addition to specific sports teams, ranging from high school athletes to professional athletes, providing consulting on areas related to strength and conditioning, nutrition, and recovery. His primary research interests include sport nutrition as well as the biochemical, cellular, and molecular adaptations relative to various forms of exercise and nutrition interventions. Specifically, his research continues to combine applied and basic science techniques to examine changes in skeletal muscle and the resulting impact on metabolic health, sarcopenia, muscle hypertrophy, and prevention of muscle atrophy in healthy as well as clinical populations.

Contributors

Elizabeth M. Broad
Sports Nutrition
Australian Institute of Sport
Belconnen, Australia

Louise M. Burke
Sports Nutrition
Australian Institute of Sport
Belconnen, Australia

Amanda Carlson-Phillips
Athletes' Performance Institute
Phoenix, Arizona, USA

Tyler Churchward-Venne
Exercise Metabolism Research Group
Department of Kinesiology
McMaster University
Hamilton, Ontario, Canada

Vincent J. Dalbo
Institute for Health and Social Science
    Research
School of Medicine and Applied Sciences
Central Queensland University
Rockhampton, Queensland, Australia

Kristin Dugan
Department of Exercise and Sport
    Science
University of Mary Hardin-Baylor
Belton, Texas, USA

Craig Friedman
Athletes' Performance Institute
Phoenix, Arizona, USA

Mark Haub
Kansas State University
Manhattan, Kansas, USA

John A. Hawley
Exercise Metabolism Group
School of Medical Sciences
RMIT University
Bundoora, Victoria, Australia

Nikki A. Jeacocke
Sports Nutrition
Australian Institute of Sport
Belconnen, Australia

Leonidas G. Karagounis
Exercise Metabolism Group
School of Medical Sciences
RMIT University
Bundoora, Victoria, Australia

Chad M. Kerksick
Health and Exercise Science
    Department
University of Oklahoma
Norman, Oklahoma, USA

Nicholas D. Luden
James Madison University
Department of Kinesiology
Harrisonburg, Virginia, USA

William Lunn
Exercise Science Department
Southern Connecticut State University
Human Performance Lab
New Haven, Connecticut, USA

Stu Phillips
Exercise Metabolism Research Group
Department of Kinesiology
McMaster University
Hamilton, Ontario, Canada

Chris N. Poole
Health and Exercise Science
  Department
University of Oklahoma
Norman, Oklahoma, USA

Michael D. Roberts
Department of Biomedical Sciences
University of Missouri-Columbia
Columbia, Missouri, USA

Nancy R. Rodriguez
University of Connecticut
Storrs, Connecticut, USA

Michael J. Saunders
Department of Kinesiology
James Madison University
Harrisonburg, Virginia, USA

Bob Seebohar
Fuel4mance, LLC
Littleton, Colorado, USA

Jeffrey R. Stout
Health and Exercise Science
  Department
University of Oklahoma
Norman, Oklahoma, USA

Kyle Sunderland
Health and Exercise Science
  Department
University of Oklahoma
Norman, Oklahoma, USA

Lem Taylor
University of Mary Hardin-Baylor
Belton, Texas, USA

Kevin D. Tipton
Department of Sports Studies
University of Stirling
Stirling, Scotland, UK

Colin Wilborn
University of Mary Hardin-Baylor
Belton, Texas, USA

Robert Wildman
Department of Food and Nutrition
Texas State University
San Marcos, Texas, USA

Oliver C. Witard
Exercise Metabolism Research Group
School of Sport and Exercise Sciences
University of Birmingham
Edgbaston, Birmingham, UK

1 The Basis of Nutrient Timing and Its Place in Sport and Metabolic Regulation

Louise M. Burke and Nikki A. Jeacocke

CONTENTS

1.1 TACKLING THE TOPIC OF NUTRIENT TIMING

Although sports nutrition goals are specific to each sport and each individual athlete, there are some common themes. The goals of the training diet include helping the athlete to get or stay "in shape," in terms of their physique and health, as well as maximizing the adaptive response to the stimulus of each exercise session. The culmination of these adaptations is to prepare the athlete to be better able to undertake future exercise

1

tasks, particularly competitive events. Competition nutrition goals focus on further identifying the physiological limitations to the performance of a sport and organizing nutrient intake to try to reduce or delay the onset of such "fatigue factors."

The aim of this book is to explore the ways in which nutritional strategies or intakes of nutrients can be timed to best achieve training, nutrition, as well as more health-aligned goals. Different aspects are highlighted in depth in the following chapters. The specific goal of this chapter is to provide a brief introduction to the concept of periodization or timing of nutrient intake. To do this, a number of ways are summarized in which athletes may be guided to manipulate the timing of nutritional strategies and nutrient intake to achieve the ultimate goal of peak performance on the day of important competitions. This moves from a global view of periodizing nutrition goals over the training and competition year; to the specific timing of nutrient intake before, during, and after an exercise session; and finally, to the general spacing of food and fluid intake over the rest of the day in the life of the athlete. Provided is an overview of each issue with direction to sources of further information within this text and elsewhere. Although the chapters focus on the benefits of the specific timing of intake of nutrients or nutritional strategies for elite athletic performance, there may be spin-offs of well-timed nutrition on the metabolic and health benefits of exercise for those who undertake recreational exercise, recovery needs, the aged, military, and metabolic complications.

1.2 PERIODIZING NUTRITION GOALS WITHIN THE ATHLETE'S YEARLY PLAN

Sports nutrition has evolved since the 1970s from a series of disjointed ideas and practices into an established and integrated science. This is evidenced by the substantial number of peer-reviewed studies that are published annually on nutritional themes for athletes or the interaction of nutrition and exercise, the establishment of professional bodies dedicated to career pathways for sports nutritionists and dietitians, and the promotion of position stands on nutrition for sports performance by prestigious bodies such as the American College of Sports Medicine (Rodriguez et al. 2009), the International Olympic Committee ("IOC Consensus Statement" 2004), and most recently, the International Society of Sports Nutrition (Buford et al. 2007; Campbell et al. 2007; Kerksick et al. 2008). Modern guidelines for sports nutrition have the sophistication of being underpinned by a strong base of evidence and the cognizance that dietary practices need to be event specific, suited to each individual athlete, and periodized to meet differences in goals across time, ranging from a training microcycle to a whole sporting career. A brief summary of goals for different issues in sports nutrition is provided in Table 1.1, with these divided into themes for the training and competition phases.

1.2.1 NUTRITIONAL NEEDS ACCORDING TO TRAINING AND COMPETITION LOAD

Although an athlete's major goals and preparation may span a longer period such as the four-year Olympic cycle or the years of a college scholarship, the annual plan

TABLE 1.1
Goals of Sports Nutrition

Training Phase

- Meet the energy and fuel requirements needed to support a training program
- Achieve and maintain an ideal physique for their event; manipulate training and nutrition to achieve a level of body mass, body fat, and muscle mass that is consistent with good health and good performance
- Enhance adaptation and recovery between training sessions by providing all the nutrients associated with these processes
- Refuel and rehydrate well during each training session to perform optimally at each session
- Practice any intended competition nutrition strategies so that beneficial practices can be identified and fine-tuned
- Maintain optimal health and function, especially by meeting the increased needs for some nutrients resulting from heavy training
- Reduce the risk of sickness and injury during heavy training periods by maintaining healthy physique and energy balance and by supplying nutrients believed to assist immune function (e.g., consume carbohydrate during prolonged exercise sessions)
- Make well-considered decisions about the use of supplements and specialized sport foods that have been shown to enhance training performance or meet training nutrition needs
- Eat for long-term health by following healthy eating guidelines
- Enjoy food and the pleasure of sharing meals

Competition Phase

- In weight division sports, achieve the competition weight division with minimal harm to health or performance
- Fuel up adequately before an event by consuming carbohydrate and tapering exercise during the days before the event according to the importance and duration of the event; use carbohydrate-loading strategies when appropriate before events of greater than 90 minutes duration
- Top up carbohydrate stores with a pre-event meal or snack during the 1 to 4 hours before competition
- Keep hydration at an acceptable level during the event by drinking appropriate amounts of fluids before, during, and after the event
- Consume carbohydrate during events of greater than 1 hour in duration or if body carbohydrate stores become depleted
- Achieve fluid and food intake before and during the event without causing gastrointestinal discomfort or upsets
- Promote recovery after the event, particularly during multiday competitions such as tournaments and stage races
- During a prolonged competition program, ensure that competition eating does not compromise overall energy and nutrient intake goals
- Make well-considered decisions about the use of supplements and specialized sport foods that have been shown to enhance competition performance or meet competition needs

Source: Adapted from Burke, L.M., ed. Training and Competition Nutrition. Edited by Burke, L.M., *Practical Sports Nutrition.* Champaign, IL: Human Kinetics, 2007.

provides a convenient template to examine the concept of periodization. Typically, the centerpiece of this plan is the important competition at which the athlete wishes to perform at a peak level; depending on the event and the prevailing philosophies in a sport, the coach and athlete may plan for a single or double peak for the year. Peaking is a challenge for team sports, for which the competitive season lasts several months and players need to be at their peak for the final series over the last weeks but to play well enough over the duration of the season to ensure their inclusion among the teams chosen for the playoff.

The annual calendar varies considerably between sports according to factors such as the nature of competition (e.g., longer-term fixtures versus short-term tournaments); the level of the athlete (e.g., opportunities to compete will vary between developmental, recreational, and elite athletes); and the type of event (how much recovery is needed). However, common elements in the periodized training calendar include a generalized preparation phase, a period of training that is more specific to the competition event, competition itself, and transition between phases, including an off-season or rest period. Figure 1.1 provides a summary of the typical phasing of training periods in the preparation of a middle-distance athlete (Stellingwerff, Boit, et al. 2007), noting guidelines for the energy and macronutrient intake needed to support the workloads at each different phase. In such a scheme, nutrient periodization is clearly driven by the fuel cost of the prevailing exercise program with energy and carbohydrate intakes increasing at times of high volume and intensity, during both training phases and the racing season.

We have further evolved the concept of nutritional periodization to identify two driving goals of the nutritional support underpinning each phase:

- To provide nutritional support for the specific training undertaken during that phase
- To prepare the athlete to achieve the physical, physiological, and behavioral characteristics needed for peak performance phases (competition)

Figures 1.2 and 1.3 provide a simplistic view of the periodized calendar for two different types of sports, incorporating key features of the training focus across a year. Figure 1.2 illustrates the changing goals of a swimmer who needs to peak for selection into a national team then undertake another training cycle before racing at a major international competition, such as the Olympic Games or world championships. A lengthy phase of general training with high-volume work is interspersed with race-specific training cycles involving greater focus on training intensity, specialized training at altitude, or competition at world cups or minor meets. Significant training tapers, which involve a substantial reduction in training volume but maintenance of training intensity, are undertaken to achieve a performance peak at the selection trials and the international competition. Of course, even within these macrocycles and microcycles, there will be a periodizing of the training week with fluctuations of training modes (pool work, gym and other "dry land" training) as well as volume and intensity. A major break of three to four weeks is undertaken at the end of the international competition, while smaller breaks (four to seven days) may also be included within the training year.

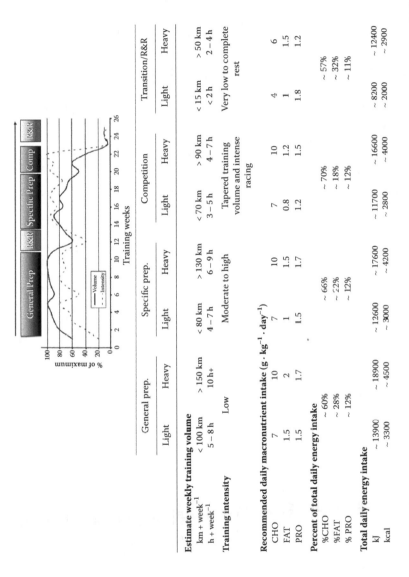

	General prep.		Specific prep.		Competition		Transition/R&R	
	Light	Heavy	Light	Heavy	Light	Heavy	Light	Heavy
Estimate weekly training volume								
km + week⁻¹	< 100 km	> 150 km	< 80 km	> 130 km	< 70 km	> 90 km	< 15 km	> 50 km
h + week⁻¹	5 – 8 h	10 h+	4 – 7 h	6 – 9 h	3 – 5 h	4 – 7 h	< 2 h	2 – 4 h
Training intensity	Low		Moderate to high		Tapered training volume and intense racing		Very low to complete rest	
Recommended daily macronutrient intake (g · kg⁻¹ · day⁻¹)								
CHO	7	10	7	10	7	10	4	6
FAT	1.5	2	1	1.5	0.8	1.2	1	1.5
PRO	1.5	1.7	1.5	1.7	1.2	1.5	1.8	1.2
Percent of total daily energy intake								
%CHO	~60%		~66%		~70%		~57%	
%FAT	~28%		~22%		~18%		~32%	
%PRO	~12%		~12%		~12%		~11%	
Total daily energy intake								
kJ	~13900	~18900	~12600	~17600	~11700	~16600	~8200	~12400
kcal	~3300	~4500	~3000	~4200	~2800	~4000	~2000	~2900

FIGURE 1.1 Training and nutritional periodization for middle-distance running. Prep = preparation; R&R = rest and recovery; CHO = carbohydrate; PRO = protein. (From Stellingwerff, T., M.K. Boit, and P.T. Res. Nutritional Strategies to Optimize Training and Racing in Middle-Distance Athletes. *J Sports Sci* 25 Suppl 1:S17–28, 2007.)

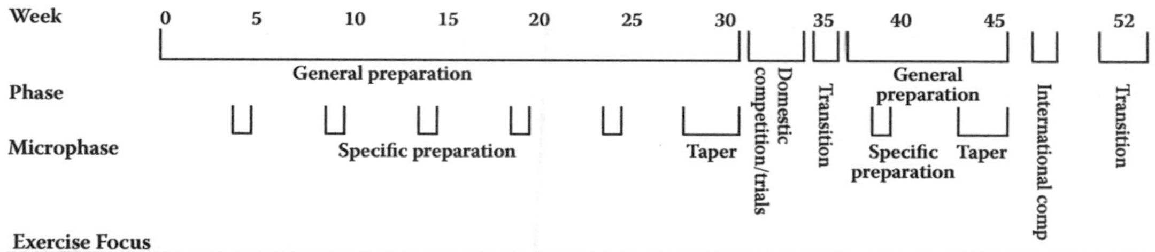

Week | 0 | 5 | 10 | 15 | 20 | 25 | 30 | 35 | 40 | 45 | 52

Phase: General preparation | Specific preparation | General preparation | Taper

Microphase

Transition — Domestic competition/trials — Transition — International comp — Transition

Specific preparation

Exercise Focus

General preparation	• high volume • mixed training modalities including resistance training, core stability, cross-training
Specific preparation	• race practice • increase in intensity • decrease in volume • could include specialized training (e.g., altitude training) • may include shorter domestic/international competitions (e.g., World Cups)
Taper	• reduction in training leading into competition
Competition	• competition racing

Nutrition Focus

General preparation	• support desired changes in body composition • general recovery after each session
Specific preparation	• support change in training focus • specific support/recovery for key sessions or specialized training
Taper	• support high intensity training but avoid unnecessary weight gain associated with a decrease in training volume
Competition	• support racing but avoid unnecessary weight gain associated with a decrease in training

FIGURE 1.2 Training and nutritional periodization for swimming.

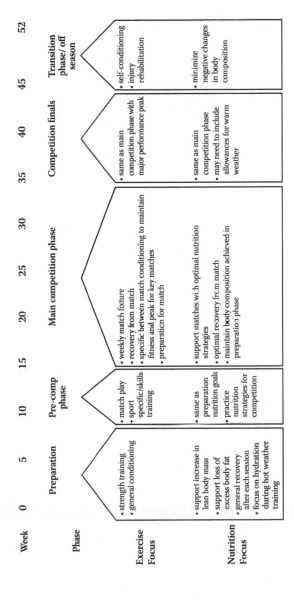

Week	0	5	10	15	20	25	30	35	40	45	52

Phase	Preparation	Pre-comp phase	Main competition phase	Competition finals	Transition phase/ off season
Exercise Focus	• strength training • general conditioning	• match play • sport specific/skills training	• weekly match fixture • recovery from match • specific between match conditioning to maintain fitness and peak for key matches • preparation for match	• same as main competition phase with major performance peak	• self-conditioning • injury rehabilitation
Nutrition Focus	• support increase in lean body mass • support loss of excess body fat • general recovery after each session • focus on hydration during hot weather training	• same as preparation nutrition goals • practice nutrition strategies for competition	• support matches with optimal nutrition strategies • optimal recovery from match • maintain body composition achieved in preparation phase	• same as main competition phase • may need to include allowances for warm weather	• minimize negative changes in body composition

FIGURE 1.3 Training and nutritional periodization for team sports.

Some of the elements of the periodized nutrition support for this training plan are summarized in Figure 1.2. These include an emphasis on manipulating body composition at the beginning of the season to reduce any body fat gains associated with the previous break as well as to increase muscle mass and strength over the general training phase. Specific fueling for prolonged high-intensity sessions should be built into the training week, as well as recovery after key pool workouts and gym sessions. Opportunities to practice specific race day nutrition strategies such as the prerace meal or use of ergogenic aids (bicarbonate for buffering or caffeine for fatigue resistance) might be built into specific preparation periods, including races at minor meets. Although minitapers may be built into these cycles, the swimmer may only undertake a substantial taper prior to the main competitions for their year. Such tapers will involve a significant reduction in training volume for most swimmers and necessitate an appropriate reduction in energy intake so that a gain in fat mass is avoided. This often requires a specific eating plan since the reduction in training volume often coincides with factors that can promote an increase in energy intake, such as having more free time in the day for social activities or residence in an athlete village with an "all-you-can-eat" or buffet-style dining facility.

Different periodization of training and nutrition can be seen in the annual calendar of a team sport player (Figure 1.3). This player is scheduled to have a longer off-season "break" or freedom from organized training activities. Depending on the level of play, the individual motivation of the player or the need for corrective surgery/rehabilitation for chronic injuries, this can be a time of minimal activity leading to substantial deconditioning of fitness and physique characteristics. Although this code might be a "winter" team sport, the preparation phase, involving general conditioning activities that may occur in summer months, requires players to practice hydration strategies suited for hot weather. Manipulations of physique are a key focus of this general phase. During the specific conditioning phase, there is an increase in skill-based and match-intensity training, including match practice and a preseason minifixture (i.e., minicamps) competition. Players will be expected to fine-tune match practices such as preevent eating, use of game day ergogenic aids, and intake of fluid and carbohydrate during a game. Recovery eating strategies will have been practiced after key training sessions during conditioning and specific preparation phases but will now need to include tactics that can be practiced "on the road." These periods of time are important to allow for athletes and coaches to determine what food types, sizes, and mixtures best suit individual needs.

The lengthy competition period in this team sport involves a weekly game, interspersed with a training program that juggles a changing priority of postmatch recovery, maintenance of conditioning, and some minipeaks for important games. Daily nutrition support will change according to the phase of the weekly cycle as well as the particular goals of the phase but may also need to consider requirements for interstate travel lasting three to four days. The final series may be played in warmer weather, again necessitating an alteration in the game day fluid and fueling practices. There will be individualization of daily and game day nutrition practices according to the specific requirements of a player's activity patterns during a match as well as any individual nutrition goals. The concept and case histories of training and nutritional periodization are covered in more detail in Chapter 13.

1.2.2 Opportunities to Alter Physique

Physique characteristics such as muscle mass and body fat levels play an important role in the performance of many sports, and athletes achieve their ideal levels as a result of the genetic potential that has made them gravitate to their sport in the first place as well as the conditioning effects of training and nutrition. Loss of body fat is underpinned by a chronic implementation of a moderate energy deficit, which can be achieved by an increase in energy expenditure, a decrease in energy intake, or a combination of both strategies. Ideally, this should be achieved without compromising hormonal and general body function, sacrificing bone and immune health, or interfering with training capacity or adaptations. Loucks (2004) has coined the term of *energy availability*, which is defined operationally as the difference between energy intake and the cost of the daily exercise program. Tracking energy intake and expenditure so that net energy availability is above 30 kilocalories per kilogram body mass (kcal/kg) should allow an energy deficit with modest impact to body homeostasis (Loucks 2004). Even so, the athlete should consider the overall timing of weight loss projects within the sporting calendar, limiting it to the preseason or the early phase of general preparation, when it will have the least impact on training capacity and adaptation. In addition, all athletes and coaches should understand that the best option is to minimize the amount of excess body fat gained during periods of inactivity, such as injury recovery or the off-season, so that the need for, or duration of, periods of fat loss are reduced.

Within a fat loss eating plan, the athlete should also periodize daily energy intake or the macronutrient contribution to energy intake to prioritize nutrition support for the most important workouts within the weekly training microcycle. Chapters 6 to 10 describe nutritional practices before, during, and after endurance and resistive training sessions that promote training capacity, adaptation, and recovery. The athlete will often need to balance the dual priorities of restricting energy intake while practicing some or all of these strategies to promote training outcomes. Most research on weight loss in sports nutrition has focused on the needs of athletes who "make weight" immediately prior to the competition weigh-in for a weight division sport, and curiously, we lack investigations of different approaches to fat loss during the early phase of a conditioning or injury rehabilitation program. Whether it is better to achieve weight loss quickly but still within healthy guidelines or over a longer period that provides more flexibility to meet nutritional goals for optimal training is a topic of great interest to many athletes.

As well as directing energy intake toward nutrition support for specific training sessions, there may be issues of timing of energy intake over the day or the promotion of certain nutrients within a fat loss diet that directly affect body fat levels. For example, there is some evidence of a relationship between the spread of energy intake within a day and body fatness in athletes (a concept discussed in greater detail regarding weight loss in Chapter 16); runners and gymnasts who experienced long periods of a lack of energy intake over the day had higher body fat levels than counterparts who spread their intake more evenly over the day and around training sessions (Deutz et al. 2000). The hypothesized benefits of incorporation of dairy products into fat loss diets (Major et al. 2008) also merit investigation in athletic populations.

Gain of muscle mass and strength is an additional goal of physique manipulation by athletes and is achieved by the interaction of resistance training and dietary intake, particularly the timing, type, and amount of dietary protein after a workout and over the day (Burd, Tang, et al. 2009). Nutrient timing to enhance the outcomes of such training is covered in great detail in Chapters 9, 10, and 12. In most sports, the main period of muscle gain is scheduled for the general conditioning phase, although a resistance program will typically be continued to maintain (or minimize the loss of) muscle mass and strength during the competition phases of a season.

1.2.3 "TRAIN LOW" TO ENHANCE THE TRAINING RESPONSE

The nutritional guidelines for training currently promote practices that provide nutrition support for each exercise session with the goal of maximizing training capacity (the "train hard" or "train better" principle). However, there is a new hypothesis that exercising within an environment of low nutritional support might stimulate greater adaptation to the same training stimulus (a "train smarter" or "train low" approach). This has been explored in relation to carbohydrate intake.

The current sports nutrition guidelines, while no longer promoting a high-carbohydrate intake for all athletes per se, recommend that the daily eating patterns of athletes provide sufficient amounts of carbohydrate to meet the fuel requirements for training/competition and recovery (Burke 2010b). However, some studies have found that when exercise is undertaken with low muscle glycogen content, the transcription of a number of genes involved in training adaptations is enhanced (for review, see Baar and McGee 2008). This has led to a paradigm that athletes should train with low-carbohydrate availability to enhance the training response but compete with high fuel availability to promote performance. There are a number of potential ways to reduce carbohydrate availability for the training environment, including doing two training sessions in close succession without opportunity for refueling or training in a fasted state with only water intake. Furthermore, it should be pointed out that these do not always promote a low-carbohydrate diet per se or restrict carbohydrate availability for all training sessions.

The study underpinning the interest in the train low idea involved a clever design in which untrained participants trained one leg for an hour each day, then performed the same training sessions with their other leg, except training was scheduled as two workouts in close succession on one day, then a rest day before the next two workouts. Since subjects consumed a carbohydrate intake designed to refuel on a daily basis, the study was able to compare outcomes of a leg that "trained high" against a leg that "trained 50% of the time low." Both legs were found to improve their maximal power equally as a result of training, but the "low leg" showed a greater increase in various muscle enzymes and glycogen synthesis and a bigger improvement in its exercise capacity (time to fatigue at a set power). Naturally, this study created a buzz in the sports world despite its lack of direct application to trained athletes undertaking more conventional exercise activities according to the training principles of progressive overload.

Further studies in subelite athletes have confirmed that train low strategies can increase metabolic enzymes and markers in the muscle—suggesting that there is an amplification of the training response (Cox et al. 2010; Hulston et al. 2010; Yeo et al. 2010). However, none has found evidence that this leads to performance enhancements. Indeed, there are potential disadvantages to the health and performance of the athlete, including the not insignificant likelihood that training low may interfere with the volume or intensity of training (Hulston et al. 2010; Yeo et al. 2010).

Clearly, more research is needed, but the current position is that we have insufficient proof to provide guidelines to athletes for incorporating train low strategies into their training programs. In real life, however, we note that most elite athletes periodize their carbohydrate environment for training; either by intent or for practicality, some training sessions are undertaken with low-carbohydrate status (overnight fasting, several sessions in the day, little carbohydrate intake during the workout), while others are undertaken using strategies that promote carbohydrate status (more recovery time, postmeal, carbohydrate intake during the session). It makes sense that sessions undertaken at lower intensity or at the beginning of a training cycle are most suited or perhaps, least disadvantaged by, train low strategies. Conversely, "quality" sessions done at higher intensities or in the transition to peaking for competition are likely to be best undertaken with better fuel support (or hydration levels). Athletes may, by accident or design, develop a mix-and-match of nutrition strategies that achieves their overall nutrition goals, suits their lifestyle and resources, and maximizes their training and competition performances. Finding this optimal balance may be the art of coaching as much as it is the science of sport.

Although the train low model—that is, deliberate exposure to an exercise stimulus in a suboptimal physiological status to enhance the adaptive response—is best explored in relation to fuel availability, it is possible that it may apply to other areas of the training adaptation. For example, specialized heat acclimation or acclimatization protocols are undertaken to prepare athletes to tolerate exercise in hot and often humid environments, with the desired adaptations including increased sweat rate with lower sodium concentration, lowered heart rate, lowered resting and exercise core temperature, an expansion of plasma volume, and decreased ratings of perceived exertion and thermal sensation (Wendt et al. 2007). Acclimatization protocols to achieve such adaptations range from daily exposure to a hot environment with prolonged low-intensity exercise to intermittent exposure with higher-intensity exercise, with various programs lasting from one to three weeks. Of course, athletes and coaches would like to minimize the interruption to the athlete's training program and the need for specialized heat chambers/environments by finding the most physiologically effective protocol that requires the least amount of time and commitment. In this regard, there is preliminary support that a five-day acclimation protocol involving daily exercise in a heat chamber was most effective in achieving cardiovascular adaptations and performance enhancements when subjects deliberately refrained from drinking fluids during the sessions to allow dehydration to occur (Garrett et al. 2004).

Further investigation of this observation is warranted, but any findings of enhanced adaptation to heat exposure through exercising while deliberately dehydrated must be balanced against the potential for increased risk of illness or injury arising from exercising when fatigued or from a reduction in training intensity. Unlike the train low protocols applied to fuel, which might be periodized into the athlete's calendar for periods in which there is less potential for, or impact of, such side effects, it is

likely that train low fluid protocols will need to be undertaken in the period immediately before the athlete is exposed to the hot competition environment. In such a
case, the penalties of any negative outcomes will be greater.

1.2.4 NUTRITIONAL NEEDS FOR SPECIAL PHASES

The athlete's annual calendar may include some other specialized periods of altered
nutritional need or change in access to food. To optimize training and performance
outcomes, the athlete needs to understand the challenges involved and to plan ahead
to meet nutritional needs as adequately as possible during these phases.

1.2.4.1 Altitude and Heat Training

Many athletes take on specialized training such as exposure to altitude or heat. This
can be undertaken with various models, including continual exposure for several
weeks at a time via relocation to a hot climate or suitable venue at a moderate location
or intermittent exposure each day via the use of heat chambers or altitude-simulating
nitrogen houses. The exposure may be planned as "acclimatization" prior to competing
in a similar environment or simply as a period of specialized conditioning offering an
amplified training response. Although the program and its goals may vary, the common elements are likely to be a change in exercise patterns and an increase in requirements for some nutrients. Relocation from the athlete's home base may also add the
nutritional challenges associated with travel (see the next section).

The primary nutritional challenges an athlete faces while training/competing
at altitude or in a hot climate will be determined by the demands of the exercise
program. Since the period of exposure may involve either an intensified training
stimulus or a competition taper and the event itself, the athlete will need to alter
total energy and fuel intake accordingly. Such changes should also accommodate
the additional fluid losses associated with increased sweating in a hot environment
or loss of moisture from the respiratory tract into the dry air at altitude. The contribution of carbohydrate to exercise fuel is typically increased in hot weather or at
altitude, so refueling strategies may also need to be adjusted. Since the adaptation to
altitude includes the synthesis of new red blood cells, the athlete should ensure that
he or she has adequate iron status. A more extensive review of the nutritional needs
for training at altitude is provided by Febbraio and Martin (2010).

1.2.4.2 Travel

Travel, both the process and the period of relocation from an athlete's home base,
provides a significant nutritional challenge to the athlete. The challenge arises from
the combination of a number of factors, including altered exercise patterns, an altered
physical environment that may expose the athlete to a different climate or altitude,
differences in water and food hygiene standards, and a change in access to food and
fluid. The change in food availability can arise simply because the athlete's 24-hour-
per-day access to his or her own kitchen is replaced by a rigid menu from a caterer
supplying three meals a day; alternatively, an athlete's supervised meals within a
family situation can be replaced by unmonitored access to food. Different food cultures at a new location may mean the absence of foods that are habitually eaten and

the requirement to eat foods that are unusual or unknown. Each athlete will need a careful approach to ensure that his or her nutrition goals are met in the face of these challenges. Strategies that may be valuable include taking a supply of key food and sports products from home to replace habitually consumed items that are likely to be missing. In some locations, the athlete will need to practice hygiene precautions such as avoidance of water that is not bottled or boiled or foods that have not been cooked or peeled. Organization of catering needs ahead of time, careful attention to menu choices at restaurants and takeouts, and appropriate eating behavior in village dining halls and other buffet dining venues can also help to keep eating patterns on track. A more extensive review of nutritional practices for travel is provided by Cummings and colleagues (2010).

1.2.4.3 Fasting—Ramadan

Fasting—the abstention from eating or drinking—is a practice that most of us experience each day for at least eight hours while we sleep. Many aspects of our body's regulatory processes are designed for, or at least able to cope with, such interruption to intake of food and fluids. However, a further absence of intake as occurs with the fasting practices within various religions and cultures can add extra nutritional challenges. The intermittent fasting associated with Ramadan has received recent attention due to the overlap that will occur in 2012 between the month of Ramadan (July 20–August 18) and the schedule of the London Olympic Games (July 27–August 12).

Fasting during Ramadan, the ninth month of the lunar calendar is one of the five pillars of the Muslim faith. Briefly, such fasting involves the abstention from all fluid and food intake during the period from first light to sunset (*Itfar*), as well as rituals involved with the breaking of the fast and various prayer and feasts throughout the night. Such fasting can result in prolonged periods without intake of nutrients or food volume, inflexibility with the timing of eating and drinking over the day and around an exercise session, and changes to usual dietary choices due to the special foods involved with various rituals (Burke 2010a). Changes to sleep patterns are also part of the picture with the shift in dietary intake from daytime to night. Depending on the timing of their specific events within the Olympic Games program, Muslim athletes may be scheduled to fast during a reasonably heavy training load, a precompetition taper, or competition itself. Of course, many other fasting practices occur in various cultures and religions, and many Muslim athletes train and compete in a variety of sports or events during the month of Ramadan each year. Nevertheless, it is likely that the high profile of the Olympic Games will focus attention on the challenges of combining sports nutrition goals within a practice that places limits on access to food and fluid intake.

Several reviews (Burke 2010a; Chaouachi et al. 2009; Maughan et al. 2010) and coordinated studies (Zerguini et al. 2008) have been recently undertaken to investigate how Ramadan fasting may affect the performance and health of the athlete. Although it is easy to identify ways in which fasting alters an athlete's ability to follow sports nutrition guidelines, particularly in relation to nutritional practices before, during, or after exercise, the currently available evidence suggests that the effects are small. However, small effects on performance are of key importance in elite sport, where margins between winning and losing are often very tight. In addition, it is noted that the sparse body of research has not yet included sporting events with the most challenging nutritional issues (e.g., marathons, triathlons, road cycling events). Therefore, further research is encouraged to allow athletes to make well-informed decisions about fasting practices. When athletes intend to fast during sporting events, they may be assisted to minimize any potential negative effects by strategies such as optimizing the choice and timing of intake of fluid and food during the hours of darkness (Burke 2010a), altering the timing of exercise sessions to better suit their opportunities for nutritional support, and choosing pacing strategies that match their altered fluid and fuel status (Maughan et al. 2010).

1.3   SPECIFIC TIMING OF NUTRIENT INTAKE AROUND EXERCISE SESSIONS

A highly topical issue in current sports nutrition is the impact of the supply of nutrients or the athlete's nutritional status in close proximity to a session of exercise. Such is the depth and importance of this aspect of the "nutrient timing"; an entire section of this book and several additional chapters of this book are devoted to an in-depth review of recent and emerging information on nutrition strategies immediately before, during, and after exercise. In the competition scenario, well-timed eating can enhance performance by reducing or delaying the onset of fatigue. In the training situation, the goal is to be able to complete sessions as well as possible and to recover quickly.

1.3.1   PRECOMPETITION GLYCOGEN-ENHANCING PROTOCOLS

In many prolonged sporting events, performance is limited by the depletion of muscle glycogen stores. Adaptations resulting from training help to protect the athlete from this source of fatigue: The trained athlete has both an increase in resting muscle glycogen concentration and an enhanced ability to oxidize fat as a fuel substrate, thus sparing these muscle glycogen stores. Other strategies undertaken in the period immediately prior to an endurance event may further enhance such advantages.

1.3.1.1   Glycogen Supercompensation

Glycogen supercompensation protocols date to the 1960s and the pioneering work of Scandinavian sports scientists, who used the percutaneous biopsy technique to identify diet and exercise strategies that could manipulate muscle carbohydrate concentrations. The first protocol involved a seven-day preparation, consisting of a depletion phase (three days of hard training in conjunction with a low-carbohydrate intake) followed by a loading phase (three days high-carbohydrate intake in conjunction with a tapering of training) (Bergstrom et al. 1967). The doubling of muscle glycogen stores achieved by this protocol was shown to extend exercise capacity. Later studies found that trained individuals were able to successfully supercompensate muscle glycogen content without the need to "prime" glycogen synthetase via a depletion phase; instead, muscle carbohydrate content was achieved by tapered exercise and three days of carbohydrate-rich eating (Sherman et al. 1981). A recent and more practical refinement comes from evidence that glycogen supercompensation can be achieved, at least for well-trained athletes, with as little as 36 hours of rest and a diet rich in carbohydrate (10 grams of carbohydrate per kilogram body mass per 24 hours) (Bussau et al. 2002). Most endurance athletes should be able to program such a strategy prior to at least their most important competitive events, although some athletes may need expert assistance to formulate a dietary plan to reach these carbohydrate targets. Chapters 6 and 8 provide further discussion of these and other glycogen supercompensation strategies.

1.3.1.2   Fat Adaptation Prior to Glycogen Supercompensation

Although well-trained athletes have an enhanced capacity for fat oxidation during exercise, their ability to utilize fat as an exercise fuel is clearly not at maximal capacity since it can be further upregulated by switching to a high-fat diet. Indeed, we have described a short-term fat adaptation protocol in which athletes consume a diet high in fat (~65% of energy) and low in carbohydrates (~2.5 grams of carbohydrate per kilogram body mass) for five days while continuing to train with both high-volume and high-intensity sessions (Burke et al. 2000). The retooling of the muscle to increase fat utilization during exercise is so robust that it persists even when the athlete supercompensates muscle glycogen stores with 24 hours of rest and a high-carbohydrate intake (Burke et al. 2000) or even further promotes carbohydrate availability by consuming a carbohydrate-rich preevent meal and carbohydrate during exercise (Burke et al. 2002).

This is a promising preparation consideration just prior to an endurance or ultra-endurance event if it could provide both high-carbohydrate stores and an ability to use them more slowly. However, we and others have failed to find that the fat adaptation-carbohydrate restoration protocol enhances the performance of subsequent prolonged exercise (Burke and Kiens 2006). One of the apparent explanations is that, rather than sparing glycogen utilization, the fat adaptation phase causes a downregulation of carbohydrate oxidation (Stellingwerff et al. 2006), impairing subsequent glycogen utilization and its ability to fuel exercise at higher intensities (Havemann et al. 2006). This might be expected to impair the athlete's ability to undertake the critical activities within most prolonged sporting events—the breakaway, the surge up a hill, the sprint to the finish line—that determine the overall outcome. Therefore, this protocol of dietary periodization is not recommended for the typical endurance event in which a range of exercise intensities is required, even for brief periods. However, there may be some atypical events involving only low- to moderate-intensity activity that could benefit from further investigation of a fat adaptation phase prior to carbohydrate loading.

1.3.2   Preexercise Meal

A principle goal of food or fluid intake in the hours prior to exercise is to maintain gut comfort throughout exercise. Other goals are to address the final opportunity to top up fuel and fluid levels in recovery from any previous exercise and in anticipation of the specific needs of the upcoming event. Therefore, the timing, amount, and type of food that is consumed will need to be individualized to the practicalities and the needs of this event, as well as the specific likes and tolerances of each athlete.

For sports and activities involving prolonged exercise, the preexercise meal offers an opportunity to top up body carbohydrate stores. This is important for exercise conducted in the morning after an overnight fast or if it has been difficult to refuel from prior exercise bouts. General guidelines to increase net carbohydrate availability during exercise—or more specifically to consume enough carbohydrate to counteract the increase in carbohydrate utilization that results from the insulin response to carbohydrate intake—are to consume carbohydrate-rich foods and fluids to provide at least one gram of carbohydrate per kilogram body mass during the period one to four hours prior to the start of exercise. Some individuals appear to suffer from hypersensitivity to, or an exaggeration of, this counterregulatory response to carbohydrate intake, especially when carbohydrate is consumed in the hours prior to the commencement of the session (Kuipers et al. 1999). Such individuals may respond to strategies such as experimenting to find the critical time before exercise that carbohydrate intake should be avoided, choosing carbohydrate sources with a low glycemic index and have an attenuated and sustained blood glucose and insulin response, including some high-intensity sprints during the warmup to the event to stimulate hepatic glucose output, and consuming carbohydrate during the event (Burke 2007).

In any case, the intake of carbohydrate during prolonged exercise promotes carbohydrate availability throughout the session, and the combination of pre- and during-exercise fueling strategies is likely to provide the most effective strategy overall. Despite some promotion of carbohydrate sources with a low glycemic index as the preferred preevent choices, there is no evidence of clear-cut benefits, especially when carbohydrate is consumed during exercise. Further information on preexercise nutrition is provided in Chapter 6.

1.3.3 DURING EXERCISE

During most exercise lasting more than 30 to 60 minutes, there is opportunity and the potential for benefits from the intake of fluids to offset sweat losses and carbohydrate to provide an additional fuel source for the muscle or central nervous system. Optimal amounts and types of fluids and foods that can be consumed during exercise will vary according to characteristics of the exercise and the individual athlete (see Chapter 7). Fluid intakes should be based on a variety of factors, such as thirst, rates of sweat losses, and gastrointestinal comfort; carbohydrate intake can benefit performance in amounts ranging from simply tasting a carbohydrate source (sustained high-intensity events lasting approximately 60 minutes) to 80 to 90 grams per hour (for events three hours or longer) (Jeukendrup 2008). A detailed account of the background and guidelines for carbohydrate intake during exercise is provided in Chapter 7.

Critical factors in determining the timing of nutrient intake during exercise are the individual characteristics of the event, which influence access to food and fluids and the opportunity to consume these. Theoretically, this can range from continuous availability in sports in which the athlete carries personal supplies but must consume them "on the move" (e.g., cycling races), to intermittent availability in events supplied by a network of aid stations (e.g., marathons). Other sports can allow participants to consume food and fluid during breaks in play, with opportunities ranging from often but unpredictable (e.g., time-outs and rotational substitutions in some team games) to infrequent but scheduled (e.g., halftime break in soccer matches or quarter and half breaks for basketball). Even when there is a likely benefit from making use of these opportunities, actual practice will vary according to individual tolerance and habituation. Even when practicalities make it challenging to consume fluid or foods during exercise, sports nutrition guidelines encourage athletes to develop a personalized plan that works for their specific event and situation (Sawka et al. 2007).

1.3.4 POSTEXERCISE

Recovery after exercise involves a complex array of processes that help to restore homeostasis or allow the body to adapt to physiological stress. The better-understood processes include restoration of muscle and liver glycogen stores, replacement of fluid and electrolytes lost in sweat, protein synthesis for repair or adaptation, and responses of the immune and antioxidant systems to help the athlete stay healthy. Many of these processes are highly dependent on the provision of nutrients in the hours after the session.

To enhance refueling, athletes are advised to consume carbohydrate as soon as possible after the completion of a workout or event. There is a potential for higher rates of muscle glycogen storage during the first two to four hours after exercise, but even in the face of carbohydrate intake, refueling rates decline after two to four hours (Ivy, Katz, et al. 1988). This observation has created the idea of a "window of opportunity" for glycogen storage during the early period of postexercise recovery. The true value of postexercise carbohydrate intake, however, comes more from the provision of a substrate to promote effective refueling than the feature of the few hours of moderately enhanced glycogen synthesis (Burke et al. 2004). The outcome of delaying carbohydrate intake means that there will be very low rates of glycogen restoration until feeding occurs. Any delay is important when there are only four to eight hours between exercise sessions, but it may have less impact over a longer recovery period as long as sufficient carbohydrate is consumed (Burke et al. 2004). There is indirect evidence that maximal glycogen storage during the first four hours after exercise is achieved by a pattern of small but frequent meals providing a total carbohydrate intake of approximately one gram per kilogram of body mass per hour (Burke et al. 2004). Further information on postexercise refueling is found in Chapter 8.

After exercise or other situations producing a significant fluid deficit, many people fail to drink sufficient volumes of fluid to restore fluid balance, even when fluids and opportunity are available. Rehydration can only commence with the intake of fluids; however, the simultaneous replacement of electrolytes via the intake of sodium-containing drinks or the coingestion of salt-containing foods or meals is required to promote effective restoration of body fluid status. The amount of fluid that should be consumed after exercise will obviously depend on the magnitude of the net fluid deficit; however, a volume equivalent to approximately 125% to 150% of this deficit will need to be consumed in the four to six hours after exercise to compensate for ongoing sweat losses and urine production. A summary of postexercise fluid need is provided by Shirreffs and colleagues (2004) and is not a concept specifically addressed by this text as many books, chapters, reviews, and position stands have been devoted to the topic.

Although previous interest on the protein requirements of athletes has focused (sometimes rather controversially) on areas of total daily protein requirements for nitrogen balance or enhanced athletic performance, it now seems it may be more important to consider the type of protein that is consumed and its timing of intake in relation to exercise. Protein balance is a product of muscle protein synthesis minus muscle protein breakdown, and over a day the direction and magnitude of the balance continually alter according to factors such as intake of dietary protein, exercise, and periods without food. In the period immediately after exercise, a substantial increase in rates of muscle protein synthesis occurs, especially in trained individuals (Tang et al. 2008). This is most evident in the hours immediately after the exercise bout, and in trained subjects, it may not return to basal levels until at least 24 hours of recovery (Tang et al. 2008). However, while exercise reduces the degree of negative protein balance that occurs between meals, the response remains negative (i.e., breakdown > synthesis) unless the athlete consumes a source of protein (Biolo et al. 1997), or more specifically, essential amino acids. The maximal protein synthetic response to a resistance exercise bout is achieved with the intake of approximately 20 to 25 grams of high-quality protein, and protein consumed in excess of this stimulates increased rates of irreversible oxidation (Moore, Robinson, et al. 2009). The increase in muscle protein synthesis that occurs in the hours after exercise and protein feeding is still evident in the 24-hour picture of net protein balance (Tipton et al. 2003) and leads to measurable differences in protein gain and functional outcomes in the chronic training situation (Hartman et al. 2007).

The maximal protein synthetic response to exercise occurs when there is good availability of plasma essential amino acids in the period around exercise, but there is some confusion with regard to the relative benefits of feeding before, immediately afterward, or in the hour postexercise. Further research is needed on this issue, but it is likely that feeding in any of these periods can be useful and may be further optimized by manipulating the digestibility of the protein source so that a favorable plasma amino acid response, yet to be determined, is achieved. A thorough discussion of the benefits of protein feeding in the immediate recovery period, particularly alongside resistance training, is provided by Chapters 9, 10, and 12.

Finally, the recovery period will involve some adaptation to the exercise-induced stress to the body's immune and antioxidant status, but specific nutritional strategies to promote or preserve optimal antioxidant and immune function in athletes are not well described. Reduced carbohydrate availability during exercise induces larger increases in stress hormones and greater perturbation of immune function parameters in the "window" of immunosuppression after the exercise bout (Gleeson 2007). However, detecting a link between changes in nutritional status, decreases in concentration or activity of various immune system parameters, and the incidence of common illnesses such as upper respiratory tract infections is exceedingly complicated. The body's antioxidant system is a similarly complicated arrangement, and further work is required to determine whether supplementation with antioxidants or plant phytochemicals can promote antioxidant status, reduce muscle damage, promote mitochondrial biogenesis, and enhance sports performance (Reid 2008).

Of course, even when goals for an optimal nutrient intake immediately after exercise can be clearly specified, there may be practical issues that delay or reduce the athlete's capacity to consume appropriate amounts or types of foods and fluids to achieve such guidelines. Eating and drinking during the recovery period may be interrupted by the scheduling of other events (e.g., media obligations, drug testing, postevent debriefing) or by a loss of appetite. Access to suitable foods and drinks may be limited in some exercise environments, and the culture of some sports may promote detrimental eating practices, such as excessive intake of alcohol. In some cases, such practical issues may be more challenging to optimal nutrient timing than the lack of clear guidelines.

1.4 SPACING OF MEALS AND SNACKS OVER THE DAY

Although the hours immediately surrounding exercise have become the focus of most of our current attention, the timing of nutrient intake over the rest of the day may also play a role in achieving sports nutrition goals. There are several themes by which the spacing of meals and snacks over a whole day may assist or detract from the achievement of the athlete's individual goals:

- Achievement of total nutrient goals, especially when desired intakes are at the low or high end of the spectrum of requirements
- Additional assistance in continuing goals of rehydration, refueling, protein synthesis, and immune or antioxidant status during the extended recovery period
- Assistance to play "catch-up" during the extended recovery period if optimal nutrient intakes were not achieved in the immediate recovery phase

Further study is needed to identify exact guidelines for the optimal timing and frequency of nutrient intake over the day, but some observations and suggestions are provided next. Information on this "periodicity" of real-life intakes of energy and nutrient by athletes is limited and is clouded by differing methodologies used to describe occasions of eating and drinking, with "meals" and "snacks" described by cultural terms rather than objective criteria (Hawley and Burke 1997). However, we have undertaken a dietary survey of the self-reported intakes of a variety of Olympic-level athletes and commented on their spread of intake of energy and macronutrients over a typical training day, based on identified time points and in relation to training sessions (Figure 1.4) (Burke et al. 2003). This study identified differences in the number of occasions of eating and drinking over a day and in the macronutrient and energy content of the foods and drinks consumed at these occasions.

1.4.1 Energy Goals

Energy intake is a key issue for many athletes, with direct effects on issues such as body composition and hormonal function, as well as indirect effects on the athlete's

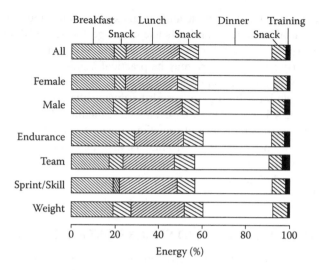

FIGURE 1.4 Proportion of reported daily energy intake consumed at various periods of the day by 167 Australian Olympic athletes, grouped by sex and by type of sport (endurance, team sports, weight sensitive, and sprint/skill). Data are mean values for all athletes and groups of athletes. Standard deviations are breakfast, lunch, and dinner: 7; snacks: 5; training: 3. Clear-cut differences: breakfast intake: endurance > sprint/skill, team. Dinner intake: sprint/skill, team > endurance. Training intake: males (3%) > females (1%); endurance, team (3%) > weight (0.5); male team (5%) > all other groups. (Reprinted with permission from Burke, L.M., G. Slater, E.M. Broad, J. Haukka, S. Modulon, and W.G. Hopkins. Eating Patterns and Meal Frequency of Elite Australian Athletes. *Int J Sport Nutr Exer Metab* 13(4):521–38, 2003.)

ability to meet his or her macronutrient and micronutrient goals (Burke 2001). It can be difficult for athletes to achieve their energy requirements or targets; this is especially the case for those at the low end of the spectra of energy intakes (e.g., athletes in a low-energy-expenditure sport or those experiencing a period of low activity levels or requirement for weight loss) or at the high end (e.g., athletes with high training or competition volume, those experiencing growth or a period of lean mass gain). Athletes may experience either hunger or "overfilling" discomfort when consuming their total daily food/energy needs, and the manipulation of the spacing of foods and drinks (as well as the choice of appropriate types, of course) in the daily diet is a common strategy advised by sports nutritionists/dietitians to assist the achievement of energy and physique goals (Burke 2001).

A lower or reduced energy intake may be marked by strategies to reduce purposeless or unnecessary snacking and perhaps incorporate some strategic or some well-timed snacks between meals. However, it is generally high-energy intake that is associated with an increase in the frequency of occasions of eating and drinking over the day since consuming a series of small meals, snacks, or energy-dense fluids over the course of the day appears to be a practical strategy to increase energy intake while minimizing the gastric discomfort that may be associated with infrequent large meals. Although the systematic relationship between energy intake and frequency of eating has not been well studied in athletes, there have been a number of dietary surveys that identified a "grazing" food pattern or high frequency of food consumption in athletes who report large energy intakes (Burke et al. 2003). In our study of the pattern of dietary intake of various types of Olympic athletes, we found that athletes typically reported consuming a significant source of energy on approximately five separate eating occasions each day, with energy intake from "snacks," defined as energy consumed between identified "main meal periods," which provided approximately 23% of total energy intake across the group. However, there were systematic differences between athletes from different types of sport in the spread of energy intake across the day, and we found a significant positive correlation between energy intake (kJ/kg) and the number of eating occasions each day (Burke et al. 2003). The pattern and timing of daily nutrient intake over the day by athletes are recommended as topics for further investigation. Similarly, the concept of increased meal frequency and its ability to modulate increases in body mass and adiposity are discussed outside athletic competition and are commonly used as a pillar of nutritional guidelines for general weight loss. A further discussion of this concept and associated research can be found in Chapter 16.

1.4.2 CONTINUED RECOVERY NEEDS

Although sufficient amounts of carbohydrate intake and timing of administration are the key issues underpinning glycogen storage, it is of interest to consider whether the pattern and timing of meals affected glycogen synthesis. In this regard, muscle glycogen storage over the 12 to 24 hours following exercise has been found to be similar when carbohydrate intake based on refueling targets is divided into two or seven meals (Costill et al. 1981) or consumed as four large meals compared to 16 hourly snacks (Burke et al. 1996). The question of whether there is a better feeding pattern to promote refueling from a suboptimal carbohydrate intake has not been addressed, but it remains that if adequate carbohydrate is provided, the impact of timing is likely lessened.

Rehydration requires the intake of fluids and electrolytes; however, only a few studies have investigated the effect of the pattern of fluid intake on restoration of fluid balance. Kovacs and colleagues (2002) compared the intake of a large volume of fluid in the immediate postexercise period with the same total amount of fluid being spread equally over five to six hours of recovery. Early replacement of large volumes of fluid was associated with better restoration of fluid balance during the first hours of recovery despite an increase in urinary output; however, differences in fluid restoration between hydration patterns disappeared by five to six hours of recovery. In another investigation, spacing fluid intake over several hours of recovery after exercise reduced urine losses and was more effective in restoring fluid balance than consuming the fluid as a large bolus immediately after the exercise (Archer and Shirreffs 2001). The spacing of fluid intake to maximize fluid retention is important not only for the restoration of fluid balance but also to reduce the potential inconvenience of large losses of urine. For example, consumption of large volumes of fluid following an evening exercise session may cause an interruption to sleep and recovery if the athlete needs to urinate during the night. In such cases, restful sleep may be the priority, with fluid balance restored in the morning.

Finally, although protein synthesis is elevated for at least 24 hours following a training session, no studies have examined the issue of regular protein feedings over the whole day following an exercise bout. Therefore, there are no firm guidelines regarding the best way to spread protein intake over meals and snacks for the remainder of the time during which muscle protein synthesis is stimulated. However, it makes sense to arrange regular feeding over the day, with 20 to 25 grams of high-quality protein remaining a benchmark for the maximum protein needed at any single feeding.

1.5   SUMMARY

Nutrition and exercise interact powerfully to promote physiological adaptations and to enhance capacity for exercise. There are a number of ways in which the timing of intake of nutrients over the day, in relation to exercise, and as part of the periodization of the athlete's training and competition calendar can enhance the outcomes of this interaction. Nutrient timing poses an exciting new area of sports nutrition in which there is an evolving base of evidence and an appreciation of the practical aspects of consuming foods and fluids around exercise as well as through the individual athlete's lifestyle.

2 Carbohydrates
The Fuel Currency in Skeletal Muscle

Chris N. Poole and Chad M. Kerksick

CONTENTS

2.1 INTRODUCTION

Carbohydrates function as a primary energy source during both endurance and high-intensity bouts of exercise. Thus, their availability is essential to generate adenosine triphosphate (ATP) within the anaerobic and aerobic metabolic systems so exercise performance can be performed at an optimal level. It is well recognized that as

23

carbohydrate stores become depleted during prolonged strenuous exercise, a sense of fatigue becomes evident that is accompanied by the termination or a significant reduction in exercise intensity (Hermansen et al. 1967; Karlsson and Saltin 1971). For this reason, researchers have found and are continuing to find various nutritional regimens and interventions that are favorable for maximizing muscle glycogen stores for athletes who participate in endurance-related activities. Before discussing the nutrient requirement aspect of carbohydrates, we must first place an emphasis on the carbohydrate molecule itself. This chapter is intended to reinforce knowledge of the function, structure, form, and sources of carbohydrates. The focus then transitions to digestion and absorption of carbohydrates, storage sites of carbohydrates, and carbohydrate metabolism. The last part of this chapter is more practical in nature and emphasizes the determinants of fuel utilization as well as provides carbohydrate recommendations for all types of athletes.

2.2 FUNCTIONS OF CARBOHYDRATES IN THE BODY

Carbohydrates carry out several functions that are associated with creating ATP via energy metabolism and fueling exercise performance. First and foremost, glucose in the blood, which during exercise comes most predominantly from muscle glycogen, is a primary energy source used to stimulate biological work. In this respect, the percentage of ATP derived from carbohydrate stores increases as exercise intensity rises. In fact, as intensity reaches near-maximal levels, carbohydrate utilization reaches near-exclusive levels of contribution as a fuel source during high-intensity exercise. Dietary carbohydrate intake must meet the activity level of an individual so the limited glycogen stores in the body are adequately maintained. When glycogen stores attain their maximum capacity, excess sugars are often converted to other energy-providing nutrients, such as fat. This principle should be explained to those individuals who believe consuming excessive amounts of carbohydrates and refraining from fat intake will improve body composition and weight control. The body's ability to transform one macronutrient into another to regulate energy storage explains how body fat can increase despite little or no dietary fat intake assuming that overall caloric intake exceeds expenditure.

When dietary carbohydrate intake is sufficient to maintain glycogen stores, tissue protein is conserved. Protein is responsible for the maintenance, repair, and building or growth of tissue, particularly the body's primary reservoir of protein, skeletal muscle. In contrast, when glycogen stores are depleted, such as in cases of starvation, low-carbohydrate dietary intake, and strenuous or exhaustive exercise, the mixture of substrates being metabolized is altered, resulting in a marked increase in fat metabolism and an increase in glucose synthesis by way of the available amino acid pool. Consequently, the body's protein levels are sacrificed, and a subsequent loss of lean tissue (muscle mass) can occur, causing kidney strain and excretion of nitrogenous by-products through urination.

Glucose serves as the primary energy source of the central nervous system (CNS), particularly the brain. Glycogenolysis by the liver aids in maintaining a narrow blood glucose range (around 100 milligrams per deciliter [mg/dL]), which permits glucose to provide energy for both nerve tissue metabolism and red blood cells. In hypoglycemic situations (blood glucose < 45 milligrams/deciliter), a lack of fuel substrate exists for the CNS, often resulting in feelings of fatigue, dizziness, hunger, weakness, and a decrease in exercise performance. Prolonged hypoglycemia can prompt unconsciousness, seizures, and even brain damage in extremely rare cases. Hypoglycemia is most commonly treated by ingesting carbohydrate foods that are easily digestible into glucose, which promotes quick restoration of blood glucose to normal levels.

2.3   STRUCTURE AND KINDS OF CARBOHYDRATES

Carbohydrates are composed of carbon, hydrogen, and oxygen atoms, with the most basic form of carbohydrates, monosaccharides, represented with the formula $(CH_2O)_n$. Although a few exceptions do exist, plants provide the majority of dietary carbohydrates that humans consume on a daily basis. Carbohydrates are most often classified as monosaccharides, oligosaccharides, and polysaccharides (see Figure 2.1) and are differentiated as such by the number of simple sugars (monosaccharides) that are linked together in these molecules.

2.3.1   MONOSACCHARIDES

Monosaccharides are the simplest form of carbohydrates, consisting of three to seven carbon atoms and one sugar subunit. From a nutritional perspective, glucose, fructose, and galactose are the three most important monosaccharides. Glucose is considered the most basic monosaccharide as other forms of sugars are broken down through digestive processes into glucose for an immediate energy source or

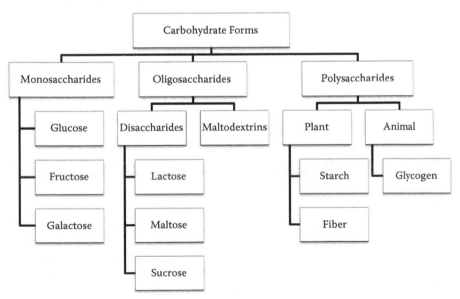

FIGURE 2.1   Forms of carbohydrates.

for uptake by the liver and skeletal muscle for glycogen synthesis. As mentioned, glucose can be converted into a triacylglycerol (fat) for a long-term energy reserve when a general abundance of energy reserves is signaled by the body.

Fructose is found abundantly in fruits, vegetables, and honey and is regarded as the sweetest-tasting sugar. As it is found in food, fructose can stand alone as a monosaccharide or bind to glucose, forming the disaccharide sucrose. The ingestion of high-fructose corn syrup, which is highly comprised of fructose, has been a criticized artificial sweetener in recent years and is thought to contribute to the overweight and obesity epidemic in the United States. It has been shown that ingesting 1,150 grams of soda per day (approximately 40 fluid ounces or between three and four cans of soda) containing high-fructose corn syrup over a three-week period increases caloric intake and body weight in males and females (Tordoff and Alleva 1990). Contrary to this notion, it is thought that high-fructose corn syrup does not contribute any longer to being overweight and developing obesity more than any other potentially harmful nutrients (Forshee et al. 2007).

Galactose is a monosaccharide that is most commonly found in lactose (milk sugar) combined with glucose. Galactose in its free form can be broken down into glucose by the liver and used during metabolic processes to generate ATP.

2.3.2 OLIGOSACCHARIDES

Carbohydrate molecules consisting of 2 to 10 monosaccharides linked together are called *oligosaccharides*. The most common oligosaccharides are *disaccharides*, which are two monosaccharides (one of these being glucose) linked together. Monosaccharides and disaccharides collectively are referred to as *simple sugars*. Sucrose (glucose + fructose) is the most common disaccharide and is typically referred to as table sugar or cane sugar. Sugar cane is grown in over 110 countries worldwide and can be sold in purified forms (i.e., brown sugar, powdered sugar) at grocery stores. Like high-fructose corn syrup, sucrose consumption is linked to the current obesity epidemic, although studies have found mixed results related to its effects on overall health and weight gain (Raben et al. 2002; Surwit et al. 1997).

Lactose (glucose + galactose) is another disaccharide that does not exist in plants as it is exclusively found in the milk of lactating animals. Lactose intolerance, the inability to digest lactose due to a deficiency in the quantity of the lactose-digesting enzyme lactase, is a common occurrence affecting diverse populations worldwide. These individuals are instructed to refrain from lactose consumption in an effort to avoid gastrointestinal discomfort.

Maltose (glucose + glucose) is the last of the common disaccharides and is present in beer, cereals, and germinating seeds. Maltose plays an important task in the process of creating fermented barley, which in turn is used to brew alcoholic beverages. If additional glucose units are bonded with maltose, a maltodextrin results. Maltodextrins, or glucose polymers, are complex carbohydrates that are easily broken down into glucose subunits through digestive processes. Maltodextrins are commonly added to many foods and beverages in addition to being a common addition to dietary and nutritional supplements. For this reason, they have been used a great deal in practice and research involving sports nutrition.

2.3.3 POLYSACCHARIDES

Polysaccharides contain anywhere from 11 to thousands of monosaccharides linked together and therefore are considered to be complex carbohydrates. They can take on a linear structure or a highly branched configuration, which increases the digestion rate of the carbohydrate (a highly branched structure creates more opportunities for hydrolytic enzymes to interact and cleave chemical bonds). The composition of polysaccharides can be made of a single monosaccharide or (which is more likely) a combination of two or more monosaccharides and thus are termed *homopolysaccharides* and *heteropolysaccharides*, respectively. Polysaccharides of both plant and animal origin provide these sizable chains of bonded monosaccharides.

2.3.3.1 Plant Polysaccharides

The primary plant polysaccharides are starch and fiber. Starch is the storage form of carbohydrates in plants, and it is found copiously in seeds; many grains, such as pasta, cereal, and bread; and vegetables such as corn, peas, beans, and potatoes. Starch can be further divided into two forms: amylose and amylopectin. Amylose is a linear chain of monosaccharide units that are twisted in a helical fashion, where amylopectin is a highly branched configuration of monosaccharides. The structures of these two forms of starch determine their digestion rate. The linear structure of amylose limits digestive enzymes to only a handful of locations to break down the starch, which consequently slows the digestive process. Conversely, the highly branched structure of amylopectin enables digestive enzymes to break down many areas of the starch simultaneously, resulting in a faster digestion rate. The digestive properties of amylose and amylopectin, to be expected, reflect their respective glycemic indexes (a topic to be covered).

Fiber is a nonstarch, structural polysaccharide that is thought to be the most plentiful organic molecule on earth. Fibers are resistant to digestive enzymes of the stomach and small intestine, thereby classifying this carbohydrate as an indigestible foodstuff. This nonstarch polysaccharide is found solely in plants and is mainly constituted of cellulose, hemicelluloses, pectin, lignin, mucilages, and gums. Fiber can be categorized into two types: soluble and insoluble. Soluble fiber dissolves in water to form a gel-like substance. Sources of soluble fiber include oats, legumes, apples, bananas, citrus fruits, barley, and psyllium. Insoluble fiber is incapable of dissolving in water, therefore increasing the movement of material through the digestive tract and increasing stool volume. Sources of insoluble fiber include whole wheat foods, nuts, seeds, and the skin of various fruits and vegetables. A balanced diet with adequate fiber intake can lower low-density lipoprotein (LDL) cholesterol, regulate blood glucose and insulin levels, and provide a sense of satiety, making fiber an effective modality to treat cardiovascular disease, type 2 diabetes, and obesity and has been used as an agent to promote weight maintenance (Marlett et al. 2002). The effects of fiber consumption on the risk, prevention, and ability to decrease colon cancer are unclear as studies have shown both positive and negative results (Slavin 2008). Daily recommendations of fiber intake include 14 grams per 1,000 calories, or 25 grams for women and 38 grams for men (Slavin 2008).

2.3.3.2 Animal Polysaccharides

Glycogen is the primary polysaccharide found in animals. Glycogen synthesis is initiated by the protein glycogenin, and the enzyme glycogen synthase is responsible for adding additional glucose units to an existing glycogen chain. A glycogen molecule is densely branched, allowing numerous enzymes to cleave glucose units in an efficient, timely manner to match any increase in energy demands. Thus, the higher and more densely branched a glycogen molecule is, the greater the capability it has to quickly supply energy to working muscles (Brooks et al. 2000). It has been reported that a 70-kilogram, nonobese man stores approximately 350 grams of muscle glycogen and 40 to 50 grams of liver glycogen (Felig and Wahren 1975). Since each gram of carbohydrate, in this case glycogen or glucose, supplies 4 calories of energy, a 70-kilogram man eating a normal diet can store roughly 1,600 calories of energy in the form of glycogen. Considering that caloric expenditure rates can easily reach 12 to 20 calories per minute, muscle glycogen can provide fuel for an estimated 80 to 130 minutes, making it a rather limited fuel source. For this reason, a great appreciation has developed for nutritional regimens before and during exercise that can help to limit its utilization and thereby may go on to have an impact on performance.

2.4 DIGESTION AND ABSORPTION OF CARBOHYDRATES

The process of digestion begins the moment food is ingested and can take up to six hours to complete. Each macronutrient has designated enzymes accountable for the breakdown of food particles. Many factors can influence the digestion and absorption of carbohydrates, including the structure of the sugar, the size of food particles, fiber content, and the presence of other macronutrients.

2.4.1 DIGESTION

The onset of carbohydrate digestion takes place in the mouth when saliva is added to ingested food. Saliva is secreted from the parotid glands, sublingual glands, and the submandibular glands at a rate of 800 to 1,500 milliliters daily. When the salivary glands are stimulated, a 10-fold increase in saliva secretion can occur to aid the digestive process. The primary component of saliva is water, but other important constituents of saliva such as amylase, an enzyme that breaks down starch into smaller units, and enzymes and antibodies that fight oral bacteria have significant roles in the early stages of digestion. When chewing begins, the food particles are mixed with saliva, which increases the number of areas where amylase can attach and start breaking apart the long glucose chains of starches.

The food is then swallowed and enters the stomach, where the gastric conditions (approximate pH 2.0 to 3.0) significantly decreases amylase activity and subsequently slows the digestive process. The contents in the stomach then travel into the duodenum, where the contents are referred to as chyme. The acidity of the chyme stimulates secretin, which then stimulates the release of sodium bicarbonate from the pancreas to neutralize the acid. Amylase from the pancreatic juice acts on the chyme in the same manner as that of salivary amylase by producing maltose, maltotriose, and polysaccharides called α-limit dextrins (average of eight glucose units). The ingested starches are almost completely hydrolyzed as the chyme reaches the ileum. The disaccharides and α-limit dextrins are further broken down by enzymes situated in the brush borders of intestinal epithelial cells. The disaccharides are acted on by lactase, sucrase, and maltase. Lactase catalyzes lactose into glucose and galactose, sucrase catalyzes sucrose into glucose and fructose, and maltase catalyzes maltose into two glucose units.

Predicaments can arise when one or more of the enzymes designated for disaccharide catabolism (lactase, sucrase, and maltase) are deficient. When lactose, the main carbohydrate of milk, is unable to be digested, gastrointestinal problems transpire (i.e., diarrhea and flatulence). Lactose-intolerant individuals are advised to stop all consumption of milk products to alleviate these issues; however, supplementation with lactase can help to improve the functionality of this process.

A fraction of carbohydrates that are ingested into the body are not digested, absorbed, and used for energy production and storage. Fiber is predominantly composed of cellulose, which is a structural element in plants that is unable to be broken down by digestive enzymes in humans. Therefore, a portion of cellulose is fermented by bacteria located in the large intestine, resulting in the production of hydrogen, carbon dioxide, and methane gases. The remaining cellulose is forced into the colon to undergo further digestion before entrance into the rectum and removal through the anus.

2.4.2 ABSORPTION

After the ingested carbohydrates are broken down through digestion and only monosaccharides remain, absorption can take place. Absorption across the intestinal walls happens via active transport, in which energy is needed to counter a concentration gradient and carrier proteins are often utilized, or by diffusion. Glucose, fructose, and galactose have specific transport proteins facilitating the absorption process. Glucose and galactose are transported through the lumen into the epithelial cell by way of a sodium-dependent carrier protein, while fructose has a separate, sodium-independent transporter to facilitate its movement into the epithelial cell. From this point, all three monosaccharides are transported from the epithelial cell to the capillary system by a common transporter protein before circulating to the liver by way of the hepatic portal vein.

2.5 GLYCEMIC INDEX

After carbohydrates are digested and absorbed into circulation, blood glucose levels elevate, followed by an increased glucose uptake in skeletal muscle or hepatic tissue that is mediated by pancreatic insulin secretion. The magnitude of this response can vary and is dependent on the digestion rate and amount of the carbohydrate and speed at which blood glucose elevates and stimulates insulin secretion. The variability of the glycemic response among different foods does not always align with structural properties of carbohydrate molecules. An example of this phenomenon can be seen when examining the glycemic responses of glucose and fructose. Both are considered simple sugars, but their digestive properties vary significantly. After ingestion, glucose is digested and absorbed quickly, causing a rapid increase in blood glucose and a return to baseline levels shortly thereafter. Fructose, on the other hand, exhibits a delayed and much lower glucose response after ingestion (a response predicated by its conversion first inside the liver before disposal into systemic circulation). Further to this point, the starches found in potatoes and white bread that are considered to be complex sources of carbohydrates actually induce a higher blood glucose response than fructose (Table 2.1). Fiber-rich foods likely have a low glycemic response because fiber impairs the rate of digestion (see Figure 2.2). Protein and fat content can also lower the digestion rate of a given food. The different glycemic responses of foods have become an important variable in the diets of individuals attempting to regulate blood glucose within a narrow range (i.e., diabetics) and in athletes trying to maximize energy stores and control fuel utilization to improve performance. To clear up the confusion surrounding the glycemic responses of foods, Jenkins et al. (1981) proposed the idea of the glycemic index and tested it on various food products. The glycemic index is a ranking of the postprandial glucose response

TABLE 2.1
Glycemic Index of Commonly Consumed Foods

Maltose (beer sugar)	105
Glucose	100
Baked potato	95
Carrots	92
Honey	87
Corn flakes	80
White rice	72
Brown rice	66
Banana	62
Sucrose	59
Potato chips	50
Peas	50
White pasta	50
Oatmeal	49
Whole wheat pasta	41
Orange	40
Apple	38
Chick peas	35
Milk	30
Lentils	29
Kidney beans	29
Sausage	27
Fructose	20
Peanuts	13
Green vegetables	0–15

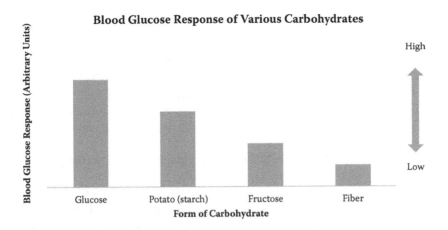

FIGURE 2.2 Blood glucose response to different carbohydrates.

of a particular food standardized to a reference food. Mathematically speaking, the glycemic index is a percentage of the area under the glucose response curve for a certain food compared to the area under the glucose response curve of the reference food (Jenkins et al. 1984) and can be determined by the following equation:

$$\text{Glycemic index} =$$
$$(\text{Blood glucose of test food/Blood glucose of reference food}) \times 100$$

The reference food is usually 50 grams of white bread or glucose, and the food of interest (also 50 grams) is measured for two hours in normal individuals and up to three hours in diabetic populations (Wolever et al. 1991). For example, a food with a glycemic index of 50 would raise blood glucose concentrations to an amount equivalent of 50% of the glycemic index for 50 grams of white bread. The glycemic index measurement itself is prone to some error, which can result from the laboratory conducting the tests to the glycemic index or quite simply subtle variations that often exist between individuals for a given food. With this being said, an analysis of many glycemic index studies demonstrated a small measurement error of 10 to 15 glycemic index units when the same foods are taken into consideration (Wolever et al. 1991).

Another important concept to understand with the glycemic index is the overall glycemic load of a particular food. While the glycemic index only takes into account the glycemic response of 50 grams of a specific food, the glycemic load measures the blood glucose response of an entire portion of food. This measurement is the product of the amount of available carbohydrate (in grams) in a food and the overall glycemic index of that food. Often, this measurement is a more practical representation of the nutrients being consumed in the diet on a daily basis. Diets consisting of a high glycemic load that are consumed over chronic periods of time have been shown to significantly increase the risk for developing type 2 diabetes (Salmeron et al. 1997).

$$\text{Glycemic load} =$$
$$\text{Glycemic index of given food} \times \text{Grams of food being consumed or tested}$$

2.6   ATP: THE FUEL CURRENCY OF THE CELL

Energy contained in food is not immediately transported to cells and utilized for biological work. Instead, energy from macronutrient catabolism is generated from hydrolysis of ATP, which fuels all of the cell's processes necessitating energy. The ATP molecule has two distinct functions involving energy transfer: 1) to remove energy contained in food macronutrients and temporarily store it within ATP bonds and 2) to remove energy stored in ATP bonds to facilitate the vast number of cellular-driven processes that make biological work possible.

ATP forms by the linkage of adenine and ribose molecules, forming adenosine, which further attaches to three phosphates. The phosphate molecules are often referred to as "high-energy phosphates" due to the high amount of energy that is released from the bonds linking the two outermost phosphates during hydrolysis. Adenosine diphosphate (ADP) is a compound that results when ATP and water are catabolized by the enzyme adenosine triphosphatase (ATPase). In some instances where a substantial amount of energy is required to meet the demands of the cell, ADP can be catabolized to form adenosine monophosphate (AMP). To replenish ATP stores, AMP and ADP attach additional phosphate ions derived from the oxidation of food macronutrients to form ATP. Thus, ATP serves as the "fuel currency" of the cell, as all of the energy-requiring processes are dependent on high-energy phosphates for fuel.

The body is capable of maintaining ATP stores within a narrow range through various metabolic processes that are situated within the cell's cytosol or mitochondria. ATP derived anaerobically through the breakdown of phosphocreatine (PCr), glucose, glycerol, and the carbon skeletons of deaminated amino acids is done so in the cell's cytosol. Aerobic production of ATP occurs in the cell's mitochondria through the tricarboxylic acid cycle, β-oxidation, and electron transport chain. The primary metabolic pathway relevant to this chapter is glycolysis, which is discussed in the next section.

Cells in the human body have a limited storage capacity for ATP; thus, ATP synthesis must occur at a rate that equals its use for energy. This limited ATP supply allows the body to tightly regulate metabolic processes involved with energy production. Any sudden alteration in ATP concentration due to cellular metabolism creates an imbalance between ATP and ADP. The imbalance stimulates metabolic processes to quickly begin resynthesizing ATP from stored energy compounds (macronutrients that were previously ingested, catabolized, and stored for later use). Such an imbalance between ATP and ADP would occur when transitioning from a jog into a sprint. ADP concentrations would quickly rise, as ATP would quickly decrease. An imbalance between these compounds initiates ATP production, so ATP levels can be maintained, allowing the new intensity of biological work to continue.

2.7   CARBOHYDRATE METABOLISM

Glycogen and glucose are the only stored energy substrates that can generate energy anaerobically. Glycolysis is the metabolic pathway responsible for glucose breakdown as it is capable of producing ATP at a fast rate for approximately two minutes during high-intensity exercise. At the onset of exercise, whether it is aerobic or anaerobic in nature, the phosphocreatine system fuels the working muscles for 10 to 20 seconds before glycolysis begins to be a significant contributor by breaking down ATP. The phosphocreatine system is the other primary metabolic pathway capable of producing ATP anaerobically; however, its importance to this chapter is minimal and is not discussed further.

2.7.1 GLYCOLYSIS

Glycolysis is the breakdown of a glucose molecule to its end product, pyruvate. Glycolysis generates ATP via substrate-level phosphorylation and produces cytosolic reducing equivalents in the form of nicotinamide adenine dinucleotide (NADH). NADH can be transported to the mitochondria, where it enters the electron transport chain for aerobic production of ATP. Glycolysis occurs in the cytosol of the cell and is initiated when glucose enters the cell via a glucose transporter (GLUT). Most notable is the fourth isoform of the glucose transporter (GLUT4), which is sensitive to any elevation in insulin secretion from the pancreas and is found in high amounts in skeletal muscle. GLUT4 translocates from intracellular vesicles to the cell membrane, where it promotes glucose entrance into the cytosol of a skeletal muscle cell. Once glucose enters the cell, ATP acts as a phosphate donor to phosphorylate glucose to glucose-6-phosphate. This reaction commits the glucose molecule to the cell, where it continues throughout the glycolytic pathway or is polymerized with other glucose molecules and stored as glycogen. Glycogen synthesis is discussed in the next section of this chapter. Glucose-6-phosphate is catabolized by an enzyme known as hexokinase. The rate at which hexokinase regulates glucose breakdown is determined by the concentration of glucose-6-phosphate. When glucose-6-phosphate concentration increases too much, it binds to a site on the hexokinase enzyme, thereby slowing the previous reaction process, thus allowing glucose to be transported to other tissue beds. This regulatory mechanism is termed product inhibition.

Glycolysis proceeds when glucose-6-phosphate changes to fructose-6-phosphate under enzymatic control of glucose phosphate isomerase. Fructose-6-phosphate is then phosphorylated (phosphate from an ATP molecule is used) and catabolized by the enzyme phosphofructokinase to form fructose-1, 6 bisphosphate. Phosphofructokinase largely regulates the speed and productivity of glycolysis as a whole since this step commits the cell to degrade glucose. Several compounds and by-products present inside the cell during resting and exercising conditions can affect the activity of phosphofructokinase and thus control the extent it will catabolize this key regulatory reaction. Table 2.2 displays the compounds that regulate the activity of phosphofructokinase.

From this point, fructose-1, 6 bisphosphate splits into two phosphorylated molecules that catabolize into pyruvate in five successive reactions. The last of these reactions, the phosphoenolpyruvate conversion to pyruvate via the enzyme pyruvate kinase, is another key regulatory step of glycolysis that generates an ATP at the substrate level (Figure 2.3). A total of four ATPs is synthesized during substrate-level phosphorylation of glycolysis; however, one or possibly two ATPs are utilized to phosphorylate the initial glycolytic reactions (two ATPs if the glucose molecule

TABLE 2.2
Regulators of Phosphofructokinase (PFK) Activity

Molecule	Effect on PFK
AMP	Increase
ADP	Increase
ATP	Decrease
H^+	Decrease
Pi	Increase
Citrate	Decrease

originates from the blood and one ATP if the glucose molecule originates from intramuscular stores), resulting in a net total of two to three ATPs. Pyruvate has two fates once it is generated during the final glycolytic step: (1) It enters the mitochondrion and is oxidized via the tricarboxylic acid (TCA) cycle or (2) it can be reduced to lactate. If the latter occurs, a number of possible outcomes may arise. Lactate can leave the cell in which it was produced, travel through the blood, and enter other tissues, where it can be oxidized to pyruvate and subsequently converted to acetyl-coenzyme A (CoA) for oxidation in the TCA cycle (Figure 2.4). In a similar manner, lactate can be transported from one muscle fiber to an adjacent fiber for oxidation. Lactate in circulation can enter the liver and be used to synthesize glucose via gluconeogenesis, or it can be used or stored as energy (in the form of glycogen) in the cell it was produced. Therefore, lactate serves as a valuable and efficient fuel source even though it is typically thought of as a negative by-product during anaerobic bouts of exercise.

2.7.2 GLYCOGENESIS AND GLYCOGENOLYSIS

Glycogenesis, or glycogen synthesis, occurs primarily in the liver and skeletal muscle, even though this metabolic process transpires throughout all animal tissues. Glucose units are added one at a time to an existing glycogen molecule, building a linear, unbranched chain configuration. Then, a branching enzyme creates bonds within the linear glycogen molecule that allow its formation to branch outward. The synthesis of a glycogen molecule can be summarized in the following steps:

1. Glucose enters the cell and is phosphorylated to glucose-6-phosphate.
2. The phosphate group on glucose-6-phosphate is relocated to a position on the first carbon in a reaction catalyzed by phosphoglucomutase, creating glucose-1-phosphate.
3. The glucose unit on glucose-1-phosphate is then activated by uridine triphosphate (UTP), creating uridine diphosphate (UDP)-glucose. This reaction is under enzymatic control of UDP-glucose pyrophosphorylase.
4. The final step includes the addition of a glucose unit to an existing glycogen molecule. Glycogen synthase adds glucosyl units from UDP-glucose to the nonreducing end of the glycogen molecule (Shearer and Graham 2004), and this reaction is irreversible.

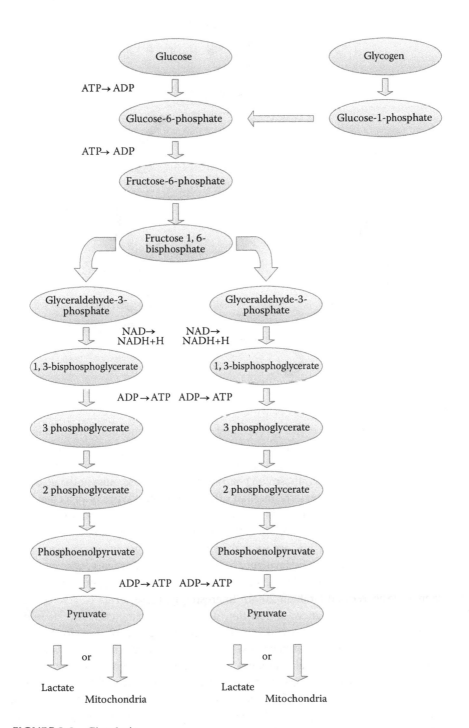

FIGURE 2.3   Glycolysis.

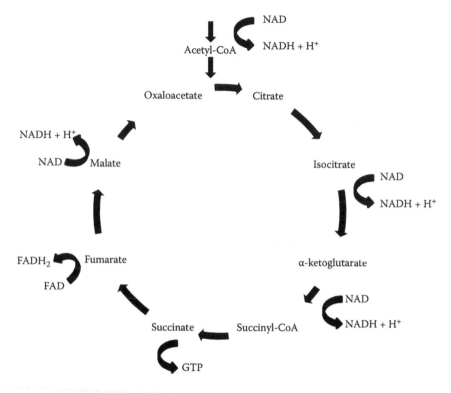

FIGURE 2.4 TCA cycle.

The primer required to create glycogen molecules is glycogenin. This primer has the capability of transferring glucose units to itself from UDP-glucose until approximately 7 to 11 glucose units have been added to its base structure (Houston 2006). From this point, glycogen synthase can continue to add glucose units to the glycogen molecule where the glycogenin primer left off. Two different types of glycogen have been recognized, and it is uncertain whether they differ based on structural size or the kinds of glycosomes they are altogether. Proglycogen is the smaller of the two types, as it contains fewer glucose units than the much larger macroglycogen molecule. Proglycogen seems to be favorably used during muscular work, whereas macroglycogen begins to donate glucose to the working muscle during prolonged bouts of exercise (Shearer and Graham 2004). Interestingly, these forms of glycogen are synthesized in a similar pattern to how they are utilized during exercise. Therefore, proglycogen molecules are restored initially after glycogen depletion, followed by macroglycogen restoration that becomes apparent a few hours later (Battram et al. 2004). In recent years, much attention has been placed on the timing of glycogenesis or the replenishment of glycogen stores in the acute time period following various exercise regimens. A discussion focused on this literature can be found in Chapter 8.

Glycogenolysis, or glycogen breakdown, is closely linked with glycolysis. During this process, glycogen molecules are cleaved of individual glucose units, which are then entered into the glycolytic pathway to eventually produce substrate-level ATP,

NADH, and pyruvate, which can enter the mitochondria to generate additional energy. The cleaving of glucose units from a glycogen molecule is made possible by inorganic phosphate (Pi). Pi and glycogen phosphorylase break the α-1-4 bond between two glucose units, causing the release of a terminal glucose unit in the form of glucose-1-phosphate. Debranching enzymes are necessary to cleave glucose units from the branch-like glycogen structure because glycogen phosphorylase is limited to cleaving glucose units that are arranged linearly. The numerous branch-like structures of a glycogen molecule increase its exposure area to enzymatic activity, allowing glucose cleaving to occur at rapid rates when metabolic demands are high. Glucose-1-phosphate is then converted to glucose-6-phosphate by phospho-glucomutase. Glucose-6-phosphate produced by glycogenolysis in the muscle enters glycolysis for breakdown and energy generation, while glucose-6-phosphate produced in the liver is subsequently dephosphorylated and fed into the blood for uptake by other tissues.

2.7.3 ROLE OF CARBOHYDRATE IN AEROBIC METABOLISM

Carbohydrates consumed through the diet not only provide glucose for anaerobic breakdown during glycolysis but also fuel aerobic metabolism via pyruvate entrance into the mitochondria. The TCA cycle, or Krebs cycle, works inside the mitochondria and uses a pyruvate molecule and CoA when sufficient oxygen is present to form acetyl-CoA. This acetyl-CoA molecule must be present to react with oxaloacetate, an intermediate of the TCA cycle, to allow this metabolic process to proceed and eventually yield two guanine triphosphate (GTP) molecules, six molecules of NADH, and two molecules of reduced flavin adenine dinucleotide ($FADH_2$) per molecule of glucose. As soon as NADH and $FADH_2$ molecules are created, they transport hydrogen atoms to the electron transport chain, where ATP is produced by phosphorylating ADP through a process referred to as oxidative phosphorylation (McArdle et al. 2007). β-Oxidation, a process involved with the catabolism of free fatty acids, provides the acetyl group necessary to form acetyl-CoA for entrance into the TCA cycle. However, TCA cycle intermediates, such as oxaloacetate, are regenerated from pyruvate during carbohydrate breakdown under enzymatic control of pyruvate decarboxylase. Therefore, if these intermediates are not continually replenished from pyruvate, oxaloacetate will not be available to react with acetyl-CoA and the TCA cycle comes to a standstill. At this point, the acetyl groups supplied from fatty acid breakdown are virtually useless as a source of potential energy. In this regard, "fat burns in a carbohydrate flame."

2.8 DETERMINANTS OF CARBOHYDRATE USE FOR ENERGY

The energy supply relied on during anaerobic and aerobic exercise is largely based on the intensity and duration of the exercise bout. Exercise bouts considered to be aerobic in nature will likely consist of a moderate-to-long duration with low-to-moderate levels of power output (e.g., intensity). Alternatively, anaerobic exercise consists of short-to-moderate durations driven by moderate- to high-power outputs (e.g., intensity). Aerobic exercise primarily relies on fat metabolism, as oxygen is consumed at low-to-moderate levels. However, as the exercise bout increases in intensity and the body transitions to anaerobic metabolism, oxygen consumption increases as well. When exercise intensity reaches a certain point or threshold, oxygen consumption can no longer increase and match the demands of the exercise bout. Therefore, the body must utilize energy stores that are broken down during anaerobic metabolism (phosphocreatine and glycolytic energy systems) in an attempt to meet the demands of the activity. If high-intensity exercise continues for several minutes, a point will be reached when the intensity of exercise will inevitably decline because the body's anaerobic energy systems are not able to produce ATP at a high enough rate to fuel exercise. Resultantly, fat metabolism plays a larger role as exercise intensity decreases. In effect, a trade-off is constantly at play between exercise and duration, an effect and transition that can only be manipulated with diligent training.

2.8.1 ANAEROBIC EXERCISE

During acute anaerobic activities, including resistance exercise (Robergs et al. 1991), maximal cycling sprints (Spriet et al. 1989), and running sprints (Cheetham et al. 1986), glycogen stores can become significantly reduced. Researchers have shown that even after a 45-minute resistance exercise bout, muscle glycogen stores can be significantly decreased. In particular, a resistance exercise bout consisting of two lower-body exercises performed at 75% of the participants' one-repetition maximums (1-RMs) depleted glycogen in type IIa and type IIb fibers of the vastus lateralis by 40% and 44%, respectively (Koopman et al. 2006). The exercise bout depleted 23% of the muscle glycogen in type I muscle fibers, which was considerably less than the muscle glycogen losses experienced in type II fibers. Robergs et al. (1991) investigated the effects of performing six sets of knee extensions at 35% and 70% of 1-RM and found that glycogen stores were preferentially depleted in type II muscle fibers compared to type I fibers. Cheetham and colleagues (1986) demonstrated that muscle glycogen of the vastus lateralis muscle can be depleted by 25% as the result of a 30-second treadmill sprint. Collectively, these studies show that muscle glycogen stores are depleted more so within type II muscle fibers when compared head-to-head with type I fibers during anaerobic exercise. Surprisingly, the volume of the exercise bout, in terms of resistance exercise or sprinting time, does not have to be overwhelming by any means to see a significant reduction in muscle glycogen. Athletes generally train and compete at much higher volumes, intensities, and durations than the protocols utilized in these studies. Therefore, depletion of muscle glycogen can occur at higher rates and over extended periods of time in athletic populations, which poses a significant threat to exercise intensity and overall performance (Haff and Whitley 2002).

2.8.2 AEROBIC EXERCISE

Two primary factors contribute to muscle glycogen utilization, and thus glycogen depletion, during aerobic exercise: the intensity of the exercise bout and the duration of the exercise bout (Figure 2.5). A direct, linear relationship exists between exercise intensity and the amount of glycogen utilized during an exercise bout (Figure 2.6) (Romijn et al. 1993). A classic example of this phenomenon can be observed in the

Exercise Intensity - Duration Relationship

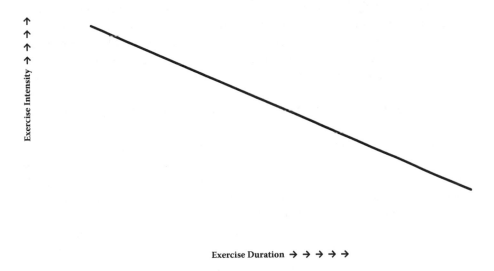

FIGURE 2.5   Relationship between exercise intensity and duration.

Exercise Intensity - Fuel Utilization Relationship

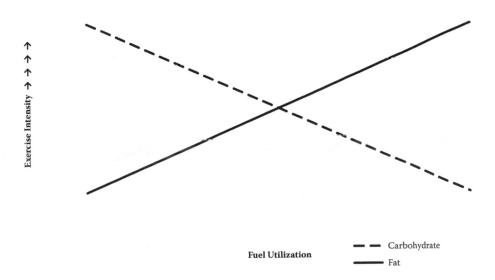

FIGURE 2.6   Relationship between exercise intensity and fuel utilization.

study conducted by van Loon et al. (2001). This research group monitored substrate utilization in cyclists at rest and during three consecutive 30-minute periods of exercise at approximately 45%, 57%, and 72% VO₂Max (maximum oxygen consumption). A significant increase was seen in both carbohydrate and fat utilization between rest and the exercise bout at 45% VO₂Max. During this stage (45% VO₂Max), 35% of the energy used by cyclists was a combination of muscle glycogen and plasma glucose (carbohydrate stores). During the second stage, when riders cycled at 57% VO₂Max, carbohydrate utilization increased to 38% of total energy expenditure. Finally, the third stage, completed at 72% VO₂Max, revealed that 58% of total energy expenditure came in the form of carbohydrate stores. Therefore, as exercise intensity increases in terms of VO₂Max, the amount of carbohydrate or glycogen stores used for producing ATP to fuel exercise also increases. More specifically, when exercising at intensities above 70% of VO₂Max, carbohydrates are primarily used to supply energy for exercise, whereas exercise intensities below 60% VO₂Max likely rely on fat stores to generate the majority of ATP to fuel exercise (Hultman 1995).

When aerobically exercising for extended periods of time, the use of muscle glycogen is highest at the onset of exercise, decreasing over time to a point at which fat becomes a significant energy contributor (McArdle et al. 2007). The transition of energy substrates can occur rather quickly during an extended exercise bout because glycogen stores have been shown to be significantly depleted within one to two hours of moderate- to high-intensity aerobic exercise (Figure 2.7) (Blom et al. 1986; Coyle et al. 1986). As the transition of substrate utilization from carbohydrate to fat occurs, it is accompanied with a decline in performance or a decrease in exercise intensity

Fuel Utilization - Exercise Duration Relationship

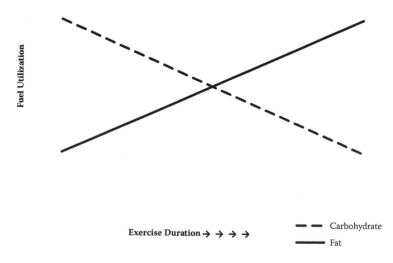

FIGURE 2.7   Relationship between exercise duration and fuel utilization.

(Bergstrom et al. 1967). The prevalence of this situation is a central theme to the importance of nutrition and more recently the timing of nutrients.

2.9 CARBOHYDRATE REQUIREMENTS FOR ATHLETES

Carbohydrates should provide the greatest proportion of total daily energy intake and are considered to be essential for peak athletic performance. Anaerobic and aerobic athletes alike use carbohydrate stores to fuel exercise, and when those stores become significantly depleted, detriments in performance and possibly to overall health can result. All athletes are encouraged to seek specific recommendations based on their own body weight and specific sporting activities, and not just typical macronutrient percentage recommendations. In addition, brief and general recommendations are provided in subsequent sections of this section; however, more specific recommendations regarding timing and exercise mode are provided in other chapters in this text (Chapters 6–10).

2.9.1 ANAEROBIC ATHLETES

Male anaerobic athletes reported consuming intakes of 3.3 to 5.4 grams of carbohydrates per kilogram of body mass per day, while female counterparts reported consuming 2.9 to 3.4 grams of carbohydrate per kilogram of body mass per day (Economos et al. 1993). Based on these data, anaerobic athletes in general are not meeting their carbohydrate recommendations on a daily basis. Dietary practices of this specific population of athletes should be to maximize internal glycogen stores in an effort to augment athletic performance. This can be achieved if athletes consume 6 to 10 grams of carbohydrate per kilogram of body mass per day or if 55% to 60% of their total daily energy intake is in the form of carbohydrates while undergoing intense training on a daily basis (Economos et al. 1993). The majority of these carbohydrates should come from complex, low-glycemic sources, with the remaining simple, high-glycemic carbohydrates to be ingested during the recovery phase immediately following training at a rate of 1 to 1.5 grams of carbohydrate per hour (Economos et al. 1993).

2.9.2 AEROBIC ATHLETES

Aerobic athletes tend to meet their carbohydrate requirements on a daily regimen more so than anaerobic athletes, which may be linked to the nature of their respective sports. Male aerobic athletes reported consuming 5.3 to 11.5 grams of carbohydrate per kilogram of body mass per day, although female aerobic athletes fell far short of their male equivalents, with carbohydrate intakes equaling 4.4 to 6.4 grams of carbohydrate per kilogram of body mass per day (Economos et al. 1993). Just as for the carbohydrate dietary recommendation for anaerobic athletes, aerobic athletes are recommended to maximize glycogen stores to enhance performance. Burke et al. (2004) suggest that carbohydrate recommendations for aerobic athletes should be determined by the intensity of exercise performed by each individual athlete. Thus, when an athlete is training with a moderate duration, low-intensity exercise, five to seven grams of carbohydrate per kilogram of body mass per day are recommended. As the intensity and volume of training increase, these higher exercise demands can be met by consuming 7 to 12 grams of carbohydrate per kilogram of body mass per day. If an athlete is undergoing extreme endurance training (four to more than six hours per day), then carbohydrate requirements should increase to 10 to 12 grams of carbohydrate per kilogram of body mass per day. Once an athlete determines his or her activity level, a carbohydrate prescription can be made to match the energy demands of the activity, thus optimizing performance.

2.10 CONCLUSION

Carbohydrates serve many important functions in the body, many of which are highly important to athletes and physically active individuals. Grasping an understanding of the different types of carbohydrates, how they are digested and stored, and how they are metabolized to form ATP for energy generation help an athlete to plan and implement an effective nutrition program for enhancing performance. After reading this chapter, one should be more prepared and able to understand subsequent chapters related to carbohydrate timing strategies structured before, during, and after exercise.

3 Proteins and Amino Acids
The Repair Blocks and Their Place in Growth and Recovery

Nancy R. Rodriguez and William Lunn

CONTENTS

3.1 INTRODUCTION

This chapter establishes the basis for nutrient timing initiatives aimed at maximizing protein utilization by the body and by the muscle for optimizing health, performance, and recovery. As an essential macronutrient, protein is defined and its role in the body and in the diet presented with specific regard for human health and performance. Following a brief overview of protein as a nutrient, protein digestion, absorption, and utilization are presented. The remainder of the chapter focuses on the role of amino acids in muscle growth and recovery. In this context, the function of amino acids in muscle recovery following resistance and endurance exercise is introduced as a foundation for further chapters that target specific mechanisms and practical application of this material.

Distinct from carbohydrate and fat, protein is unique as a macronutrient because nitrogen is a critical component of its constituent amino acids, and certain amino acids are essential nutrients that must be provided in the diet. Like carbohydrate and fat, protein contains carbon, hydrogen, and oxygen. However, the presence of the amino group in the structural template of all amino acids constitutes the unique nitrogen-containing characteristic of this macronutrient. Approximately 16% of protein is nitrogen. This particular distinction provides the opportunity to assess the utilization of protein by the body via nitrogen balance (i.e., nitrogen intake-nitrogen output). This particular method of evaluating the use of protein by the body remains the "classic" technique, while more contemporary approaches employ stable isotope methodology. The former gives a general overview of use of protein by the body, and the latter allows for characterization of organ-specific protein metabolism. Further chapters explore the application of this methodology in the context of nutrient timing in more depth.

The Recommended Dietary Allowance (RDA) for protein is 0.8 grams of protein per kilogram of body mass (Panel on Macronutrients et al. 2005). This particular value lies within the acceptable macronutrient distribution range (AMDR) for protein. The AMDR is the amount of energy from a macronutrient that is considered healthful. The range of energy intake, or AMDR, for protein is 10% to 35% of calories consumed (Panel on Macronutrients et al. 2005). Protein is needed in the diet to support numerous functions in the body. While these include transport proteins, hormones, enzymes, and neurotransmitters, it is the structural role that protein has specific to skeletal muscle that provides a rationale for dietary protein in nutrient timing initiatives directed at increasing, repairing, or maintaining muscle mass. The growth, maintenance, and repair of muscle require various amounts of the individual amino acids that comprise protein.

3.2 PROTEINS

3.2.1 Protein Structure and Function

Amino acids are the infrastructure of proteins. These single molecules consist of an amine group, a carboxylic acid, and a side chain that is commonly referred to as an R-group. These R-groups vary and have been classified as neutral, acidic, and basic, as well as aromatic. In addition to possessing a charge at a particular pH, these R-groups can be characterized as large or small. Of significance to this discussion is the fact that the charge or the size of the R-group can affect the ultimate structure of the protein. Overall, changing the structure of the protein or changes in the resulting polypeptide chain that comprises the protein has an impact on the stability and functionality of the protein in a physiological environment.

There are four levels of protein structure: primary, secondary, tertiary, and quaternary. The primary structure of protein is the polypeptide chain that consists of individual amino acids joined by covalent peptide bonds. This level of structure is specific for each protein in the body because the amino acid sequence has been "coded" for by a respective gene. Therefore, it is at the primary level of protein structure that protein function is determined. Clearly, amino acid availability for forming the polypeptide at the primary level is critical for the synthesis of proteins. The secondary structure of proteins involves hydrogen bonding and the spatial arrangement of the amino acids without respect for the R-groups. The α-helix, pleated sheet, and random coil are the major configurations for the secondary structure of proteins. At the tertiary level of protein structure, R-groups are involved, and the protein becomes three dimensional. Hydrophobic interactions occur and salt bridges are formed resulting, in a more stable protein. Hydrogen and sulfide bonding also contribute to the protein becoming thermodynamically stable in its respective physiological environment. Quaternary protein structure involves at least two polypeptide chains, or subunits, which are typically held together by hydrogen bonds and electrostatic salt bridges.

The resulting protein can be classified as either dynamic or structural. Examples of dynamic proteins include transport proteins (i.e., albumin, transferrin); regulatory proteins (i.e., enzymes, peptide hormones); contractile proteins (i.e., actin, myosin); and immunoproteins (i.e., antibodies). Structural proteins provide a matrix for bone and connective tissue (e.g., skeletal protein, collagen, elastin, keratin) and give structure and form to the body. Regardless of whether a protein is dynamic or structural, its function is determined at the primary level where the specific amino acid sequence has been dictated. Therefore, it is critical that a constant supply of amino acids be readily available so that the initial polypeptide can be synthesized.

3.2.2 ESSENTIALITY

Amino acid pools throughout the body are replenished from endogenous (e.g., muscle) or exogenous (i.e., diet) proteins (Figure 3.1). Skeletal muscle is a primary reservoir for amino acids in the body and as such is subjected to various levels of metabolic regulation of protein synthesis and protein breakdown (Wolfe 2005, 2006). Amino acid availability is central to these processes of regulation. Simply put, when dietary intake of amino acids is adequate to habitually replenish free amino acid pools, the reliance on endogenous protein breakdown for provision of amino acids to support protein synthesis is reduced. Conversely, when dietary intake of amino acids is insufficient, there is increased dependence on endogenous proteolysis to supply amino acids to the body's pools for protein synthesis.

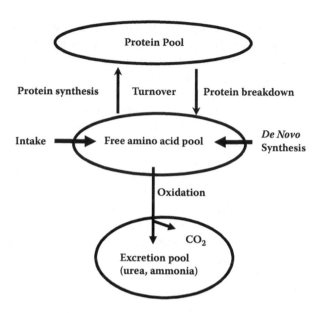

FIGURE 3.1   Amino acid movement among body pools.

While all amino acids are needed for synthesis of various proteins in the body, these nutrients can be further classified as indispensable and dispensable amino acids (Table 3.1). The classic definition of an *indispensable amino acid* is "one which cannot be synthesized by the animal organism out of materials ordinarily available to the cells at a speed commensurate with the demands of normal growth" (Reeds 2000). Indispensable amino acids are essential nutrients, therefore, that must be provided in the diet. In contrast, dispensable amino acids can be produced by the body and are nonessential to the diet. Although outside of the scope of this chapter, it is important to note that a more functional classification system for amino acids has evolved over recent years to accommodate various physiological scenarios and clinical conditions that have an impact on the need for certain amino acids, causing them to be "conditionally" indispensable (Laidlaw and Kopple 1987).

3.2.3 PROTEINS IN THE BODY

Proteins in the body can be generally classified as visceral and somatic proteins. Visceral proteins are nonskeletal proteins found in tissues and organs as well as those proteins that circulate in the blood; somatic protein is skeletal muscle. Reeds (2000) further delineated body protein into four systems that coincide with maintenance and health: the intestine (digestive), the immune system and other defense systems in the body, the nervous system, and skeletal muscle (muscular). Regardless of how these proteins and their respective systems in the body are characterized, it is clear that maintenance of these systems is central to optimal human performance and health. Therefore, routine consumption of a diet that provides essential nutrients, particularly the indispensable amino acids, should be a priority.

TABLE 3.1
Amino Acid Classification

Indispensable (Essentlal) Amino Acids (IDAAs)
Isoleucine
Leucine
Lysine
Methionine
Phenylalanine
Threonine
Tryptophan
Valine
Histidine

Dispensable (Nonessential) Amino Acids (DAAs)
Alanine
Arginine
Aspartic acid
Asparagine
Glutamic acid
Glutamine
Glycine
Proline
Serine

Branched-Chain Amino Acids (BCAAs)
Isoleucine
Leucine
Valine

3.2.4 PROTEINS IN THE DIET

Dietary protein can be characterized as complete or incomplete and therefore having high versus low biological value, respectively, depending on the indispensable amino acid content of a particular food. Protein quality is a measure of how efficiently dietary protein can be used by the body for protein synthesis. Although several methods exist for evaluating the protein content in food, the chemical score remains a standard for measuring protein quality by comparing the amino acid content, particularly the indispensable amino acid content, of food to that of a reference protein (e.g., egg). Often, protein evaluation will focus on the limiting amino acid of the protein being evaluated. The limiting amino acid is whatever indispensable amino acid is present in the lowest quantity in a food or protein relative to other indispensable amino acids. For example, if a test protein has a limiting amino acid that is present at 75% of the level found in egg, a chemical score of 75 will be assigned to the test protein. Proteins that contain all of the indispensable amino acids in a profile that is similar to a reference protein are considered complete proteins. These proteins will have higher chemical scores than those proteins with lower amounts or some, but not all, of the indispensable amino acids. This concept has been extended to protein utilization of a particular food in that the higher the chemical score, the better the biological value or quality of a protein and therefore the more efficiently the protein is utilized by the body. This view has been refined with a newer method of protein quality known as the protein digestibility corrected amino acid scores (Schaafsma 2005). By factoring in the digestibility of the protein being evaluated, protein digestibility corrected amino acid scores go one step beyond chemical score in evaluating dietary proteins. Regardless, the principle remains the same: Proteins that provide a complete profile of the indispensable amino acids are of higher quality than those that contain some, but not all, of these essential nutrients.

3.3 FORMS OF PROTEIN

3.3.1 INTACT PROTEIN SOURCES

3.3.1.1 Whole Food

Whole food is the most natural source of protein in the diet. Dietary protein is readily available in diets rich in animal flesh and milk. Animal sources, such as beef, poultry, fish, eggs, and dairy (milk, yogurt, and cottage cheese), provide an abundance of high-quality protein that can ensure an adequate amino acid intake. Plant-based foods such as grains, vegetables, and beans also provide protein and, in some diets, can be the predominant source of dietary protein. The protein density, as well as quality, of plant versus animal sources varies.

From a practical perspective, a three-ounce serving of beef or poultry contains approximately 25 grams of protein, whereas a single serving of grains or vegetables has only two grams. The former is considered a complete, high-quality protein, while the latter may be incomplete protein of lesser quality. Individuals choosing to obtain their dietary protein solely from plants must be vigilant in eating a variety of plant-based foods throughout the day to ensure adequate intake of indispensable amino acids. While most individual plants may not be a sufficient source of indispensable amino acids, soy is a plant protein considered to be complete and therefore a good-quality protein. Protein found in whole foods is considered intact protein. Protein can also be provided in the diet as protein isolates or individual amino acids.

3.3.1.2 Isolates

Protein isolates have become a common source of dietary protein supplementation. Soy and bovine milk protein whey are the most prevalent protein isolates and are typically available in powder form. Soy protein isolate is approximately 90% protein by weight, produced from dehydrated soy flour that has been defatted and stripped of any plant carbohydrates. Vegans, vegetarians, and individuals who choose to limit animal protein intake frequently depend on soy protein to meet their daily requirement. Soy protein isolate is approximately 93% to 97% digestible (Liu 1997), a value similar to the digestibility of animal protein such as whey.

Whey protein isolate is found in the liquid remnant generated during the coagulation of cow's milk for cheese production. A collection of proteins, whey is a mixture of β-lactoglubulin, α-lactalbumin, and serum albumin. Like soy, whey isolate is dehydrated, and fat and any nonproteinaceous components are removed. The exceptional digestibility and indispensable amino acid content of whey make it a popular choice for protein supplementation. Whey is abundant in branched-chain amino acids (Table 3.1), and the branched-chain amino acid leucine is known for its ability to stimulate protein synthesis at the molecular level (Fujita et al. 2007). In addition, whey contains another important amino acid, cysteine. The biosynthesis of glutathione, an important antioxidant by virtue of its ability to reduce disulfide bonds in reactive oxygen species, requires cysteine linkage at the amine group to the carboxyl group of glutamic acid (Courtney-Martin et al. 2008; Zavorsky et al. 2007).

Although whey is the more-favored milk protein as a commercial protein supplement, casein is the most abundant, representing 80% of protein in cow's milk. Casein isolate is water insoluble, present in milk as micellar particles of protein. Casein is an attractive protein isolate from a digestibility standpoint. The insolubility of the molecule results in the formation of a gel in the stomach following ingestion, which allows a slow, steady release of hydrolyzed amino acids into the gut. It is this characteristic of casein, combined with the high digestibility of whey, that influenced the generation of the "slow" and "fast" protein nomenclature for the respective proteins (Boirie et al. 1997).

Use of casein as a safe dietary protein supplement is controversial. The protein can hydrolyze into the casomorphin peptide, an opioid that can compete with serotonin at opioid receptors at neural synapses in the brain. The resultant sedation and insensitivity to pain suggests brain biochemistry as a mechanism, and casein consumption as a suspected cause of autistic behavior in children. However, only anecdotal evidence is available demonstrating positive effects of casein avoidance on behavior improvement (Elder et al. 2006), and limiting milk proteins in the diet in otherwise healthy, exercising individuals for this reason alone is not recommended.

3.3.2 HYDROLYSATES

Hydrolyzed proteins (protein hydrolysates) are fractions of intact animal or plant proteins that have been cleaved into smaller polypeptides, oligopeptides, and individual amino acids. Cleavage occurs by hydrolysis of peptide bonds within the intact, polymeric protein by treatment with acid, alkaline, heat, or enzymes. Enzymatic proteolysis (breakdown of proteins) is a common avenue of hydrolysate production, and the enzymes used are common digestive components from animals, such as pepsin, chymotrypsin, and trypsin or plant-based, food-grade enzymes. Microorganismic enzymes are also used in hydrolysate production, and although sources include strains of *Bacillus* and *Escherichia coli*, no health risks following consumption of protein hydrolysates cleaved via these organisms have been reported (Schaafsma 2009).

A wide variety of whole foods is used in the preparation of protein hydrolysates. Milk (whey and casein), fish, beef, collagen, egg, pea, bean, soy, rice, and potato are common food sources for hydrolysate production and subsequent application to functional foods and nutritional supplements. The advantage of protein hydrolysates over intact proteins is not clear. However, application to the sports and exercise milieu is prevalent. Intestinal absorption of hydrolysates is accelerated compared to intact protein (Koopman et al. 2009) and free amino acids (Bilsborough and Mann 2006). Predominantly composed of truncated polypeptides, hydrolysates are better absorbed by way of the greater transport efficiency of di- and tripeptides across the brush border into the enterocyte (intestinal cell) than amino acids.

3.3.3 INDIVIDUAL AMINO ACIDS

Individual amino acids are readily available for consumption in powder or liquid form in many health food stores and from dietary supplement providers. Free, monomeric amino acids do not require the biochemical reactions that occur during digestion. Like the end products of protein digestion that they are, free amino acids can be absorbed in the intestine and transported directly into the blood. For healthy men and women with an intact digestive system, there is little, if any, advantage to consuming free amino acids. However, documentation of benefits of certain amino acids to specific metabolic events has fueled supplement production, as well as research targeting potential physiological outcomes subsequent to amino acid consumption in isolation or in combination with other nutrients. Several of these are discussed in greater depth in subsequent chapters.

3.4 PROTEIN DIGESTION

Digestion of dietary protein begins in the stomach. Inactive enzyme precursors called zymogens are activated after secretion for protein digestion. Pepsinogen is the first zymogen involved in protein digestion; it is synthesized by chief cells in the stomach and is autoactivated. Because pepsinogen is activated by acidic pH conditions, the hydrochloric acid in the stomach causes pepsinogen to cleave itself, forming the active protease (protein enzyme) pepsin. The acidic stomach pH denatures, or unfolds, the protein, allowing pepsin to cleave peptides and amino acids from the intact protein.

The denatured, truncated protein, with the newly cleaved peptides and amino acids, enters the small intestine. Bicarbonate ions are secreted from the exocrine pancreas, a collection of ducts from the pancreas that lead into the intestine. The bicarbonate begins to neutralize the acidic contents from the stomach, raising the pH. The increased alkalinity promotes secretion of pancreatic enzymes, inactive proenzyme zymogens that are initially secreted, then activated. The first intestinal zymogen secreted is trypsinogen, cleaved into the active form trypsin by an intestinal secretion of enteropeptidase. Trypsin is the central enzyme in protein digestion. Not only does trypsin continue to break peptide bonds from the original dietary protein, but also this enzyme activates other intestinal zymogens. Trypsin cleaves the zymogenic proenzymes chymotrysinogen, proelastase, and procarboxypeptidase into chymotrypsin, elastase, and carboxypeptidase, respectively. Trypsin, chymotrypsin, and elastase are collectively known as endopeptidases according to their enzymatic action on proteins. Endopeptidases specifically hydrolyze peptide bonds within a polypeptide chain. Conversely, exopeptidases such as carboxypeptidase, produced by both the exocrine pancreas and intestinal epithelial cells, cleave individual amino acids from the end of the polypeptide chain, typically at the C-terminus of the polymer. In brief, endopeptidases continue to break down the dietary protein into smaller peptides within the intestinal lumen, and exopeptidases continue to produce individual amino acids in the intestinal lumen and within the intestinal cell.

3.5   AMINO ACID ABSORPTION

Once in the intestinal lumen, hydrolyzed amino acids and di- and tripeptides require transport into the enterocyte (intestinal cell) and bloodstream so that they can be used by different compartments in the body. Transport of amino acids into the enterocyte is indirectly a process dependent on ATP (adenosine triphosphate). Although the actual transporter on the intestinal brush border membrane is a Na^+ cotransporter, transport is driven by a Na^+ concentration gradient that is set up by the Na^+/K^+-ATPase (adenosine triphosphatase) transporter on the basolateral cell membrane (adjacent to the portal vein) of the enterocyte. The ATPase transporter pumps Na^+ into the intestinal lumen, allowing amino acids to follow Na^+ down the gradient into the cell. Di- and tripeptides are also readily absorbed via H^+ cotransport similar to the Na^+ system. The peptide fragments are then hydrolyzed into amino acids by exopeptidases described previously.

Amino acids accumulate in the enterocyte and are subsequently transported into the bloodstream via the portal vein adjacent to the cell. Because of the Na^+ concentration gradient, cotransport with Na^+ to exit the cell will not work. Facilitated transport of the amino acid down its own concentration gradient enables efflux into the portal vein. Once in the bloodstream, amino acids do not require a carrier protein and travel freely in the systemic circulation to different body tissues. Na^+-dependent cotransport is the primary mechanism of entry into cells once amino acids are distributed to specific tissues.

3.6   AMINO ACID UTILIZATION

After consumption and completion of hydrolysis, amino acids are released and ready for distribution throughout the body to various amino acid pools. These pools can be general, such as the systemic circulation as a whole, or specific among organs and tissues, such as amino acids bound within skeletal muscle protein or free amino acids in the cytoplasm of individual cells. Although amino acids can be used for ATP resynthesis for cellular energy, their primary role is for structural integrity of somatic, visceral, and globular proteins that give body tissues shape and function. Comprehensive utilization of amino acids on uptake from circulation, then, is an expansive topic and beyond the breadth of this chapter. This discussion focuses on skeletal muscle protein utilization, and the concept of protein turnover is explained. Further, the role of amino acids is elucidated in the context of skeletal muscle tissue.

3.7 AMINO ACIDS IN MUSCLE GROWTH AND RECOVERY

3.7.1 Skeletal Muscle Protein Turnover

Skeletal muscle is a dynamic tissue. Muscle protein is constantly broken down and rebuilt in sensitive, yet constant, processes. Paramount to these processes is the flux of amino acids into and out of amino acid pools that influences the maintenance of skeletal muscle tissue. Certain body proteins, such as globular proteins (enzymes, hemoglobin) have short half-lives and therefore high amino acid flux rates. Somatic proteins, such as skeletal muscle, turn over amino acids at a relatively slower rate. The rate of amino acids incorporated, or bound, into muscle protein is protein synthesis; the rate of decay, or release, of amino acids from protein into intracellular or plasma pools is protein breakdown, and the difference between the two processes is net protein balance, or turnover (Figure 3.1). Positive net turnover values indicate an anabolic condition, or protein growth. Negative values indicate catabolism, or a condition promoting protein loss. Transient catabolic states are a normal part of daily maintenance of muscle tissue. Protein balance (synthesis = breakdown) promotes protein retention and maintenance of muscle mass.

3.7.1.1 Protein Synthesis

The source of amino acids incorporated into muscle protein during synthesis can be either free amino acids from dietary protein digestion and absorption or amino acids released from skeletal muscle tissue itself during breakdown. Synthesis starts inside a muscle cell, where translation occurs. Translation involves the transfer of the genetic message in messenger RNA (mRNA) transcribed, or copied, from DNA into an intact protein. The mRNA is then *translated* into an intact protein on ribosomes via amino acid incorporation. In brief, translation is the process of protein synthesis. Translation consists of three steps: (1) initiation of a ribosome complex that can be translated into protein, (2) elongation of the nascent polypeptide, and (3) termination and release of the polypeptide from the ribosome.

Initiation is the major regulatory step of translation and consists of five primary components: (1) eukaryotic initiation factors (eIFs), which bind other initiation-related components to form complexes; (2) ribosomal subunits, which act as a structure on which a new polypeptide can be created; (3) transfer RNA (tRNA), which recognizes and incorporates amino acids into the new polypeptide; (4) mRNA, which contains the genetic message; and (5) guanosine triphosphate (GTP), the energy source needed for dephosphorylation of initiation factors during translation. Synthesis begins with formation of the 43S preinitiation complex, which contains the small 40S ribosomal subunit, GTP, two eIFs, and methionyl-tRNA. For an initiation complex to be fully capable of synthesizing protein, the 43S complex needs additional ribosomal subunits and mRNA. The next step involves unraveling and incorporating mRNA into the 43S preinitiation complex. The binding of mRNA to the 43S complex is the second regulatory step of initiation. Another complex of initiation factors (eIF4F) forms, and its function is to unwind and bind to mRNA. Formation of this complex is essential for initiation to proceed, as the amount of this complex has been positively correlated to protein synthesis rate (Vary et al.

2001). Availability of eIF4E to bind to eIF4G depends on activity of the translational repressor protein eIF 4E-binding protein 1 (4E-BP1). 4E-BP1 occupies the same binding site on eIF4E as eIF4G (Stipanuk 2007) and prevents association of the two initiation factors. However, when hyperphosphorylated, 4E-BP1 releases from eIF4E and allows eIF4G to bind to eIF4E, forming the eIF4F complex that allows mRNA to bind to the ribosome, driving translation. Phosphorylation of eIF4G also enhances eIF4F complex formation, evidenced by increased skeletal muscle protein synthesis rates (Vary and Lynch 2006). The translationally active eIF4F complex allows unwinding, binding to, and activation of mRNA in the 43S preinitiation complex to form the 48S preinitiation complex. The complex is nearly ready to start synthesis of new protein. The only deficiency is a complete ribosome. A 60S ribosomal subunit associates with the 48S complex, hydrolysis of bound GTP releases more initiation factors, and an elongation-functional 80S ribosome is assembled.

Elongation is the process of incrementally adding amino acids to the developing polypeptide chain. The sequence of codons in the mRNA determines the order of addition of amino acids, and protein eukaryotic elongation factors (eEFs) are required for elongation catalysis. Initially, GTP-bound eukaryotic elongation factor 1 (eEF1) complexes with incoming amino acids bound to tRNA. The eEF1-GTP complex associates with the 80S ribosome, where the Met-tRNA is located. The anticodon of the incoming amino acid-tRNA is matched to the mRNA codon, and amino acids unable to make a match are ejected from the ribosome. Only 20 three-base-pair combinations of mRNA are recognized by tRNA, so only 20 different amino acids are incorporated into protein within the body. Eukaryotic elongation factor 2 (eEF2) translocates the ribosome along mRNA by one codon, and the tRNA is shunted along the ribosome so the next mRNA codon can match with a new incoming amino acid-tRNA anticodon. Hydrolysis of GTP bound to eEF2 is required for ribosomal translocation. Inactivation of eEF2 kinase stimulates protein synthesis, as dephosphorylated eEF2 is required to shunt the ribosome along mRNA.

Finally, the process is terminated when the ribosome encounters a UAG stop codon, a termination factor protein releases the polypeptide chain to the cell, and GTP hydrolysis facilitates the separation of the 48S and 60S ribosome subunits. The released ribosomes can then be recycled for use in a new elongation cycle. The process of elongation and termination underscores the energy-consuming nature of protein synthesis. Three molecules of GTP are hydrolyzed during the two processes: one to place tRNA on the mRNA codon, one to shunt the ribosome along mRNA, and one to dissociate the ribosomal subunits.

3.7.1.2 Protein Breakdown

Just as synthesis of skeletal muscle protein is influenced by translational pathways in eukaryotic cells, molecular mechanisms also have an impact on protein breakdown. There are four systems that are largely responsible for the degradative mechanisms of skeletal muscle protein: the lysosomal, the calcium-dependent calpains, the cysteine protease caspases, and the ubiquitin (Ub)-proteasome pathway. The translational pathways of protein synthesis are well characterized and commonly supplement synthesis kinetic outcomes in discussions of muscle protein turnover. However, protein breakdown, also known as proteolysis, is less well understood and has received less attention in the scientific literature. This review provides a mechanistic understanding of the four proteolytic systems as they relate to skeletal muscle protein.

Lysosomes, the primary constituents that comprise the lysosomal proteolytic system, are constitutively expressed in mammals and bound in cell membranes as vesicles containing acid hydrolases consisting of enzymes specific to cellular degradation. The most abundant proteases in lysosomes are cathepsins, given the nomenclature L, B, D, and H (Bechet et al. 2005), and are synthesized in the rough endoplasmic reticulum (ER) as pre-proenzymes. Once in the lysosome, procathepsins are cleaved from the phosphate receptors by the mildly acidic lumen into an active enzyme when the pH drops in the mature lysosome. To maintain the necessary acidic pH in the lumen, ATP-proton pumps in the lysosomal membrane supply protons from the cytosol, a biochemical consideration that underscores the energy-consuming nature of lysosomal protein degradation. Cathepsins L, B, D, and H are all peptidases that, despite their ubiquitous expression in mammals, are distributed within the body in varying abundances among the tissues. Expression is highest in high-protein-turnover tissues, such as kidney and liver, while relatively slow-turnover skeletal muscle protein exhibits modest cathepsin expression (Bechet et al. 2005). Nonetheless, the proteases are characterized in adult skeletal muscle (Bechet et al. 1996), but this expression is much more present in fetal muscle tissue (Bechet et al. 2005). Each cathepsin possesses specific proteolytic activity with respect to targeted myofibrillar proteins. Cathepsin L cleaves almost every protein in the myofibril except troponin C and tropomyosin (Matsukura et al. 1981). Cathepsin B degrades troponin T, troponin I, and tropomyosin (Noda et al. 1981) and myosin heavy chain (Schwartz and Bird 1977). Cathepsin H hydrolyzes troponin T only (Ebashi and Ozawa 1983).

Calpains are nonlysosomal cysteine proteases found in the cytosol and are primary constituents of the Ca^{2+}-dependent calpain system. There are three calpains expressed in muscle protein; two are ubiquitously expressed (calpains 1 and 2), and calpain 3 is highly expressed. Calpains are tightly controlled and kept inactive under most conditions to regulate their great potential for intracellular protein degradation. The calpains initiate degradation by cleaving the actin and myosin constituents of the myofibril, a key initial step that provides these proteins as substrates for their removal by the proteasome from the cytosol. The ubiquitous calpains, specifically calpain 1, function by dismantling the Z-disk and associated proteins titin, nebulin, filamin, and desmin (Williams et al. 1999). Actin and myosin can then release to the cytosol for proteasomal processing. Because myofibrillar fragments tend to accumulate as a result of calpain action, a positive-feedback effect on protein degradation can occur. Proteasome activity can increase in response to cytosolic protein fragments associating with Ub ligases (Li et al. 2004).

Caspases are cysteine proteases that execute physiologic cell death through activation by intracellular signaling pathways. In mammals, at least 14 caspases have been identified, numbered 1 through 14. Because caspases act either upstream or downstream based on their site of action in the proteolytic cascade, they are classified as either initiator or effector caspases (Nunez et al. 1998). Initiators are caspases 2, 8, 9, and 10, and they have longer prodomains than the effectors, caspases 3, 4, 5, 6, 7, 11, 12, and 13 (Nunez et al. 1998). Similar to calpains, caspases are needed to provide actin and myosin fragments for the Ub-proteasome pathway. Apoptotic analysis reveals that actin is a caspase 3 substrate (Mashima et al. 1997), and Western blot analysis confirms accumulation of a characteristic 14-kDa actin fragment associated with enhanced caspase 3 activity in in vitro skeletal muscle cells (Du et al. 2004). Specifically, caspase 3 influences turnover of skeletal muscle protein by way of intracellular signaling. Deactivation of the phosphoinositide-3-kinase (PI3K)/Akt pathway induces caspase 3 activation (Du et al. 2004; Jackman and Kandarian 2004; Kandarian and Jackman 2006).

Although not recognized as a separate system of protein degradation, the forkhead box subgroup O (FOXO) family of transcription factors is implicated in the proteolytic process and is also controlled by PI3K/Akt regulation. Activation of the PI3K/Akt pathway (a well-accepted "growth" response) promotes FOXO phosphorylation, which causes association with intracellular proteins that prevent its movement to other cellular compartments (Tran et al. 2003). In the absence of the insulin signal survival factor, Akt is dephosphorylated and in turn induces dephosphorylation of FOXO. The FOXO protein can then translocate into the nucleus, where it transcribes atrogenes responsible for protein disassembly (Tran et al. 2003). Specifically, FOXO3a has been demonstrated to stimulate transcription of the skeletal muscle-specific Ub ligases MAFbx/atrogin and MuRF1 (Sandri et al. 2004). An overview of proteolytic suppression induced by PI3K/Akt pathway activation is depicted in Figure 3.2.

It has been established that active proteolytic enzymes are responsible for initiating the destruction of skeletal muscle protein by hydrolyzing peptide bonds of myofibrillar proteins to produce fragments. The fragments must then be "cleaned"

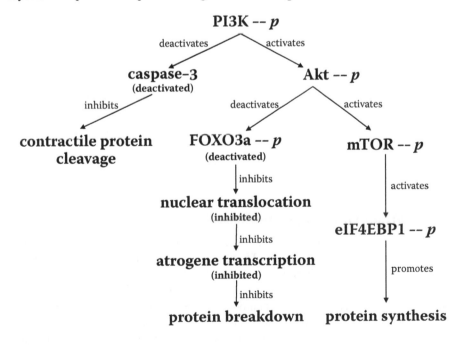

FIGURE 3.2 Proteolytic suppression by PI3K/Akt pathway activation. Italicized p indicates a phosphorylated protein.

from the intracellular space, a process reserved for the Ub-proteasome pathway. In brief, proteins targeted for degradation must encounter the Ub-proteasome pathway to complete the process of proteolysis in eukaryotes. The Ub-proteasome pathway is implicated primarily in skeletal muscle protein breakdown due to its association with myofibrillar degradation (Jagoe and Goldberg 2001). The constitutively expressed ubiquitin-proteasome pathway consists of five major components: (1) the tagging of polypeptide Ub, (2) Ub-activating enzyme E1, (3) Ub-conjugating enzyme E2, (4) the Ub-protein ligase E3, and (5) a multicatalytic proteinase complex, the 26S proteasome. The process is simple, as the two required steps are covalent bonding of Ub to the protein targeted for destruction and recognition of the ubiquitinated protein by the proteasome. Once proteolytic enzymes have hydrolyzed muscle proteins, the cytosolic fragments are prepared for proteasomal disposal by ubiquitination-covalent bonding of the protein fragment to at least four molecules of Ub. Polyubiquitination begins with ATP hydrolysis driving E1 activation of Ub by covalently binding the two proteins via a thioester bond. E1 transfers the activated tagging protein to E2, which monoubiquitinates the targeted protein fragment via a peptide bond. However, further ubiquitination depends on E3, which recognizes the fragment. The Ub-protein ligases are either really interesting new gene (RING) finger enzymes (MuRF1) or U-box-containing enzymes (MAFbx/atrogin). Once a fragment has been tagged with a minimum of four Ub molecules, it can be processed by the proteasome. The second step is recognition and degradation of the Ub-tagged fragment by the 26S proteasome. The proteasome structure has two components: the 20S catalytic core and 19S regulatory "caps" on either end of the core. The proteolytic activity of the proteasome resides in the cylindrically shaped core, while the 19S cap recognizes and prepares the Ub-tagged fragment (Wolf and Hilt 2004). Stacked rings of protease complexes comprise the 20S core architecture; two rings of seven inactive α-subunits sandwich two inner rings of seven proteolytically active β-subunits (Lowe et al. 1995). Enzymatic specificity of each β-subunit defines the core. Subunit $\beta7$ possesses chymotrypsin-like activity and is the most active degradation site (Heinemeyer et al. 1997). The trypsin-like activity of $\beta2$ and acidic activity of $\beta1$ are next in the hierarchy of degradation power (Heinemeyer et al. 1997). Following entry into the core, the unraveled fragment is cleaved into smaller fragments of oligopeptides, on which the remnants are ejected back into the cytosol. Final degradation by cellular peptidases releases amino acids to be used by the cell or disposed as cellular garbage.

3.7.1.3   Kinetic Measures

Amino acid entry into and exit from body pools is the rate of appearance (Ra) and rate of disappearance (Rd), respectively. These rates represent muscle protein synthesis and breakdown. Isotopic labeling of amino acids infused intravenously allows kinetic measurement, as an amino acid tracer is differentiated from the native, nonisotopic amino acid (the tracee). A three-pool model of turnover specifies the body of protein where synthesis and breakdown rate calculation is desired. Because the venous pool is complemented with the bound protein and intracellular pool sources of amino acids, Ra and Rd, or synthesis and breakdown, for skeletal muscle protein can be determined. This model adequately describes skeletal muscle protein turnover and

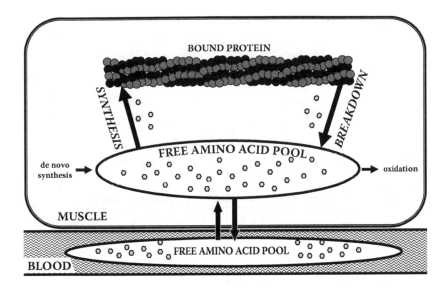

FIGURE 3.3 Three-pool model for skeletal muscle protein turnover.

consists of the bound amino acids in the myofibrillar contractile unit; the intracellular pool of free amino acids either released from bound protein or transported from the blood; and the plasma pool of free amino acids in the blood, derived from either dietary protein or skeletal muscle protein breakdown (Figure 3.3).

Additional routes of amino acid entry and exit into and out of the intracellular free pool are de novo synthesis and oxidation within the cell. When assessing skeletal muscle protein turnover, choosing an isotopic tracer that can neither be synthesized nor oxidized is logical because correcting for amino acid loss or gain in the intracellular free pool is mitigated. The indispensable amino acid phenylalanine satisfies both requirements. Thus, any appearance of phenylalanine tracer in the intracellular or plasma-free pools is indicative of skeletal muscle protein breakdown, and tracer disappearance from the pools reflects synthesis. Administration of the isotope for kinetic measurement is possible by either bolus ingestion or continuous venous infusion. The idea paramount to muscle turnover kinetics determination using stable isotope infusion is achievement of isotopic steady state, or equilibrium. That an isotopic steady state exists during kinetic determination is one of several assumptions of the three-pool model. This implies that when isotopic phenylalanine is infused, isotopic steady state is achieved when exogenous amino acid (the tracer) and endogenous amino acid (the tracee) appear and disappear from the free pools of the model (intracellular and plasma) at equal rates. As long as the infusion rate is constant, there will be a time when the concentrations of each of tracer and tracee in the free pools remain static, the enrichment of the tracer in the pool of tracee plateaus, and steady state is reached. Synthesis of skeletal muscle protein can be calculated at isotopic steady state by measuring incorporation of tracer into the bound protein pool (product) from the intracellular pool (precursor) over time. This rate is called the *fractional synthetic rate* (Figure 3.4).

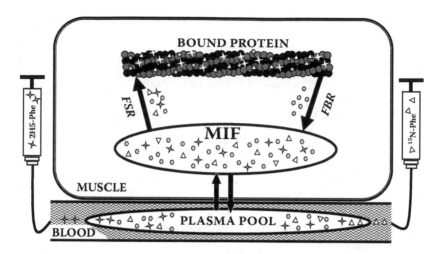

FIGURE 3.4 Tracer methodology for estimates of skeletal muscle fractional synthetic rates (FSRs) and fractional breakdown rates (FBRs).

To fully characterize skeletal muscle protein turnover, a description of the measurement of protein breakdown needs to supplement the fractional synthetic rate. In a catabolic state, breakdown exceeds synthesis, but both synthesis and proteolysis increase because amino acids released during breakdown provide the precursor for synthesis. Therefore, both synthesis and breakdown require assessment when making determinations about turnover. Logically, measuring the decay of the same tracer back into the precursor pool would seem an appropriate approach to measure breakdown. However, healthy adult humans have a maximum protein breakdown rate of 2% per day (Wolfe et al. 2005), making an accurate measurement of tracer release to the precursor pool in the relatively brief infusion duration not feasible using standard analytical techniques. A more viable approach is to measure dilution of the tracer in the intracellular pool by the release of tracee from the bound protein. The simplicity of using a single precursor and product pool for fractional synthetic rate becomes more complicated in breakdown calculations with the addition of another pool, blood plasma. Because breakdown is the topic, the roles of the pools are reversed. The bound protein and plasma pools become precursors, and the intracellular compartment becomes the product pool into which amino acid flux is measured. Cessation of the infusion once isotopic steady state is obtained allows generation of decay curves of tracer enrichment in the product pool due to tracee release from the bound precursor and tracee transit from the plasma precursor into the product pool. Inclusion of the third pool in the precursor-product model for breakdown requires breakdown rate calculations that are intrinsically more complex than for fractional synthetic rate. The equation calculates the rate at which a fraction of unlabeled amino acid releases from the bound precursor into the product pools over time, resulting in a fractional breakdown rate (Figure 3.4). Once both fractional synthetic rate and fractional breakdown rate have been determined, net skeletal muscle protein turnover, or protein balance, can be calculated easily by subtracting fractional breakdown rate from fractional synthetic rate. For detailed descriptions of isotopic tracer methodology, refer to the text by Wolfe and colleagues (2005).

3.7.2 Exercise and Muscle Recovery

Physical exercise, muscular contraction specifically, is considered a potent regulator of skeletal muscle protein metabolism. Since the inception of investigations evaluating physiologic measures of muscle protein turnover in response to exercise interventions, the most common mode of exercise employed has been resistance training. There are myriad original studies that elucidate the impact of the resistance exercise stimulus on molecular and kinetic outcomes of human skeletal muscle protein synthesis and proteolysis.

3.7.2.1 Resistance Exercise

After the discovery of enhanced amino acid transport within skeletal muscle tissue after a bout of resistance exercise (Biolo et al. 1995), the road was paved for researchers to demonstrate that molecular signaling and kinetic events of protein synthesis are suppressed during the bout (Dreyer et al. 2006; Rennie and Tipton 2000) and subsequently stimulated during postexercise recovery (Dreyer et al. 2006; Mayhew et al. 2009; Phillips et al. 1997; Rennie and Tipton 2000; Sheffield-Moore et al. 2005; Trappe et al. 2004). Further, proteolysis is enhanced both during and following exercise (Mascher et al. 2008; Phillips et al. 1997; Raue et al. 2007; Rennie and Tipton 2000; Yang et al. 2006). Despite the advancements in muscle protein turnover determination made with resistance exercise models, only recently have researchers probed endurance exercise. Interest in regulation of muscle protein by endurance exercise has grown markedly.

3.7.2.2 Endurance Exercise

Similar responses by skeletal muscle to endurance exercise have been observed. At the translational level, suppression of intracellular signaling in the PI3K/Akt pathway during endurance exercise and stimulation during recovery occurs in both preinitiation (Frosig et al. 2007; Mascher et al. 2007; Rose et al. 2009; Vary et al. 2001) and elongation (Frosig et al. 2007; Mascher et al. 2007; Rose et al. 2005, 2009). To that end, the skeletal muscle protein fractional synthetic rate measured during recovery from endurance exercise has been observed to increase relative to the preexercise and during-exercise measurements (Harber et al. 2009; Imoberdorf et al. 2006; Sheffield-Moore et al. 2004). Concomitant to increased skeletal muscle protein synthesis during recovery is elevated molecular activity promoting proteolysis (Coffey et al. 2006; Feasson et al. 2002; Harber et al. 2009; Louis et al. 2007; Mahoney et al. 2005; Thompson and Scordilis 1994).

Regarding kinetic adaptations of skeletal muscle proteolysis to endurance exercise, few examples exist in the literature, and data are limited to chronic training effects. Pikosky et al. (2006) showed a tendency for skeletal muscle protein fractional breakdown rate to increase at rest following four weeks of aerobic training consisting of running bouts at 65% of VO_2Peak. (VO_2Peak is the peak oxygen consumption achieved during maximal aerobic exercise.) The proteolytic effect resulted in a reduction of net protein balance, indicating a more catabolic state at rest after the training period. In total, these studies underscore the important role of amino acids in muscle recovery from exercise. Most of the previous studies cited were conducted with subjects in the postabsorptive (fasted) state, so the only amino acids available to induce a fractional synthetic rate increase are likely derived from breakdown of the muscle protein itself. The quintessential effect of an exercise bout on muscle protein turnover is an increase in synthesis and breakdown following exercise, but breakdown exceeds synthesis (Phillips et al. 1997). Therefore, unless exogenous amino acids are provided (i.e., dietary protein intake), muscle protein turnover will remain negative. This role of dietary protein and amino acids in muscle growth and recovery is highlighted in the context of nutrient timing for optimal health and human performance in further chapters.

3.8   SUMMARY AND RECOMMENDATIONS

Nutrient timing initiatives aimed at maximizing protein utilization by the body and by the muscle for growth and recovery are a reality. As an essential macronutrient, protein, as well as individual amino acids, remains a pivotal nutrient in the nutritional supplement industry and is consistently considered in strategies for maintaining, increasing, or repairing muscle. Timing of protein ingestion, particularly in the proximity of an exercise bout, is one approach to maximizing the maintenance and deposition of lean body mass. Intact proteins, particularly those found in whole foods, are well utilized by the body and the muscle. In addition, food sources of good-quality, or complete, protein typically provide other essential micronutrients (i.e., vitamins and minerals) as well. The body is well equipped to digest and absorb intact protein and protein isolates. For most healthy men and women, there appears to be little advantage to consuming individual amino acids or amino acid mixtures with specific regard to digestion and absorption. The more significant observation is the role of individual amino acids, specifically leucine, in metabolic regulation. Habitual consumption of good-quality protein within the AMDR will replenish the body's amino acid pools and contribute to increased protein synthesis and decreased protein breakdown, eventually achieving a positive net protein balance. When combined with an exercise bout, resistance or endurance based, this anabolic scenario is enhanced. In this context, good-quality protein and indispensable amino acid consumption during the time frame associated with muscle recovery following resistance or endurance exercise can be one option in a nutrient timing plan that targets specific mechanisms to enhance protein utilization by employing realistic and practical approaches to diet designs targeting optimal performance and health.

4 Lipids
A Dense Fuel Supply and Important Cellular Component

Kristin Dugan and Lem Taylor

CONTENTS

4.1 INTRODUCTION

Dietary fat is a dense fuel source that is essential for normal cellular physiology and daily activity (Table 4.1). Internal fat depots throughout the human body comprise more than 50 times the amount of stored energy compared to stored carbohydrate, and for this reason alone fat becomes a critical fuel source for many types of athletic activities, particularly those of prolonged duration. In fact, typical body fat stores could allow a runner to run at least 800 miles (or more than 130 hours if running at a pace of six miles per hour) before depletion of fat depots will occur—although this concept is only accepted in theory when considering the rate-limiting steps of fat metabolism to be discussed further in this chapter. Fat has somewhat of a paradoxical role for competing athletes. On one end, its role in providing invaluable constituents to allow for hormone production, nutrient transport, and so on necessitates its intake, while its relatively high energy density often leads to concern over excessive energy intake, which can lead to undesired changes in body mass and body composition. In specific regard to nutrient timing, fat ingestion is a carefully approached topic as studies that have explored some aspect of fat loading or supplementation consistently report unfavorable gastrointestinal responses. Dietary fat intake throughout the day is essential, but from the standpoint of trying to promote ideal adaptations by manipulating food choices, fat intake can inhibit these adaptations under certain conditions. This chapter first discusses lipids from a basic nutrition perspective and then outlines their role in metabolism during various exercise scenarios.

TABLE 4.1

Functions of Fat

A. Primary fuel source both at rest and during prolonged aerobic exercise

B. Protects vital organs from trauma

C. Essential for the absorption and transport of important nutrients

    1. Beta-carotene

    2. Vitamins A, D, E, K

D. Structural component of cell membranes

E. Necessary in the formation of bile

F. Precursor to sex hormones

    1. Estrogen

    2. Testosterone

4.1.1 NATURE OF LIPIDS

Fat is an essential nutrient that when provided in deficient levels would dramatically compromise several physiologic processes. A diet too low in fat can inhibit muscle building since fat is a necessary component in the production of sex hormones (e.g., testosterone). In addition, dietary fat provides an abundant energy source for endurance athletes; this macronutrient becomes a primary fuel source during prolonged, submaximal aerobic exercise. An adequate amount of dietary fat must therefore be consumed by athletes as well as general populations who restrict their caloric intake in an attempt to lose weight to sustain the physical demands of the activities involved. Determining optimal fat intake is difficult to achieve and is largely dependent on the individual, but if the athlete's specific training regimen and personal metabolic demands are considered, a healthy balance of dietary fat intake and caloric expenditure can be achieved and should be the goal.

4.1.2 ROLE OF LIPIDS IN NUTRIENT TIMING

The timing of fat consumption affects performance both directly and indirectly. Directly, a large amount of fat intake just prior to or during exercise often causes gastrointestinal problems, which may necessitate reduction of exercise intensity, decreasing performance. It takes longer for fat to be digested and absorbed in the digestive tract, so in preexercise periods or times of rest, blood flow is diverted to the stomach and intestines to accommodate this demand. If exercise commences when digestion is occurring, this prioritization of blood flow away from the muscles may slow reaction time and overall performance, and the athlete may also experience gastrointestinal stress resulting from the slow transit time of fat in the gut. Alternatively, a low intake of dietary fat could potentially limit testosterone production because of the restricted cholesterol intake that is usually present in dietary fat sources of animal origin, which could have an impact on testosterone-mediated adaptations to the exercise training.

To determine the right time and amount of fat intake in regard to performance, the process of digestion and absorption of fat must be understood and considered. It takes the digestive system a significantly longer amount of time to break down and absorb lipids than protein and carbohydrates since lipid digestion is a multistep process. Unlike carbohydrates, fat must undergo a series of transformations before the fat is able to supply the body with energy, so dietary fat intake must allow an adequate amount of time to digest and absorb prior to physical activity to optimize fat as a fuel source. Thus, in terms of nutrient timing, fat has to be dealt with in a different manner than carbohydrate and protein sources throughout the day, and this point is addressed more specifically in Chapters 6 and 7 of this text.

4.2 CLASSIFICATIONS OF FAT

Fat is classified primarily by its chemical structure, which has a profound effect on its absorption and utility in the body. Some forms of lipids, such as medium-chain fatty acids, are not typically stored in the body due to their ability to be rapidly

absorbed and utilized in the body; therefore, the function of the different classifications of fat in the body should be an important consideration for physical activity as
well as when selecting various dietary sources of fat. Different forms of fat not only
can have effects on performance, but are also linked with various health risks, so it is
important to understand the distinction between the different types of lipids to make
healthy choices in the diet.

4.2.1 GENERAL STRUCTURE

Lipids consist of hydrocarbon chains composed of oils, fats, and waxes that are typically soluble in organic solvents, such as acetone, ether, and chloroform, but are
highly insoluble in water. Like carbohydrates, lipids contain the elements carbon,
hydrogen, and oxygen; however, lipids have a small amount of oxygen relative to
carbon and hydrogen. Represented by the chemical formula $CH_3(CH_2)_nCOOH$, lipids consist of three components, a carboxyl acid (–COOH) group, a methyl (–CH_3)
group, and a hydrocarbon (–CH_2)$_n$ chain. The hydrocarbon chain separates the
methyl group and the carboxyl group, which can bind to glycerol to form mono-,
di-, or triacylglycerol to be used by cells as a fuel source for energy as well as serve
other roles in the body. From here, lipids are subdivided into simple, compound, and
derived lipids, which are outlined in Table 4.2; common dietary sources of these
types of fat are shown in Table 4.3.

TABLE 4.2
Classes of Lipids

I. Simple lipids
A. Triglycerides
   1. Short-chain fatty acid
   2. Medium-chain fatty acid
   3. Long-chain fatty acid
   4. Saturated fatty acid
   5. Unsaturated fatty acid
      a. Monounsaturated fatty acid
      b. Polyunsaturated fatty acid
      c. Trans fatty acid
B. Waxes
II. Compounds lipids
A. Phospholipid
B. Glycolipid
C. Lipoprotein
III. Derived lipids
A. Fatty acid
B. Sterols consisting primarily of cholesterol
C. Hydrocarbons

TABLE 4.3

Dietary Sources of the Different Classes of Lipids

Type of Lipid	Dietary Sources
Short-chain fatty acids	Vinegar, carob seeds, butter, parmesan cheese
Medium-chain fatty acids	Coconut oil, palm oil
Long-chain fatty acids	Fish oil
Saturated fatty acids	Beef, butter, cream, whole milk
Unsaturated fatty acids	Olive oil, canola oil, peanut oil, avocado, most nuts (excluding walnuts)
Trans fatty acids	Hydrogenated oils, processed foods

4.2.2 SIMPLE LIPIDS

Simple lipids only contain carbon, hydrogen, and oxygen molecules with the basic structure described. Examples of simple lipids are monoacylglycerol (monoglyceride), diacylglycerol (diglyceride), and triacylglycerol (triglyceride), which is the most common and composes the majority of dietary fat intake.

4.2.2.1 Triacylglycerols

Triacylglycerols are the most abundant of dietary lipids, consisting of a three-carbon glycerol backbone esterified with three fatty acids. The fatty acids typically vary in length according to the number of carbon molecules composing them.

4.2.2.2 Short-Chain Fatty Acids

Short-chain fatty acids contain six carbons or less, and representative examples include *acetic acid*, responsible for the sour taste and smell of vinegar; *isobutyric acid*, which can be found in carob seeds; *butyric acid*, commonly found in butter and parmesan cheese; *isovaleric acid*, a common occurrence in a wide variety of plants and essential oils; and *caproic acid*, a constituent of various animal fats and oils.

4.2.2.3 Medium-Chain Fatty Acids

Medium-chain fatty acids are important fuel sources found in coconut and palm oils, and they contain eight to ten carbon molecules. Medium-chain fatty acids have historically been used as a dietary supplement in athletes and bodybuilders since they are typically not transported in the same manner as longer-chain fatty acids, making their oxidation easier, reducing potential body fat gains; they are a potential alternative fuel source during extended bouts of endurance exercise. Due to the water solubility of medium-chain fatty acids, these fatty acids are quickly digested and are rapidly absorbed directly into the bloodstream by independent crossing of the intestinal mucosa. Unlike long-chain fatty acids, medium-chain fatty acids do not require chylomicrons of the lymphatic system for transport, which allows them to be immediately absorbed into the bloodstream via the portal vein. The blood then transports the fatty acids directly to the liver and muscle for potential use as energy instead of storage in adipose tissue. Once the medium-chain fatty acids reach the target cell, they diffuse first through the plasma membrane and then through the inner mitochondrial membrane for oxidation. Medium-chain fatty acids are able to diffuse freely and enter the mitochondria more quickly than longer fatty acids because they do not require a carrier to enter the organelle. This is thought to provide an advantage to endurance athletes by elevating plasma-free fatty acid concentrations, thus sparing glycogen stores. By providing a readily available energy source to working muscle, medium-chain fatty acids could ideally stimulate fat metabolism and provide an additional substrate during prolonged endurance exercise. This purported ergogenic mechanism of medium-chain fatty acid supplementation seems to exist only in theory, however, since the amount of medium-chain fatty acids an athlete can tolerate (up to 30 grams) does not appear to have a significant impact on performance and only contributes to 3–7% of total exercise energy requirements. Consuming a dose of medium-chain fatty acids greater than 30 grams has shown to be detrimental to the gastrointestinal tract, causing abdominal cramps, gas, bloating, and even vomiting during endurance training and is thus discouraged.

4.2.2.4   Long-Chain Fatty Acids
Unlike medium-chain fatty acids, long-chain fatty acids are composed of 12 carbons or more and are digested and absorbed by the digestive system to be potentially stored as triacylglycerols in adipose or muscle tissue if not immediately used as a fuel source during daily or physical activity.

4.2.2.5   Degree of Saturation
Triglycerides are also identified according to the nature of the chemical bonds connecting the fatty acids to the glycerol molecule. When double bonds are formed in the molecule, hydrogen atoms are eliminated; therefore, triglycerides are often described according to the degree of saturation of hydrogen atoms in the fatty acid components of the triglyceride molecule. The greater the number of double bonds contained in the fatty acid, or unsaturation, the more susceptible the fatty acid is to peroxidation (rancidity) and thus instability. Fatty acids that contain one or more double bonds are called unsaturated fatty acids and are thus considered unstable fats. Unsaturated fats possess a lower melting point and tend to be liquids at room temperature. Dietary sources high in unsaturated fats consist of olive oil, canola oil, peanut oil, most nuts (excluding walnuts), and avocados. Unsaturated fats that contain only one double bond are referred to as monounsaturated fatty acids, while fatty acids connected to glycerol that contain two or more double bonds are called polyunsaturated fatty acids. Polyunsaturated fats exist in two forms, either a *cis* conformation or a *trans* conformation, depending on the nature of the double bond. The *cis* isomer stacks all of the hydrogen atoms on one side of the double bond, whereas the *trans* isomer places the hydrogen atoms on opposite sides. When polyunsaturated fats possess one or more double bonds in the *trans* conformation, they are called trans fatty acids or hydrogenated fats. The larger bend angle in the molecule increases the stability of the fatty acid; therefore, *trans* fats are popular in the manufacturing of processed foods. Trans fatty acids can occur naturally in very small amounts in meat and poultry but are most often human-made by artificially adding hydrogen to oils to solidify the substance, most commonly in margarine and

shortening and subsequently foods containing these ingredients. Although trans fats were designed to increase shelf life and to add stability to processed foods, these fats can be detrimental to health since hydrogenated fat tends to decrease high-density lipoprotein ("good") cholesterol while increasing low-density lipoprotein ("bad") cholesterol levels. Artificial trans fats may also result in an increased inflammatory response, which can result in negative heart health consequences through the promotion of atherosclerosis (Harvey et al. 2008; Lemaitre et al. 2006); therefore, trans fats should be eliminated from the diet as much as possible. Unlike saturated fats, there is no physiological need for any amount of trans fat in the diet, so elimination of hydrogenated fats involves no risk of deficiency in the body.

Saturated fatty acids contain no double bonds between the molecules and are thus considered to be highly stable fats. Saturated fatty acids can be found in several animal products, such as high-fat cuts of beef, butter, cream, full-fat (whole) and 2% milk, cheese, and full-fat yogurt, as well as coconut and palm oils. Saturated fats are popular in processed foods due to their resistance to rancidity and ability to remain a solid at room temperature. The American Heart Association recommends that 7% of total calories should come from saturated fat since large amounts of saturated fatty acids can increase inflammation throughout the body as well as elevate blood cholesterol levels, which has been shown to increase the risk of coronary heart disease (Kato et al. 1973; Keys et al. 1966). Based on a 2,000-calorie diet, the American Heart Association suggests that individuals consume no more than 16 grams (equal to 140 calories) of saturated fat per day, and that individuals should attempt to replace saturated fats with mono- or polyunsaturated fats to further reduce cardiovascular heart disease risk. In fact, it has been reported that by replacing 5% of total energy from saturated fat with polyunsaturated fat, cardiovascular heart disease risk is reduced by 42% (Hu et al. 1997). It is important therefore for individuals to be conscientious of the ratio of the various classes of lipids ingested daily. The amount of dietary polyunsaturated fat relative to saturated fat intake (referred to as the P:S ratio) may actually be a more significant predictor of cardiovascular heart disease risk than the consideration of total saturated fat intake alone. Saturated fat should therefore not only be limited on the basis of grams per day based on caloric intake, but also should be limited to quantities less than that of daily polyunsaturated fat intake. The recommendations vary, but a general consensus suggests that caloric intake in the form of saturated fats should not exceed 7% and that of polyunsaturated fats should be approximately 10%, thus producing a P:S ratio of greater than 1.0 that ensures an optimal dietary fat intake.

4.2.3 COMPOUND LIPIDS

Compound lipids, like simple lipids, contain carbon, hydrogen, and oxygen atoms; however, they are combined with one or more additional elements, such as phosphorous, nitrogen, or sulfur. Compound lipids are not typically used as dietary sources of fat intake, but instead include phospholipids, glycolipids, and lipoproteins, which are each essential components of cellular structure. Although compound lipids do not directly aid the body as an exogenous fuel source, these lipids are essential in cellular structure and are thus necessary for proper biochemical functioning during daily activity.

4.2.3.1 Phospholipids

Phospholipids form cell membranes by forming a bilayer around the cell to regulate the transport of substances into and out of the cell. The role of the phospholipid bilayer is especially important to nutrition and performance since it regulates nutrient transport into the cell. The phospholipid bilayer determines and controls the rate-limiting functions of glucose, fatty acid, and amino acid entry to and from the cell, all of which are considered to have an impact on exercise capacity. The phospholipid bilayer of the cell membrane is stabilized by glycolipids, which serve as biochemical markers on the cell to act as recognition sites for specific chemicals. Glycolipids consist of fatty acids bound with carbohydrate and nitrogen and function much like lights on an airport runway—these biochemical markers show traveling chemicals where to taxi on the cell membrane and how to reach the proper terminal (i.e., receptor, transport channel, port, etc.).

4.2.3.2 Lipoproteins

Lipoproteins function to transport water-insoluble lipids in the water-based bloodstream. Lipoproteins consist of protein spheres that are formed in the liver when a protein molecule and a triacylglycerol or phospholipid molecule bind. These spheres function to provide a major avenue for transporting lipids in the blood. Without binding to a lipoprotein, the lipid would float to the surface of the bloodstream like an inner tube in a body of water instead of circulating throughout the blood homogeneously. The most well-known lipoproteins are high-density lipoproteins (HDLs) (good cholesterol) and low-density lipoproteins (LDLs) (bad cholesterol), which enable fats to travel in the blood throughout the body. HDL is produced in the liver and small intestine and contains the highest percentage of protein (~50%) and the least amount of lipid (20%) and cholesterol (20%). HDL is considered to be the good form of cholesterol since (unlike LDL) it acts as a scavenger by removing cholesterol from arterial walls, thus reducing plaque buildup and the incidence of atherosclerosis and heart disease. It is important to maximize HDL levels while minimizing LDL concentrations in the blood to reduce the risk of heart disease. A constellation of lifestyle factors, such as avoidance of tobacco smoke, increased intake of polyphenols found in red wine, increased niacin intake, regular participation in a moderate-to high-intensity exercise program, and many others, are often considered for their ability to improve circulating levels of HDL cholesterol and reduce personal risk for cardiovascular disease. A complete discussion of this topic is beyond the scope of this chapter.

4.2.4 Derived Lipids

The products of the hydrolysis of simple and compound lipids are called derived lipids. *Hydrolysis* refers to a chemical reaction of water with a specific compound to produce a new substance. The most common derivatives of hydrolysis reactions involving simple and compound lipids are fatty acids and sterols.

4.2.4.1 Fatty Acids

Fatty acids are carboxylic acids derived from the hydrolysis of a triacylglycerol, as mentioned in this chapter, but they also exist in the form of free fatty acids and essential fatty acids. Most of the fatty acids in the body are obtained from the diet and are classified into families depending on the location of the last double bond and the number of carbon atoms, such as omega-3, -6, and -9 fatty acids. On absorption, dietary fatty acids circulate in the blood and are taken up by cells either to be utilized for fuel, stored for later use by the body or incorporated as some other cellular constituent. Free fatty acids by nature are not esterified to form a monoacylglycerol, diacylglycerol, or triacylglycerol but rather circulate in the bloodstream bound to albumin (a common blood protein that allows for its transport in the blood) as a readily available energy source to working muscles. Free fatty acids are released into the bloodstream as a result of either the digestion of dietary fat or the hydrolysis of triacylglycerol stores in the body. Although excessive intake of dietary fat is discouraged, fatty acids are essential nutrients required by the body for many aspects of physiology.

The human body cannot produce essential fatty acids, so they must be obtained through exogenous fat sources. The primary essential fatty acids consist of α-linolenic acid (omega-3) and linoleic acid (omega-6), which are necessary in the production of eicosanoids, hormone-like substances that affect blood pressure, immunity, inflammation, and the contraction of smooth muscle tissue. Of the known eicosanoids, eicosapentaenoic acid (EPA) and docosahexaenoic acid (DHA) have repeatedly been shown to benefit various aspects of health. When consumed, omega-3 fatty acids replace omega-6 fatty acids in certain blood and liver cell membranes, which results in improved cell membrane function. Further, the resulting anti-inflammatory effect on blood vessels reduces blood viscosity, which goes to directly improve cardiovascular functioning. Furthermore, it has been suggested that supplementation with EPA and DHA inhibits the production of inflammatory eicosanoids produced by damaged molecules as a result of exhaustive exercise and various aspects of disease and clinical conditions. Although the immediate effect on performance remains to be clearly determined, the long-term anti-inflammatory effect could potentially benefit health and physical functioning in athletes as well as many other specialized populations, healthy or not. A small amount of each essential fatty acid should be consumed daily; however, it is recommended to balance the intake of omega-3 and omega-6 fatty acids in a two-to-one ratio (for every one gram of omega 6 ingested, two grams of omega-3 should be ingested) to balance the proinflammatory effects of omega-6 fatty acids. Sunflower, corn, soybean, and sesame oils are abundant sources of omega-6 fatty acids, while flaxseed, walnut, canola, and fish oils provide a wealth of omega-3 fatty acids and should often substitute for omega-6-rich food sources.

4.2.4.2 Sterols

A sterol is the product of a steroid and an alcohol molecule that is present in the fatty tissue of plants and animals, consisting of a ring structure instead of a chain. The most important sterol produced in the body is cholesterol, which provides many essential functions in the biochemical processes of the body. Cholesterol is a lipid found in the cell membranes of all animal tissues and is transported in the blood plasma. The primary roles of cholesterol in the body are

- Building and maintenance of cell membranes
- Regulation of membrane fluidity
- Manufacture of bile
- Metabolism of fat-soluble vitamins (A, D, E, K)
- Major precursor in the synthesis of steroid hormones, such as testosterone and estrogen

Despite the essential roles cholesterol plays in the body, excess cholesterol in the body can compromise health, so individuals must moderate their dietary intake of this sterol. Cholesterol is found only in animal-based foods, and those individuals who have elevated levels of cholesterol in their blood (particularly those with a family history of elevated cholesterol) should be aware and limit their intake.

4.3 LIPID METABOLISM

It is essential to understand the nature of lipid metabolism to optimize the processes involved to ensure maximal performance capabilities. The digestion and absorption of fat is more complicated than that of other nutrients to accommodate the resistant water-lipid gradient in the human digestive system. The body is composed of approximately 45–75% water depending on the age and body composition of an individual; therefore, the water-insoluble nature of lipids resists interaction with the water-based elements of the body. Lipids must then undergo significant transformation during the digestive process to facilitate their metabolism. This involves several additional biochemical processes that slow the rate of digestion and thus absorption, assimilation, and storage of exogenous lipid sources, which must be taken into consideration when performing physical activity.

4.3.1 Digestion, Absorption, and Assimilation of Lipids

Digestion begins in the mouth when lingual lipase, along with chewing, splits triacylglycerols into fatty acids and a glycerol molecule, which provides 10–30% of total lipid digestion before the lipids even reach the stomach. Once the lipids reach the stomach, acid-stable lipases continue to hydrolyze the triacylglycerols, but at a rate much slower due to the water fraction in which the lipase is found. Only short-chain and medium-chain fatty acids are digested in the stomach, while long-chain fatty acids wait to be digested by the small intestine, where triacylglycerols are organized into large lipid globules. In the duodenum, additional bile and pancreatic lipase enter the intestine to continue the digestion of the fatty acids. Bile salts from the gallbladder form micelles on which phospholipids and fatty acids form a bilayer and emulsify the lipids. The formation of micelles increases the total surface area of the fatty acids to be digested to better facilitate hydrolysis by pancreatic lipase. When bile salts are added to the duodenum, 97% of the fat can be absorbed, whereas only 50% of fat is absorbed without bile salts. It is therefore harder for individuals without a gallbladder to digest and absorb lipids due to the absence of bile salts.

After all micelles are formed, fatty acids are transported to the villi of the target cell to diffuse across the epithelial membrane. Some of the fatty acids are reesterified in the endoplasmic reticulum of the cell, where the fatty acids combine with cholesterol and phospholipids to form chylomicrons, while the remaining free fatty acids circulate in the bloodstream as a readily available fuel source for active muscles.

4.3.2 STORAGE OF LIPIDS

Every cell in the body contains a small amount of fat since lipids make up cell membranes, nerve sheaths, hormones, and other structures that influence body functioning; however, fat cells, or adipocytes, are specifically designed to store large amounts of fat. Energy stored as fat in the body provides a concentrated source of fuel to be used for both daily activity as well as various forms of exercise. Fat is stored with a very minimal amount of water, so fat stores are more compact and thus store significantly greater amounts of energy than carbohydrate reserves. One gram of fat yields nine kilocalories of heat energy, a value more than twice the potential energy of protein or carbohydrate (four kilocalories). In this respect, even athletes with very low body fat percentages still have a substantial caloric reserve because of this high concentration of compact energy in the form of stored fat.

The location of fat stores and the type of fat in the reserve determine the function of these lipid stores. Fat is not a dormant body tissue, but an active site contributing to energy needs, temperature regulation, cellular signaling and communication, and inflammatory responses in the body. The majority of our body fat exists as white fat, is stored in adipocytes, and relates to what is commonly thought of as body fat. White adipocytes release individual fatty acids into the bloodstream for transport to active muscle tissue corresponding with energy demands. Excess white adipose tissue should be avoided since a common consequence of enlarged white adipocytes is the manufacture and secretion of inflammatory eicosanoids in addition to insulin resistance. In contrast, the primary role of brown fat is to produce heat when activated by cool temperatures. Brown fat burns an excessive amount of energy to heat body tissues and is located in the upper back, side of the neck, along the spine, and between the clavicle and shoulder region. Babies have greater amounts of brown fat, functioning as a protective mechanism against their inability to shiver in cool temperatures; however, babies lose brown fat as a consequence of normal growth and development and in conjunction develop an ability to control thermoregulation. Although it has been established that the caloric expenditure capacity of brown fat increases in cooler climates, it is still unknown how exercise affects this capacity.

White fat is primarily stored in two locations, in subcutaneous fat stores and the muscle. Subcutaneous fat consists of the layer of fat just below the skin that provides approximately 50% of total body fat storage. Subcutaneous fat functions to conserve body heat in cold environments as a natural form of insulation. This insulation layer may be problematic in those with an excess of subcutaneous fat during warm weather since the body may have difficulty releasing the heat generated by physical activity. Trapping in body heat in hot environments increases the risk of heat stress and dehydration as the body produces an excess of sweat in an attempt to reduce body temperature. Lipids are also stored in muscle tissue as intramuscular fat, or intramuscular triglycerides, as a readily available fuel source to the active muscle fibers. Utilization of intramuscular triglycerides is maximized during moderate-intensity exercise lasting one to three hours, during which the body is known to derive 20% to 40% of its fuel from intramuscular triglyceride stores. The more often intramuscular triglyceride is utilized during prolonged physical activity, the more the muscles "remember" to store greater amounts of fat in the muscle to be used during exercise; therefore, the capacity for intramuscular triglyceride storage adapts to endurance exercise training. White fat also composes the body's visceral fat, which is body fat located deep in the body surrounding the organs; however, this storage site is not commonly used as a fuel source during exercise. Visceral adipocytes are larger and more active than other adipocytes, actively releasing free fatty acids and inflammatory eicosanoids into the bloodstream. An excessive accumulation of visceral fat around the abdomen is dangerous since large amounts of visceral fat have been found to contribute to the development of diabetes and heart disease; however, regular exercise exerts powerful prevention over this adaptation.

4.3.3 LIPID MOBILIZATION AS A FUEL SOURCE

Fatty acids are oxidized in the mitochondria of active skeletal muscle cells during physical activity from two primary sources: adipose tissue and intramuscular triacylglycerols. The muscle can oxidize fatty acids either from its own fat stores (intramuscular triglycerides) or from fatty acids transported in the bloodstream from adipose tissue to fuel activity and contribute to adenosine triphosphate (ATP) production through oxidative phosphorylation. This choice is determined primarily by the intensity and duration of the exercise involved. During low-intensity exercise at the beginning of the activity, muscles first use the free fatty acids available in the blood since they are in such great supply. As exercise reaches moderate intensity, muscles begin to use intramuscular triglyceride stores as the next immediate source to provide energy lasting about two hours. After two hours, however, muscles refer back to the free fatty acids in the blood to supply the energy, and as high-intensity exercise begins, a transition from fat utilization to carbohydrate utilization occurs.

At rest, fat is the primary fuel source for body functioning and ATP synthesis, so adipocytes release fatty acids into the bloodstream to provide a readily available fuel source to cells. As activity progresses into exercise, blood lipid levels become depleted as the muscle cells continue to use an increasing number of fatty acids as a fuel source to satisfy the demand. As these levels are depleted, the body begins to rely on the provision of fatty acids from the breakdown of stored fat to sustain activity. At the onset of exercise, the body releases catecholamines (epinephrine and norepinephrine) along with growth hormone and glucagon to stimulate lipolysis in adipose tissue and muscle. In adipose tissue, these hormones activate enzymes (hormone-sensitive lipase) that begin to split the triacylglycerol into fatty acids and glycerol molecules (lipolysis) to be released into the blood and transported to active muscles. A small percentage of the fatty acids produced are then retained by adipocytes to be used to form new triacylglycerols within the adipose tissue in a process called reesterification. The remaining fatty acids, traveling through the bloodstream as free fatty acids, are then taken up by skeletal muscle, while the glycerol molecules are transported to the liver to form new glucose molecules (gluconeogenesis) or inserted into carbohydrate metabolism to fuel glycolysis during exercise. Inside the muscle, triacylglycerols are broken down by hormone-sensitive lipase, thus increasing the availability of nutrient-dense fatty acids inside the active cell. The resulting fatty acids circulating in the cell are released to be activated by a coenzyme and carried into the mitochondria by carnitine. Once in the mitochondria, the fatty acids are used as a substrate via β-oxidation to fuel the oxidative phosphorylation processes (Krebs cycle and electron transport chain) to sustain submaximal physical activity.

4.3.4 LIMITATIONS OF FAT OXIDATION

Fat is a calorie-dense fuel source that, unlike carbohydrates, has an unlimited capacity for storage in the body. Fat utilization is typically desired to fuel daily activity and exercise to prevent excessive body weight and to spare the limited glycogen stores that deplete much faster than fat reserves. Why then can't the body burn fat all of the time? If the average 154-pound (70-kilogram) individual with a moderate amount of body fat (17%) has the potential to burn 107,000 calories using fat stores alone, why does the body not use only this energy? The answer to these questions lies in the rate-limiting steps of fat oxidation that potentially inhibit the use of fat as a fuel source at higher rates and the nature of the activity involved, particularly the exercise intensity and duration. Several key rate-limiting steps exist that control fat oxidation, including the activation of lipolysis, removal of fatty acids and their transport in the bloodstream, transport of fatty acids into the muscle, transport of fatty acids into the mitochondria, and oxidation of fatty acids in the β-oxidation pathway and Krebs cycle.

4.3.4.1 Activation of Lipolysis

Lipolysis, or the breakdown of stored fat into fatty acids, begins when triacylglycerol lipase and other enzymes split off the first fatty acid from a triacylglycerol molecule to form a diacylglycerol. Hormone-sensitive lipase is then translocated to the cell and activated to split the triacylglycerol molecules into their individual fatty acid and glycerol components. Hormone-sensitive lipase is regulated primarily by the catecholamines and insulin, which bind to the adipocyte either to stimulate (epinephrine and norepinephrine) or inhibit (insulin) hormone-sensitive lipase release. The activation of hormone-sensitive lipase is thus highly dependent on the sympathetic nervous system and circulating epinephrine. When the sympathetic nervous system is stimulated, for example, during the onset of physical activity, norepinephrine is released from the nerve endings of the sympathetic nervous system, and epinephrine is discharged from the adrenal medulla, thus eventually stimulating lipolysis in the adipocytes throughout the body. In the presence of epinephrine, the secretion of insulin (the most important antagonizing hormone of hormone-sensitive lipase) from the pancreatic islets is suppressed, allowing lipolysis to continue. If epinephrine levels are absent, elevated insulin in the blood resulting from carbohydrate absorption remains at high levels, which inhibits the release of hormone-sensitive lipase and ensuing levels of lipolysis. For this reason, insulin is considered to be an important rate-limiting hormone to consider when attempting to increase lipolysis.

74 Kristin Dugan and Lem Taylor

4.3.4.2 Removal of Fatty Acids and Transport in the Bloodstream

The removal of fatty acids from the fat cell into the bloodstream for transport depends primarily on three rate-limiting factors: (1) the blood flow to the adipose tissue, (2) the albumin concentration in the blood, and (3) the number of free fatty acids binding sites on the albumin molecule. The greater the blood flow to and from adipose tissue, the greater potential that exists for lipolysis. When blood flow increases from physical activity, lipolysis-stimulating catecholamines are transported to the adipocytes at a greater rate, and fatty acid mobilization increases. As a result, lipolysis increases to meet the energy demands of the physical activity and to replace the fatty acids that are more quickly being transported and utilized by cells. If there is inadequate blood flow to the adipocytes and muscle tissue, fat oxidation cannot occur as quickly since the activation of hormone-sensitive lipase from catecholamines and transport of fatty acids is slowed. Blood flow therefore provides a significant rate-limiting effect on fat oxidation. Blood flow is not typically a rate-limiting factor during exercise, however, since cardiac output can increase up to 500% during physical activity to accommodate the oxygen demands of working tissues.

Fatty acids cannot be transported in the blood without binding proteins to carry them to their destination. Albumin is the most abundant blood plasma protein and is responsible for the transport of fatty acids in circulating blood. Albumin is known to carry 99.9% of all circulating fatty acids; therefore, the amount of albumin in the blood determines the amount of fatty acids that can be transported and oxidized by the destination cells, thus affecting the rate of fat oxidation. Typical plasma albumin concentrations consist of 0.7 millimoles (mmol) per liter of blood (45 grams per liter of blood), so levels dipping below this concentration can inhibit fat utilization. The amount of free binding sites on the plasma albumin also affects fat oxidation. Most of the time, only a fraction of the total number of binding sites is actually occupied on the albumin carrier protein. As endurance exercise progresses, the plasma fatty acid concentration rises from 0.2 to 0.4 millimoles per liter of blood at rest to about 2.0 millimoles per liter of blood, which can approach the maximum capacity of fatty acid-albumin binding. If fatty acid concentration increases beyond this level, the amount of unbound fatty acids circulating in the blood begins to increase beyond the transport capabilities of albumin in the blood and of the carrier proteins on the sarcolemma. The inability of fatty acids to bind to albumin and the lack of available carrier proteins on the sarcolemma thus limit the rate of fatty acid mobilization and oxidation at this maximal level.

4.3.4.3 Transport of Fatty Acids into the Muscle Cell

Once the fatty acids are transported to the muscle cell, specific carrier proteins are needed to transport the fatty acids across the cell membrane and into the muscle cell. These carrier proteins are found in the sarcolemma and sarcoplasm of the muscle cell, and without these carrier proteins, fatty acids are unable to enter the cell, and fat oxidation cannot occur. Plasma membrane fatty acid-binding protein (FABPpm) and fatty acid transporter protein (FAT/CD36) located in the sarcolemma translocate to the cell membrane for fatty acid transport. As muscle contraction increases, FAT/CD36 travels to the plasma membrane, decreasing its circulation in the sarcoplasm. What stimulates the translocation of FAT/CD36 is currently unknown; however, it is suspected that this mechanism is similar to factors resulting in GLUT4 (glucose transporter 4) translocation. FAT/CD36 is responsible for the majority of fatty acid transport across the sarcolemma; however, these transporters become saturated when plasma fatty acid concentrations reach 1.5 millimoles per liter of blood, thus limiting the rate of fat oxidation at this level.

4.3.4.4   Transport of Fatty Acids into the Mitochondria

Once fatty acids enter the sarcoplasm of the muscle cell via sarcolemma carrier proteins, the next step in lipid metabolism that must occur is the transport of the fatty acids into the mitochondria, the primary site of ATP production through oxidative phosphorylation. Fatty acids are activated by the enzyme, acyl-CoA (coenzyme A) synthetase or thiokinase, to form an acyl-CoA complex, or "activated fatty acid." The acyl-CoA complex is then either used to synthesize intramuscular triglyceride or is bound to carnitine by the enzyme carnitine palmitoyl transferase I to be transported into the mitochondria. Once the activated fatty acid bonds with carnitine for entry into the mitochondria, free coenzyme A is released. The fatty acyl-carnitine complex is then transported with a translocase enzyme to be reconverted into fatty acyl-CoA, which occurs on the matrix side of the inner mitochondrial membrane by the enzyme carnitine palmitoyl transferase II. Carnitine is then released and diffused back across the mitochondrial membrane into the sarcoplasm to become available for the transport of additional fatty acids. As a result, the activation of fatty acids, the availability of carnitive palmitoyl transferase I and II, and the availability of unbound carnitine become rate limiting factors in this stage, leading to fat oxidation. The end result of the carnitine palmitoyl transferase transport process is to increase the levels of available lipid substrates able to be metabolized for energy.

4.3.4.5   Oxidation of Fatty Acids during β-Oxidation and Krebs Cycle

Fatty acids must be oxidized to produce substrates to fuel oxidative phosphorylation during aerobic exercise for submaximal types of activity to continue. This oxidation occurs in the mitochondria and is called β-oxidation. After its transport across the inner mitochondrial membrane, fatty acyl-CoA enters the mitochondrial matrix to undergo a series of reactions referred to as β-oxidation, which uses repeated cycles of four reactions to produce acetyl-CoA. Acetyl-CoA can then be plugged into the Krebs cycle to go on to produce NADH (nicotinamide adenine dinucleotide) and FADH as substrates for the electron transport chain. Fatty acid oxidation during β-oxidation is thus essential for sustaining submaximal aerobic activity since β-oxidation provides the substrates used by this aerobic metabolic pathway. The complete oxidation of fatty acids in the mitochondria depends on several factors:

1. Activity of enzymes of the β-oxidation pathway
2. Concentration of Krebs intermediates
3. Activity of enzymes in the Krebs cycle
4. Presence of oxygen

The absence or unavailability of any of these factors compromises the utilization of fat during exercise and thus controls the rate of fat oxidation.

4.4 EXERCISE EFFECTS OF LIPID METABOLISM

Carbohydrates and fats are oxidized in combination with one another; however, the nature of this mixture depends on the intensity of exercise, duration of exercise, level of aerobic fitness, and amount of available intramuscular triglycerides.

4.4.1 FAT OXIDATION AND EXERCISE INTENSITY AND DURATION

Fat oxidation increases as duration of exercise increases. It seems likely that the increase in fat oxidation is linked to decreases in muscle glycogen stores. In contrast, fat usage corresponding with exercise intensity is much more understood. Fat is usually the predominant fuel used during daily activities and low-intensity exercise, while carbohydrates become the primary fuel utilized at high intensities. Fat oxidation continues to increase as exercise intensity elevates from low to moderate levels, and reesterification is suppressed to increase the availability of fatty acids for transport in response to the elevated rate of lipolysis.

During the first 15 minutes of exercise, plasma fatty acid concentrations actually decrease as the rate of fatty acid uptake by the muscle exceeds the rate of fatty acid release from lipolysis. As the rate of lipolysis increases to compensate for the fatty acid deficit in the blood, the plasma fatty acid concentrations begin to recover and increase according to exercise intensity as a result of the increased activation of the sympathetic nervous system and corresponding elevations in serum catecholamines. During moderate-intensity exercise, fatty acid concentrations may reach one millimole per liter within the first 60 minutes of exercise as lipolysis increases to 300% of its resting rate in an attempt to provide oxidative pathways with available substrates. When transitioning from low to moderate intensity, the increase in fat oxidation is the direct result of increased energy expenditure. Blood flow to adipose tissue is doubled, and the rate of reesterification is decreased, thus delivering fatty acids to active skeletal muscle at a rate exponentially faster than that seen at rest. Once exercise reaches higher intensities, plasma fatty acid concentrations may plateau as fuel utilization begins to transition to greater rates of carbohydrate utilization.

As intensity progresses upward to greater than 70–75% of VO_2Max (maximum oxygen consumption), fat oxidation is inhibited, and the rate of fat utilization is reduced to negligible values. Blood flow to the adipose tissue is decreased by sympathetic vasoconstriction of the blood supply to the adipocytes, resulting in inhibited removal of fatty acids from the adipose tissue and consequently increased reesterification. Blood lactate accumulation further increases the rate of reesterification, which continues to decrease plasma fatty acid levels during high-intensity exercise as carbohydrate usage replaces that of fat utilization. The decreased availability of fatty acids only partially explains the decreased rate of fat oxidation observed in these conditions. For example, when blood plasma fatty acid concentrations were replenished with an infusion of intralipid triacylglycerols and heparin to ensure a plentiful supply of fatty acids during higher-intensity exercise, fat oxidation only experienced slight increases in exercising subjects (Romijn et al. 1995). Another purported mechanism for the decrease in fat oxidation seen during higher-intensity exercise can be attributed to the transport of fatty acids into the mitochondria (Sidossis et al. 1997).

It was observed in these studies that even though long-chain fatty acid oxidation was impaired during high-intensity activity, the oxidation of medium-chain fatty acids was unaffected, suggesting that differences in the ability of these fatty acids to be transported into the mitochondria may be a central factor. Further in this regard and due to their shorter hydrocarbon length, medium-chain fatty acids are less dependent on transport mechanisms into the mitochondria; therefore, the data support the possibility that carnitine-dependent fatty acid transport may be a limiting factor. While complete identification of associated mechanisms are beyond the scope of this chapter, changes in exercise intensity are known to interact strongly with the ability of the cell to oxidize fatty acids for fuel.

4.4.2 Fat Oxidation and Aerobic Capacity

Endurance training affects both substrate utilization and exercise capacity by initiating a metabolic shift to greater fat utilization and decreased glycogen breakdown during exercise. Well-trained athletes are able to burn more fat at higher intensities than untrained individuals due to hormonal and muscular adaptations to regular exercise training. Trained athletes release lower levels of catecholamines and thus have lower levels of fatty acid concentrations in the blood, enabling the athlete to better utilize intramuscular triglyceride stores, which have also increased in size as a result of endurance training. In addition, the following muscular adaptations contribute to the greater stimulation of fat oxidation in well-trained endurance athletes:

1. Increased mitochondrial density
2. Increase in the number of oxidative enzymes
3. Increased capillary density
4. Increased fatty acid-binding protein concentrations
5. Increased carnitine palmitoyl transferase I and II concentrations

The increased mitochondrial density and number of oxidative enzymes in trained muscle tissue increases its capacity to oxidize fat and synthesize ATP using oxidative phosphorylation. The increased capillary density enhances fatty acid delivery to the muscle, and increased fatty acid-binding protein concentrations facilitate a larger amount of fatty acids transported across the sarcolemma. Since trained muscle has a larger carnitine palmitoyl transferase enzyme concentration, more fatty acids can be transported across the mitochondrial membrane to be oxidized and used as fuel. One factor seemingly uninfluenced by endurance training is lipolysis in adipose tissue as shown by similar lipolysis rates at the same absolute exercise intensity after endurance training (Klein et al. 1994).

4.4.3 Role of Intramuscular Triglycerides

Intramuscular triglyceride stores are usually located adjacent to the mitochondria as lipid droplets to provide energy during exercise. The location of the droplets is important and adapts to exercise training, specifically to endurance training, and these levels of intramuscular triglycerides are elevated in the trained endurance athlete. The closer the droplets are to the mitochondria, the more efficient their utilization during exercise. In trained muscle, the lipid droplets are located next to the mitochondria, whereas in untrained muscle, the droplets are not intricately linked with the mitochondria but rather are dispersed throughout the sarcoplasm. This cellular shift in location of the intramuscular triglyceride droplet is assumed to favorably effect its ability to be oxidized, but this fact has yet to be confirmed.

4.5 SUMMARY OF KEY POINTS

- Although fat should be consumed in moderation, the macronutrient provides several functions vital to both daily activity and physical activity. These functions include
  - Providing the primary fuel source both at rest and during prolonged aerobic exercise
  - Protecting vital organs from trauma
  - Absorbing and transporting important nutrients (β-carotene and vitamins A, D, E, K)
  - Providing the structural component of cell membranes
  - Forming bile and important hormones
- Fat is classified primarily by its chemical structure and has three classes: simple, compound, and derived lipids.
- Omega-3 fatty acid ingestion is recommended on a daily basis since this form of fat has consistently shown benefits to health and reduces inflammatory responses during exercise.
- Carbohydrates and fats are oxidized in combination with one another; however, the nature of this mixture depends on the intensity of exercise, duration of exercise, level of aerobic fitness, and amount of intramuscular triglycerides.
- Fat metabolism requires significantly more time than the other macronutrients, so an athlete must allow adequate time for ingested fat to digest and absorb prior to exercise.
- Preexercise food intake should be primarily based on individual tolerance, and the following considerations should be made:
  - The food should not interfere with training.
  - The food should help prevent hunger during training.
  - High-fat foods should not take the place of high-carbohydrate foods, which are needed to fuel muscles.
- Lipid intake during exercise should be minimized to prevent possible gastrointestinal distress and to prevent the delay of other macronutrient intake during digestion and absorption. Lipid intake should be elevated during extreme exercise requiring an abundant amount of calories to sustain the activity since fat is the most energy-dense macronutrient but should only be elevated to individual tolerance.
- Minimal fat intake is suggested immediately following exercise to allow for faster carbohydrate and protein absorption and replenishment in the

body. Moderate amounts of fat should be considered after one hour to effectively replenish calorie deficits resulting from prolonged exercise without compromising carbohydrate delivery.

5 Vitamins/Minerals
Invaluable Cellular Components for Optimal Physiological Function

Michael D. Roberts and Chad M. Kerksick

CONTENTS

5.1 AN INTRODUCTION TO VITAMINS AND MINERALS

Most physically active individuals, as compared with their less active counterparts, fail to consume a diet that contains adequate amounts of vitamins and minerals which leads to marginal nutrient deficiency and results in substandard training and impaired performance.

—Lukaski (2004)

Providing dietary support to optimize athletic performance is a practice that has existed for thousands of years. As part of the Nutritional and Physical Performance: A Century of Progress and Tribute to the Modern Olympic Movement symposium given at the 96th Experimental Biology meeting, lecturer Louis Grivetti detailed the innovative practices of the Greek philosopher Pythagoras of Samos (580–500 BC), who is considered the first person to train athletes on a high-meat diet (Grivetti and Applegate 1997). While the intentions of his methods are unknown, Pythagoras clearly recognized the need for nutritional adequacy to support the demands of rigorous training. Over 2,500 years later, scientist Paul Schenk observed the dietary habits of athletes participating in the Berlin Olympics of 1936, reporting that the typical preevent meals of endurance athletes consisted of high-carbohydrate foods, including porridge, shredded wheat, cornflakes, and pasta (Grivetti and Applegate 1997). When comparing these two historical perspectives, it is apparent that coaches and athletes have always recognized the importance of adjusting macronutrient profiles to sustain peak performance levels in elite athletes. However, in the late 1930s scientists began rapidly changing the face of nutrition, and consequently sports nutrition, with the isolation and subsequent preparation of vitamin and mineral concoctions (Applegate and Grivetti 1997). As evidenced in the brilliant writings of Dr. Henry Lukaski (2004), scientists now appreciate the notion that athletes must obtain an adequate amount of dietary vitamins and minerals to effectively combat the various physiological stressors that are incurred during exercise. Simply stated, vitamins and minerals are biochemical compounds, or micronutrients, that are required by all cells of the body to maintain homeostasis. Vitamins and minerals are unable to be synthesized by the body and therefore must be adequately obtained through the diet on a daily basis. Vitamins are divided into two classes: fat soluble and water soluble. Both classes are present in the fluid portion of the body (i.e., blood serum and intracellular fluid), although fat-soluble vitamins are also stored in the lipid fraction of tissues (i.e., cell membranes, subcellular membranes, and adipose tissue), which poses toxicity risks (albeit rare) if they are consumed in abundance. Likewise, minerals are found in both bodily fluids (i.e., blood and intracellular fluid compartments) and tissue structures (i.e., iron in hemoglobin or calcium in sarcoplasmic reticulum). While comprehensive descriptions highlighting the physiological importance or dietary source of each vitamin and mineral are beyond the scope of this chapter, Table 5.1 provides such summaries.

Vitamin and mineral deficiencies were common before the twentieth century; modern-day food fortification practices in industrialized countries have effectively ensured that minimum dietary requirements are met in a majority of these populations. For instance, in 1998 the U.S. Food and Drug Administration (FDA) deemed it mandatory that grain manufacturers enrich their products with folate, a mandate that resulted in an average 100-μg increase in the consumption of this vitamin per person, which is nearly half of the daily recommended allowance (Honein et al. 2001). Similar fortification trends included the addition of iodine to salt in the 1920s, the addition of vitamin D to milk in the 1930s, wheat and flour enrichment in the 1940s, and the addition of calcium to various foodstuffs in the 1980s (Bishai and Nalubola 2002); these are trends that have led to the virtual disappearance of vitamin-deficiency-related illnesses in the United States and other industrialized

TABLE 5.1
The Physiological Importance and Food Sources of Various Vitamins and Minerals

Vitamin/Mineral (Chemical Name) and DRI[a]	Physiological Function and Other Notes	Common Food Sources[b] (1 ounce = 28 grams)
	Fat-Soluble Vitamins	
Vitamin A (retinol) Males: 900–3,000 µg/day Females: 700–3,000 µg/day	Needed for retinal metabolism (vision); promotes cellular gene expression; promotes bone and immune health and red blood cell formation; promotes overall bodily growth *Note:* dietary β-, α-, and γ-carotene are dietary derivatives that can be converted into vitamin A	Animal liver (up to 18,000 µg per ounce) Sweet potato (~1,600 µg per ounce) Carrots (~1,380 µg per ounce)
Vitamin D (ergocalciferol and cholecalciferol) Males: 200–600 IU/day Females: 200–600 IU/day	Promotes bone and immune health; cancer and cardiovascular disease prevention *Note:* Sun exposure converts 7-dehydrocholesterol stored in skin tissue into vitamin D, which increases blood levels	Salmon (~265 IU per ounce) Mackerel (~130 IU per ounce) Milk (~15 IU per fluid ounce)
Vitamin E (tocopherols and tocotrienols) Males: 15–1,000 mg/day Females: 15–1,000 mg/day	Combats oxidative stress; cancer and cardiovascular disease prevention	Enriched cereals (~10–15 mg per ounce) Sunflower seeds (~10 mg per ounce) Almonds (~7 mg per ounce)
Vitamin K (phylloquinone) Males: 80 µg/day Females: 60 µg/day	Promotes blood clotting and bone health	Green, leafy vegetables: kale, spinach, collard greens (up to 250 µg per ounce) Brussels sprouts (~50 µg per ounce)
	Water-Soluble Vitamins	
Vitamin C (ascorbic acid) Males: 90–2,000 mg/day Females: 75–2,000 mg/day	Needed for collagen metabolism (skin, bone, cartilage, and blood vessel health); combats oxidative stress; promotes immune health	Broccoli (~25 mg per ounce) Papaya (~17 mg per ounce) Strawberries (~17 mg per ounce) Oranges (~14 mg per ounce)

(continued)

TABLE 5.1 (continued)
The Physiological Importance and Food Sources of Various Vitamins and Minerals

Vitamin/Mineral (Chemical Name) and DRI[a]	Physiological Function and Other Notes	Common Food Sources[b] (1 ounce = 28 grams)
Vitamin B_1 (thiamin) Males: 1.5 mg/day Females: 1.0 mg/day	Needed for the breakdown of sugars and amino acids (energy metabolism)	Sunflower seeds (~0.65 mg per ounce) Ham (~0.27 mg per ounce) Peanuts (~0.12 mg per ounce)
Vitamin B_2 (riboflavin) Males: 1.3 mg/day Females: 1.1 mg/day	Needed for the breakdown of fats, sugars, and proteins (energy metabolism) Riboflavin (specifically FAD) is also a cofactor for tissue glutathione reductase, which is an integral endogenous antioxidant enzyme	Animal liver (up to 1.2 mg per ounce) Pork (~0.1 mg per ounce) Dairy: milk, yogurt, cottage cheese (up to 0.07 mg per fluid ounce)
Vitamin B_3 (niacin) Males: 16–35 mg/day Females: 14–35 mg/day	Needed for the breakdown of sugars and proteins (energy metabolism)	Canned tuna (3.7 mg per ounce) Animal liver (up to 3.3 mg per ounce) Poultry (up to 2.8 mg per ounce)
Vitamin B_5 (pantothenic acid) Males: 5 mg/day Females: 5 mg/day	Needed for the breakdown of sugars and proteins (energy metabolism)	Animal liver (up to 1.5 mg per ounce) Mushrooms (~0.4 mg per ounce) Lentils (~0.2 mg per ounce)
Vitamin B_6 (pyridoxine) Males: 1.3–100 mg/day Females: 1.3–100 mg/day	Needed for the breakdown of glycogen (energy metabolism) and whole-body protein synthesis (cell turnover and muscle growth)	Animal liver (up to 0.25 mg per ounce) Medium baked potato (~0.7 mg) Medium banana (~0.7 mg)
Vitamin B_7 (biotin) Males: 30 μg/day Females: 30 μg/day	Needed for the breakdown of fats and proteins (energy metabolism); blood glucose maintenance	Animal liver (up to 32 μg per ounce) Medium egg (~27 μg)
Vitamin B_9 (folate) Males: 400–1,000 μg/day Females: 400–1,000 μg/day	Needed for DNA synthesis (cell turnover); integral in red blood cell formation	Animal liver (up to 220 μg per ounce) Lentils (~45 μg per ounce) Green, leafy vegetables: kale, spinach, collard greens (up to 9 μg per ounce)

Nutrient	Function	Food Sources
Vitamin B$_{12}$ (cobalamin) Males: 2.4 µg/day Females: 2.4 µg/day	Integral in red blood cell formation	Clams (up to 28 µg per ounce) Animal liver (up to 22 µg per ounce) Canned tuna (up to 0.3 µg per ounce)

Essential Minerals

Nutrient	Function	Food Sources
Calcium Males: 1,000–2,500 mg/day Females: 1,000–2,500 mg/day	Promotes bone health; helps control blood pressure and heart rate; assists in nerve transmission and muscle contraction	Spinach (122 mg per ounce) Dairy: milk, yogurt, cottage cheese (up to 50 mg per fluid ounce) Tofu (~33 mg per ounce)
Chloride Males: 2,300–3,600 mg/day Females: 2,300–3,600 mg/day	Important electrolyte; helps control blood pressure and heart rate; assists in nerve transmission and muscle contraction; helps regulate stomach acidity (digestion)	Table salt (~3,600 mg per tsp) Ham (~310 mg per ounce) Canned soups (up to 250 mg per fluid ounce)
Chromium Males: 30–35 µg/day Females: 20–25 µg/day	Assists in insulin signaling and blood glucose maintenance; needed for fat and protein synthesis (cell growth)	Broccoli (~2.8 µg per ounce) Regular bagel (~2.5 µg) Orange juice (~0.3 µg per fluid ounce)
Copper Males: 0.9–10 mg/day Females: 0.9–10 mg/day	Integral in red blood cell formation; promotes bone health	Animal liver (up to 1.26 mg per ounce) Cashews (~0.5 mg per ounce) Shellfish: oysters, clams, crab (~0.2 mg per ounce)
Iodine Males: 120–1,100 µg/day Females: 120–1,100 µg/day	Needed for thyroid hormone production (regulates metabolic rate)	Iodized table salt (400 µg per tsp) Cod (~30 µg per ounce)
Iron Males: 8–45 mg/day Females: 18–45 mg/day	Integral in red blood cell formation	Animal liver (up to 2.4 mg per ounce) Beans: white, black, kidney (up to 1.7 mg per ounce) Beef (up to 0.6 mg per ounce)
Magnesium Males: 420 mg/day Females: 320 mg/day	Needed for whole-body ATP breakdown (energy production); maintenance of blood pressure and heart rate	Almonds (~84 mg per ounce) Tofu (~47 mg per ounce) Beans: white, black, lima, kidney (up to 15 mg per ounce)
Phosphorus Males: 700–4,000 mg/day Females: 700–4,000 mg/day	Promotes bone health; needed for DNA synthesis (cell growth)	Dairy: milk, yogurt (up to 95 mg per fluid ounce) Lentils (~89 mg per ounce) Salmon (~83 mg per ounce)

(continued)

TABLE 5.1 (continued)
The Physiological Importance and Food Sources of Various Vitamins and Minerals

Vitamin/Mineral (Chemical Name) and DRI[a]	Physiological Function and Other Notes	Common Food Sources[b] (1 ounce = 28 grams)
Potassium Males: 4,700 mg/day Females: 4,700 mg/day	Important electrolyte; helps control blood pressure and heart rate; assists in nerve transmission and muscle contraction	Beans: black, kidney (up to 100 mg per ounce) Lentils (~91 mg per ounce) Prune juice (~88 mg per ounce)
Selenium Males: 55–400 μg/day Females: 55–400 μg/day	Combats oxidative stress; promotes immune health Selenium is a cofactor for glutathione peroxidase, which is an endogenous antioxidant	Crab meat (~13 μg per ounce) Salmon (~13 μg per ounce) Halibut (~13 μg per ounce)
Sodium Males: 1,500–2,300 mg/day Females: 1,500–2,300 mg/day	Important electrolyte; helps control blood pressure and heart rate; assists in nerve transmission and muscle contraction; helps regulate stomach acidity (digestion)	Table salt (~2,400 mg per tsp) Ham (~465 mg per ounce) Canned soups (up to 375 mg per fluid ounce)
Zinc Males: 11–40 mg/day Females: 8–40 mg/day	Promotes immune health; assists in hormone production (i.e., testosterone)	Oysters (up to 34 mg per ounce) Beef (up to 1.5 mg per ounce) Lentils (~0.3 mg per ounce)

~ = approximately; μg = microgram; IU = international units; mg = milligram; α = alpha isoform; β = beta isoform; γ = gamma isoform; FAD = flavin adenine dinucleotide; DNA = deoxyribonucleic acid; tsp = teaspoon.

[a] DRIs = Dietary Reference Intakes for adults (>19 years) set forth by the Institute of Medicine and National Academy of Sciences, which are modifications to the Recommended Daily Allowance (RDA); ranges include UI (upper intake) levels.

[b] Data are from http://www.nutritiondata.com.

countries (Bishai and Nalubola 2002). However, novel exercise science research is beginning to unveil that several athletes may indeed be vitamin or mineral deficient due to the increased needs of these nutrients with vigorous physical activity. Therefore, this chapter examines scientific literature that has examined micronutrient deficiencies in athletes. This discussion transitions to current-day research that has examined the potential ergogenic benefits of explicit vitamin or mineral concoctions. Potential future considerations of this topic are then hypothesized, including how interindividual genetic differences may warrant the need for vitamin or mineral supplementation in certain individuals. Finally, general recommendations in regard to vitamin/mineral intakes to optimize performance are given.

5.2 VITAMINS AND MINERALS IN ATHLETICS: ARE ATHLETES INGESTING ENOUGH?

Vitamin and mineral intake suggestions for military personnel were first established by the Food and Nutrition Board of the National Academy of Sciences in the early 1940s in a six-page document, "Recommended Dietary Allowances." While the intention of the council for publishing these guidelines was solely in the interest of optimizing U.S. military prowess, their scientific rationale for the various micronutrient recommendations were vague and rudimentary. Various governing agencies have since amended these recommendations every five to ten years until the Institute of Medicine of the National Academies set forth in 1997 broader dietary guidelines for all macro- and micronutrients: the Dietary Recommended Intake (DRI) Guidelines, which included adequate intake (AI) and tolerable upper intake (UI) levels for all macro- and micronutrients. The definitions are provided next for clarification.

5.2.1 RECOMMENDED DIETARY ALLOWANCE

The Recommended Dietary Allowance (RDA) is defined as the average daily dietary consumption of a nutrient that is sufficient to meet nutrient requirements of 97–98% of healthy persons within particular age and sex groups.

5.2.2 REFERENCE DAILY INTAKE

The Reference Daily Intakes (RDIs) are values established by the FDA for use in nutrition labeling; values were based initially on the highest 1968 RDA for each nutrient to ensure that needs were met for all age groups.

5.2.3 ADEQUATE INTAKE

The AI is derived from DRI guidelines that recommended intakes for nutrients based on experimentally derived approximations of nutrient intake by groups of healthy individuals (used when RDAs have not been determined).

88 Michael D. Roberts and Chad M. Kerksick

5.2.4 Tolerable Upper Intake Level

The UI level is determined from DRI guidelines and is defined as the greatest amount of nutrient intake daily that will not pose a risk of adverse effects for most people in the population; these values were not offered by the old RDAs.

For simplification, recommended daily intakes (in contrast to AI or RDA values) will be referred to in regard to micronutrient intakes. While current DRI guidelines in concert with the aforementioned food fortification methods have proven to be invaluable in quelling the prevalence of micronutrient deficiencies in the United States, keep the perspective should remain that these recommendations were made for the general population. In fact, various nutritional research endeavors discussed in this chapter provide invaluable scientific evidence to suggest that, in some instances, athletes must exceed 100% (or more) of the RDI value of micronutrients to sustain acceptable vitamin/mineral status. Prior to discussing the topic of micronutrient adequacy in athletes, it is necessary to introduce the following terminology (Figure 5.1):

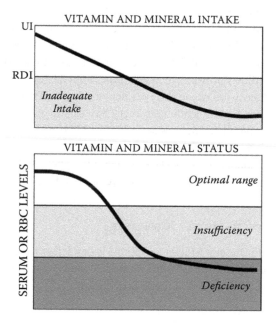

FIGURE 5.1 The relationship between vitamin/mineral intake and vitamin/mineral status. In summary, prolonged inadequate intake will likely lead to insufficiency and subsequent deficiency, a sequence that will inevitably cripple sports performance. DRI = Dietary Reference Intake for adults (>19 years) set forth by the Institute of Medicine and National Academy of Sciences, which is the modification to the Recommended Daily Allowance (RDA). UI = upper intake levels that should not be exceeded for prolonged periods. Vitamin and mineral status = blood or serum (non-red-blood-cell portion of blood) levels of a particular vitamin or mineral. Inadequate intake = habitually consuming below the RDI for one or more multiple vitamins or minerals. Vitamin or mineral insufficiency = between what is considered to be the normal and lower limit as assessed by blood or serum testing. Vitamin or mineral deficiency = lower than what is considered to be the lower limit as assessed by blood or serum testing. RBC = red blood cell.

Vitamin and mineral status: blood or serum (non-red-blood-cell portion of blood) levels of a particular vitamin or mineral

Inadequate intake: habitually consuming below the recommended daily intake for one or multiple vitamins or minerals

Vitamin or mineral insufficiency: between what is considered to be the normal and lower limit as assessed by blood or serum testing

Vitamin or mineral deficiency: lower than what is considered to be the lower limit as assessed by blood or serum testing

Modern-day research efforts have determined that an adequate vitamin and mineral intake is vital for optimizing sports performance, and in some circumstances, the supplementation of explicit vitamin/mineral concoctions may enhance sports performance or recovery. As examples of this perspective, researchers have determined the following:

- Thiamin deficiency can potentially lead to the accumulation of lactate in working skeletal muscle during prolonged exercise and exacerbate fatigue (Lukaski 2004).
- Vitamin C deficiency increases the occurrence of upper respiratory tract infections in long-distance runners (Lukaski 2004).
- Vitamin E deficiency reduces endurance capacity in rodents by 40%, an effect that ultimately leads to premature fatigue (Evans 2000). Further, severe vitamin E deficiency in rodent skeletal muscle increases the rate of muscle atrophy up 350% compared to nondeficient counterparts (Dayton et al. 1979).
- When supplemented with iron over an 80-day period, iron-deficient subjects exhibited the following attributes (Gardner et al. 1975): (1) a 61% to 97% increase in blood hemoglobin, (2) a reduction in peak exercise heart rates from approximately 150 beats per minute to approximately 120 beats per minute (signifying less fatigue), (3) a 15% increase in oxygen delivery to working muscles during exercise, and (4) a drastic reduction (50%) in blood lactate levels immediately after exercise (signifying less fatigue).
- Twelve weeks of magnesium depletion in postmenopausal women decreased tissue levels by 8% to 13% while concomitantly reducing work economy during exercise by 10% (i.e., the amount of oxygen used during a known exercise workload) (Lukaski and Nielsen 2002).

It is becoming evident that athletes need to ingest more vitamins and minerals compared to sedentary populations. Dr. Malinda Manore at Arizona State University published a scientific article stating that there is an increased need of B vitamins in athletes because (1) B vitamins, specifically B_1, B_2, and B_6, serve as cofactors (i.e., components needed for full enzyme function) for various metabolic enzymes, and physical activity increases the metabolism as well as the breakdown and resynthesis of these enzymes; and (2) chronic exercise increases muscle mitochondrial enzymes, which further increases the need for these cofactors. For instance, it has been determined that nearly one milligram of vitamin B_6 (i.e., approximately the RDI for adults)

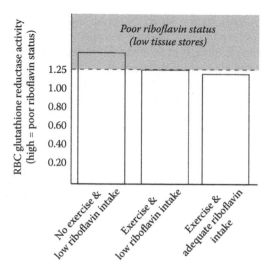

FIGURE 5.2 Interactions between dietary riboflavin intake, physical activity levels, and tissue riboflavin status. No exercise and low riboflavin = Ingested 0.58 milligrams of riboflavin/1,000 kilocalories. Exercise and low riboflavin = Ingested 1.00 milligram riboflavin for every 1,000 kilocalories in the diet (>50% RDI) and ran 25 to 60 minutes per day for six days per week over a three-week period. Exercise and adequate riboflavin intake = Ingested 1.38 milligrams of riboflavin for every 1,000 kilocalories in the diet (>110% RDI) and ran 25 to 60 minutes per day for six days per week over a three-week period. These data nicely demonstrate that athletes need to ingest greater amounts of riboflavin (and presumably other vitamins and minerals) to optimize tissue stores (and presumably athletic performance). (Adapted from the data of Belko, A.Z., E. Obarzanek, H.J. Kalkwarf, M.A. Rotter, S. Bogusz, D. Miller, J.D. Haas, and D.A. Roe. Effects of Exercise on Riboflavin Requirements of Young Women. *Am J Clin Nutr* 37(4):509–17, 1983.).

is degraded in runners during and following a marathon, as determined by a urinary B_6 by-product, due to the increased metabolic demands imposed by the exercising musculature (Manore 2000). Similarly, a clinical investigation examining dietary riboflavin intake and physical activity levels determined that riboflavin status (i.e., erythrocyte glutathione reductase activity coefficient or EGRAC) was optimized in active individuals when consuming 1.38 milligrams of riboflavin per 1,000 kilocalories consumed in the diet versus 1.00 milligrams of riboflavin per 1,000 kilocalories consumed in the diet (see Figure 5.2) (Manore 2000).

The following examples were gathered from scientific literature describing other vitamin and mineral inadequate intakes or deficiencies reported in various athletic populations (Lukaski 2004):

- Approximately 40% to 60% of endurance athletes have an inadequate tissue vitamin B_6 status.
- In male athletes, 23% of wrestlers and 20% of football players ingested less than 70% of the RDI for vitamin C. In female athletes, 13% of basketball

players, 22% of gymnasts, and 25% of cyclists consume less than 70% of the RDI for vitamin C.

- Similar trends as outlined for vitamin C were also evident for vitamin A intake.
- Approximately 53% of collegiate athletes consume less than 70% of the RDI for vitamin E.
- Approximately 25% to 44% of female runners as well as 4% to 13% of male endurance athletes were tissue iron deficient.
- According to a 1995 report, female athletes on average ingested 60% to 65% of the RDI for magnesium (Lukaski, 2004).
- According to two scientific accounts, 25% of male endurance runners and 22% of female endurance runners had depressed blood zinc levels.
- Approximately 68% of Finnish female athletes (runners and gymnasts) and nonathletes were vitamin D insufficient, and 13% of those were deficient (Willis et al. 2008). Similarly, 40% of American distance runners were vitamin D insufficient despite living in regions where their exposure to sunlight was adequate year-round (Willis et al. 2008).

Therefore, while athletes generally ingest proportionally more macronutrients to support the metabolic demands of exercise, these data suggest that athletes likely ingest an inadequate amount of one or multiple vitamins or minerals for optimal physiological processes to ensue during exercise. Interestingly, scientists have examined the effects of weeks to months of inadequate magnesium intake on serum versus tissue magnesium levels (see Figure 5.3) (Lukaski and Nielsen 2002). Simply stated, 12 weeks of consuming around 30% of the RDI for magnesium led to an 8% to 13% decrease in tissue levels while minimally affecting serum levels (i.e., a 5% decrease, which was not statistically different from predepletion levels). This finding is disconcerting due to the fact that tissue deficiencies did not mirror serum levels, which, in many instances, would make vitamin/mineral status screening difficult. More important, assuming that all vitamins and minerals behave in such a manner, it is apparent that inadequate vitamin/mineral intakes over a series of weeks have profound physiological consequences. Taking the aforementioned data into consideration coupled with the notion that athletes need more dietary vitamins and minerals makes tissue micronutrient deficiencies seemingly inevitable in physically active individuals, an effect that ultimately impairs sports performance, as discussed in previous paragraphs.

While research is lacking, it is presumed that the need for extra vitamins and minerals in athletes is a product of training volume and nutrition (Figure 5.4). For instance, well-fed recreational weightlifters performing 10 to 15 minutes of muscle work per training session (i.e., approximately 40 seconds per set × 15 to 25 sets) four days per week have not exhibited increases in strength, muscle mass, or circulating levels of magnesium or zinc when supplementing an extra 450 milligrams of magnesium and 30 milligrams of zinc per day into their diets over an eight-week period (Wilborn et al. 2004); this finding likely occurred because tissue mineral repletion with low training volumes is likely obtainable with the current RDI level. As discussed, however, increasing continuous muscle work up to 60 minutes per day

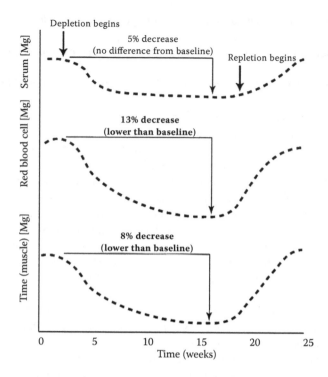

FIGURE 5.3 A hypothetical model of vitamin/mineral depletion on serum and tissue concentrations. Restricting magnesium from the diet may minimally impact serum levels while significantly impacting tissue levels. It is assumed that other vitamins and minerals follow similar trends, and that habitual physical activity coupled with dietary deficiencies exacerbate these patterns. (Adapted from the data of Lukaski, H.C., and F.H. Nielsen. Dietary Magnesium Depletion Affects Metabolic Responses During Submaximal Exercise in Postmenopausal Women. *J Nutr* 132(5):930–35.)

may require individuals to increase vitamin and mineral intake up to twice what is currently recommended (Manore 2000).

Athletes can easily remedy or prevent deficiencies through dietary means (i.e., eating more nutrient-dense foods or consuming multivitamins/minerals on a daily basis), although self-reported food surveys have indicated that a majority of the population is unaware of personal micronutrient intake levels. In response to the aforementioned research reporting that one milligram of vitamin B_6 is degraded and excreted following a marathon (Manore 2000), researcher Malinda Manore writes:

> In general, any loss of vitamin B_6 due to exercise is small and could easily be replaced by eating one to two servings of a food high in vitamin B_6. However, [most] individuals have poor plasma [B_6] concentrations while consuming self-selected, free-living diets.

Similarly, there is online testimony from a registered dietician claiming that she had become chronically lethargic due to extensive endurance training and an unbeknownst vitamin D deficiency (Ewing 2009). According to this athlete, her serum

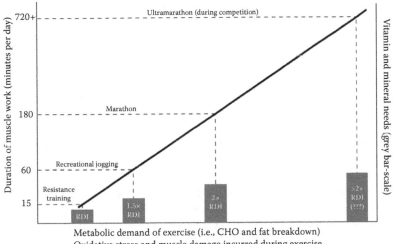

FIGURE 5.4 Hypothetical model of vitamin and mineral needs for different athletes. This model assumes the athlete is in a well-fed state. For those athletes restricting energy intake with the intent of optimizing precompetition body composition, these needs are presumably greater. CHO = carbohydrate.

vitamin D levels were 50% lower than the low-end normal value despite eating a well-balanced diet, consuming a vitamin/mineral supplement daily, and extensively training outside on a daily basis. After nearly three months of consuming 1,000 to 2,000 international units (IU) of supplemental vitamin D (up to 230% RDI), this athlete's serum vitamin D levels were restored to normal values, and she set a new personal record for a half-marathon within that same year. Again, these examples reinforce the ideas that (1) habitual exercise increases the need for micronutrients, and (2) athletes potentially are susceptible to micronutrient deficiencies because they may be unaware of personal dietary inadequacies or are not consuming enough micronutrients based on the current RDIs. Therefore, while dietary recommendations for vitamin and mineral intakes have not been formally constructed for athletes, various micronutrient ingestion strategies are discussed at the conclusion of this chapter with the intent of preventing vitamin and mineral deficiencies.

5.3 VITAMINS AND MINERALS IN ATHLETICS: IMPACT OF SUPPLEMENTATION

5.3.1 VITAMIN/MINERAL SUPPLEMENTATION FOR ERGOGENIC PURPOSES

Vitamin/mineral supplementation for ergogenic purposes is fervently debated in the exercise physiology and sports nutrition fields. For example, seven to eight months of multivitamin/mineral supplementation in 82 multidisciplinary athletes did not improve markers of sports performance (Telford et al. 1992). Similarly, well-fed athletes consuming high doses of either vitamin B_1 (thiamin), vitamin B_9 (folate), vitamin B_{12} (cobalamin), vitamin A, vitamin E, zinc, or chromium reported no improvement in performance markers of strength or endurance athletes (Lukaski 2004). Stear and colleagues (2009) authored a scientific review article in which they argued that antioxidant supplementation in athletes is frivolous. The authors state:

> Regular exercise training promotes increased enzymatic and non-enzymatic antioxidants in muscle fibers resulting in improved endogenous protection against exercise-mediated oxidative damage. Therefore, this increase in endogenous antioxidants may be sufficient to protect against exercise-induced oxidative damage.

The authors (Stear et al. 2009) also provide scientific evidence that refutes the use of antioxidant supplements because they may disrupt long-term exercise adaptations. In addition, one investigation determined that one gram per day of vitamin C supplementation to humans (approximately 10 times the RDI) reduced increases in VO_2Max (maximum oxygen consumption) (+10% in vitamin C group versus +22% in the nonsupplemented group) following eight weeks of training at three days per week for 40 minutes per session (Gomez-Cabrera et al. 2008). Follow-up molecular evidence from rodents in this same study determined that an equivalent exercise and vitamin C supplementation protocol (1) reduced the genetic expression of muscle antioxidants (superoxide dismutase [SOD] and glutathione peroxidase), (2) reduced various messenger RNAs (mRNAs) and proteins (PGC-1) needed for mitochondrial synthesis, and (3) reduced mitochondrial synthesis itself (accessed via depressed cytochrome C levels). A similar investigation determined that supplementing humans with vitamin C (one gram per day) and vitamin E (400 IU per day) prevented endurance exercise-induced increases in (1) insulin sensitivity, (2) the genetic expression of mRNAs needed for mitochondrial synthesis, and (3) the genetic expression of mRNAs needed for muscle antioxidant synthesis (SOD1 and SOD2). Interestingly, both studies concluded that oversupplementing with antioxidants disrupted the generation of intramuscular free radicals during exercise that are needed for positive training adaptations (i.e., an increase in the antioxidant system of the musculature or the amount of energy-producing mitochondria) to ensue during postexercise recovery periods. Finally, providing a supraphysiological dose of one gram of vitamin B_3 (approximately 6,300 times the RDI) one hour prior to two hours of submaximal exercise decreased circulating free fatty acid levels (Heath et al. 1993), an effect that may accelerate muscle glycogen depletion and impair performance during prolonged exercise settings.

Conversely, sparse evidence exists demonstrating that vitamin/mineral supplementation is ergogenic. For instance, administering 400 milligrams per day of vitamin E to six high-altitude mountain climbers enhanced anaerobic threshold (i.e., the amount of work able to be performed without leading to substantial fatigue) during a 10-week climbing expedition (Simon-Schnass and Pabst 1988), albeit this effect has not been observed at sea level (Williams 2004). Furthermore, numerous studies have demonstrated that iron supplementation (100 to 975 milligrams per day of ferrous sulfate or up 12,000 times the RDI) increases markers of endurance performance, albeit all of these studies administered iron to tissue iron-depleted or anemic participants (i.e., persons with a decrement in red blood cell count or hemoglobin content) (Hinton et al. 2000; Rowland et al. 1988; Stewart et al. 1984). Administering

360 milligrams per day of magnesium (85% to 115% of RDI) for four weeks to athletes has been shown to reduce lactate production and fatigue (i.e., oxygen consumption) during prolonged rowing (Lukaski 2004). Likewise, administering eight milligrams of magnesium per kilogram body mass per day decreased fatigue during endurance exercise in recreationally active individuals (Lukaski 2004). However, scientists Ian Newhouse and Eric Finstad (2000) reviewed all of the pertinent literature on magnesium supplementation in athletes and concluded the following:

> Most evidence indicates no effect of magnesium supplementation on performance (strength, anaerobic-lactic acid, and aerobic). When only peak treadmill speed during a VO$_2$Max test is examined, the strength of [scientific support] is equivocal. Trained subjects appear to benefit less than untrained subjects, but this observation requires further study. Little research has focused on physically active females who may be at the highest risk for magnesium deficiency. Research has been confounded by numerous factors.

Therefore, the current scientific literature suggests that athletes in a well-fed, non-deficient state do not derive an ergogenic benefit from vitamin or mineral supplementation. Further, recent evidence suggests that chronically supplementing with copious amounts of antioxidants in well-fed states may impair endurance performance.

5.3.2 Sodium, Potassium, and Chloride: Crucial Electrolytes for Normal Homeostasis

Electrolytes are ions that exist in a balanced state between the intracellular (i.e., within muscles and nerves) and extracellular (i.e., blood) compartments of the body. The primary mineral electrolytes include sodium, potassium, chloride, calcium, and magnesium. The balance of electrolytes is crucial because this equilibrium regulates hydration, blood acidity, and muscle and nerve function both at rest and during exercise. However, numerous studies have clearly demonstrated that mineral electrolyte balance is disrupted during prolonged exercise with heavy sweating. Specifically, sodium loss is a primary concern during endurance exercise bouts spanning more than two hours, making the ingestion of a solution containing sodium chloride crucial (Coyle 2004). Sodium loss or the dilution of blood sodium through overdrinking of water during prolonged exercise poses serious health consequences, including (1) a disproportionate increase in circulating potassium, which depresses heart rate, cardiac output, and subsequent performance; and (2) increases in the risk of contracting hyponatremia (low blood sodium levels), which can lead to tissue and brain swelling, which leads to cramping, nausea, vomiting, headache, coma, and even death. While the serious consequences of hyponatremia are rare, it has been estimated that 12.5% of marathoners contract asymptomatic hyponatremia because they overconsumed water (or any non-sodium-containing fluid) throughout the race (Kipps et al. 2009).

In regard to this type of fluid intake, it was estimated that those with hyponatremia consumed 3.7 liters (420 milliliters for every 30 minutes of activity) of fluid, whereas unaffected athletes consumed 1.9 liters of fluid (225 milliliters for every 30 minutes of activity). Thus, this study stresses the physiological importance of monitoring non-sodium-containing fluid intake during prolonged exercise in terms of affecting blood sodium levels. Recent scientific data have also studied the efficacy of carbohydrate-electrolyte drinks versus water ingestion on maintaining blood sodium levels (Anastasiou et al. 2009). In this study, participants performed a series of endurance and resistance training exercises designed to elicit calf cramps at 30°C for approximately two hours. During each trial, participants ingested a volume of fluid that matched fluid loss during exercise; the four conditions were (1) carbohydrate-electrolyte drink containing 36.2 millimoles of sodium per liter; (2) carbohydrate-electrolyte drink containing 19.9 millimoles of sodium per liter; (3) mineral water; and (4) colored and flavored distilled water (lowest sodium content). During both of the carbohydrate-electrolyte conditions, blood sodium levels were similar to preexercise values, whereas there were decreases in blood sodium during the mineral water and distilled water trials. A similar investigation reported that ingesting sodium-laden beverages during thermally stressful exercising environments has a favorable impact on fluid homeostasis (Mitchell et al. 2000). These scientists employed a protocol in which (1) subjects exercised in a 35°C environment until dehydrated by 2.9% preexercise body mass, (2) the subjects were rehydrated for 180 minutes, and (3) the subjects subsequently exercised for an additional 20 minutes. Four rehydration strategies were employed that differed in fluid volume and sodium content: (1) 100% fluid replacement lost during exercise with a 25-millimole sodium chloride solution, (2) 100% fluid replacement with a 50-millimole sodium chloride solution, (3) 150% fluid replacement with a 25-millimole sodium chloride solution, or (4) 150% fluid replacement with a 50-millimole sodium chloride solution. Each condition was tested for the effects on body mass, intracellular and extracellular fluid restoration, and cardiac stress parameters during the 20-minute postrehydration exercise period. The results from this study indicate that both 150% fluid replacement solutions promoted full fluid recovery, which was significantly greater than the two 100% solutions. Furthermore, intracellular rehydration was significantly greater in the 150% fluid replacement with a 25-millimole sodium solution compared to all other solutions.

While carbohydrate-electrolyte sports beverages typically contain 20 millimoles of sodium chloride (1.17 grams of sodium per liter), consuming too much of these drinks may not be effective at maintaining blood sodium concentrations in endurance athletes, who are known to lose large amounts of sodium during exercise (i.e., "salty sweaters"). In these rare occurrences, athletes may benefit by coingesting sodium tablets with carbohydrate-electrolyte beverages, albeit efficacious dosages differ from person to person and require interindividual experimentation. Nonetheless, it is apparent that consuming an adequate amount of a carbohydrate-electrolyte beverage that matches or slightly exceeds sweat rates (i.e., 400 to 500 milliliters per hour during cycling; Bates and Miller 2008) in endurance athletes is effective at maintaining blood mineral electrolytes during exercise.

5.3.3 Vitamin/Mineral Supplementation and Recovery Enhancement

Scientists have determined that prolonged endurance exercise can dramatically impair the body's natural antioxidant systems (summarized in Table 5.2), which help the body prevent muscle and bodily tissue damage as a result of exercise-induced oxidative

TABLE 5.2

The Two Major Antioxidant Systems Present in Skeletal Muscle

Antioxidant System	Physiological Function and Other Notes	Chemical Reaction
• Glutathione • Glutathione peroxidase (GPx) • Glutathione reductase (GRed)	• Glutathione is a two-residue amino acid (cysteine and glutamate) antioxidant that breaks down hydrogen peroxide (H_2O_2) into water (H_2O) • Selenium acts as a cofactor for GPx • Vitamin B_2 is a cofactor for GRed	
• Superoxide dismutase (SOD) • Peroxiredoxins • Catalase	• With the help of catalase, SOD breaks down superoxide (O_2) into water (H_2O) • Copper and zinc are cofactors for cytosolic SODs • Manganese is a cofactor for mitochondrial SODs	

stress (Duthie et al. 1990; Machefer et al. 2004). Dietary minerals serve as cofactors for various antioxidants. For example, several variants of SOD contain copper, zinc, or manganese as cofactors. Similarly, selenium is a cofactor for glutathione peroxidase. Thus, individuals deficient in these minerals likely possess compromised endogenous antioxidant systems that function suboptimally in response to exercise stressors.

With regard to exercise-induced oxidative stress, scientists Kelsey Fisher-Wellman and Richard Bloomer write (2009), "simply stated, any situation in which the consumption of oxygen is increased, as during physical exercise, could result in an acute state of oxidative stress." If prolonged endurance exercise repeatedly occurs in a dietary antioxidant-deficient state, such as during road cycling or ultramarathon events, then muscle and systemic tissue damage is imminent (Figure 5.5).

Dietary antioxidants include vitamin A, vitamin C, vitamin E, and selenium, albeit vitamin/mineral supplementation for antioxidant purposes is also aggressively debated in the exercise physiology and sports nutrition fields. As mentioned previously, two research groups demonstrated that the prolonged administration of vitamin C (one gram per day) or vitamin E (400 IU per day) prevent exercise-induced free radicals from activating intramuscular molecular pathways that serve to increase endogenous antioxidant and mitochondria levels (Gomez-Cabrera et al. 2008; Ristow et al. 2009). However, dietary antioxidants ingested in a prophylactic (or preventive) fashion prior to extreme endurance events have been shown to reduce excessive muscle damage. Examples include the following research findings:

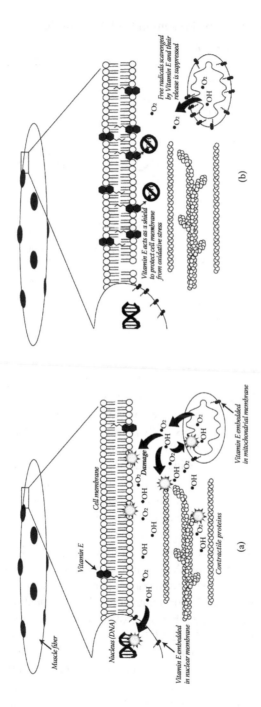

FIGURE 5.5 A summary of muscle damage as a result of oxidative stress. (A) In vitamin E-deficient states, exercise-induced free radicals (hydroxyl radicals, superoxide radicals, peroxynitrite, and lipid peroxidation products) chemically disrupt and damage various tissue structures, including DNA, cell membranes, contractile proteins, and mitochondrial structures. (B) Sufficient stores of vitamin E (and vitamin C, not shown) act to quench free radicals produced during prolonged exercise, which spares excessive tissue damage. Note that chronic oxidative stress can damage other tissues as well (e.g., tissue lining the cardiovascular system), and that long-term oxidative stress has been linked to various diseases (i.e., sarcopenia, cardiovascular disease, cancer, and dementia).

- Administering 400 milligrams per day of vitamin E to six high-altitude mountain climbers sustained pentane exhalation (a measure of cell membrane lipid peroxidation) after four weeks in the supplement group, while increasing 100% in the placebo group climbers during a climbing expedition (Simon-Schnass and Pabst 1988).
- Researchers administered 150 milligrams vitamin C, 24 milligrams vitamin E, 4.8 milligrams β-carotene, and various minerals to 17 athletes daily three weeks prior to and during the Marathon des Sables, which consists of six race days ranging from 26 to 71 kilometers per day in the desert (Machefer et al. 2007). Compared to the nonsupplemented condition, supplementation reduced blood thiobarbituric reactive substances (abbreviated as TBARSs throughout) three days into the competition and experienced increases in circulating plasma β-carotene.
- Another research group determined that supplementing endurance athletes with vitamin E (400 IU per day) and vitamin C (200 milligrams per day) 4.5 weeks prior to a marathon substantially reduced blood creatine kinase (a circulating marker of muscle damage) 24 hours following the event (Rokitzki et al. 1994).
- Administering 400 IU vitamin E, one gram vitamin C, and 90 micrograms selenium per day 14 days before and 2 days after an eccentric elbow flexor exercise bout prevented increases in circulating levels of malondialdehyde (a marker of cell membrane oxidative stress) 48 hours following exercise (Goldfarb et al. 2005). However, it is problematic to apply eccentric resistance exercise research findings to conventional resistance exercise settings due to the greater amount of force production that occurs and stress placed on individual activated motor units.

Notwithstanding micronutrient deficiencies, these research findings suggest that antioxidant supplementation up to four weeks prior to and during extremely prolonged exercise bouts (i.e., events lasting days to weeks) is beneficial in reducing oxidative stress during the bout and accelerating recovery. Applying these findings to strenuous training periods in strength and power athletes (i.e., two to three practices per day in football) remains to be determined. Furthermore, it has not been tested whether prophylactic dietary antioxidant supplementation translates into sustaining a more prolonged competitive season or career.

5.4 VITAMINS AND MINERALS IN ATHLETICS: FUTURE PERSPECTIVES

As evident in other chapters in this text, molecular biologists have determined what occurs within skeletal muscle in response to various exercise stressors. Likewise, geneticists have even begun determining how slight genetic differences dictate how humans perform during various athletic endeavors. While a comprehensive description of the interaction between exercise and genetics is beyond the scope of this chapter, those interested are encouraged to read brilliant publications highlighting these areas (Bray et al. 2009; MacArthur and North 2005; Roth 2007).

Simply stated, each cell within the body contains a nucleus or multiple nuclei. The nuclei contain DNA, which possesses an individual's unique genetic code. Based on comparative genetics estimates, approximately 99.5% of the genetic code is similar from person to person, while the 0.5% difference in genetic code endows each individual with different phenotypic characteristics (i.e., appearance, athletic capability, etc.). For this reason, some individuals may possess a unique sequence of DNA (termed a gene) that encodes an exceptionally efficient antioxidant enzyme, while others possess a slightly different gene sequence that encodes a less-efficient antioxidant (Figure 5.6). Thus, this physiological phenomenon can be likened to dietary vitamin/mineral deficiencies in that persons possessing "negative" genes are less equipped to deal with exercise-induced oxidative stress. Interestingly, this consideration alone could explain the individual differences commonly reported in vitamin/mineral supplementation literature in conjunction with exercise performance and recovery.

In addition, Table 5.3 provides examples of variant genes that exist that may impair endogenous antioxidant systems in persons expressing these genes. Based on

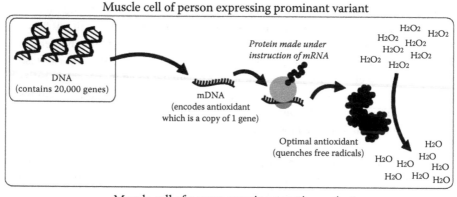

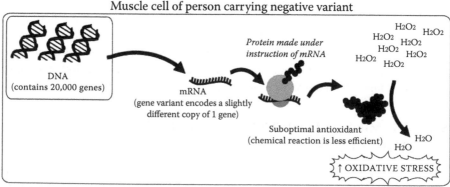

FIGURE 5.6 The concept of genetic polymorphisms affecting antioxidant systems. Each rectangle represents a muscle cell from two different individuals. CHO = carbohydrate; PRO = protein.

TABLE 5.3
Examples of Currently Known Genetic Polymorphisms of Various Antioxidant Enzymes

Gene	Polymorphisms and Characteristics
CAT	• This gene encodes the antioxidant enzyme catalase. • The *C1167T* single-nucleotide polymorphism variant (thymine is substituted for cytosine in a region of exon 9) does not change the amino acid sequence or affect protein function (Zotova et al. 2004).
GPX1	• Gene encodes the antioxidant enzyme glutathione peroxidase 1. • The C593T single-nucleotide polymorphism variant leads to the substitution of proline to leucine on amino acid residue 197 (Zotova et al. 2004). • No research to date has examined the presence of this allele in relation to exercise-induced oxidative stress.
GSTT1	• Gene encodes an isoform of glutathione S-transferase, an enzyme that conjugates glutathione to other organic structures and is prevalent in red blood cells. • A deletion variant, in which a large portion of the normal genetic code is missing, has been shown to encode a functionally inactive protein. • This allele has been observed in 38% of the population in screening studies (Zotova et al. 2004). • No research to date has examined the presence of this allele in relation to exercise-induced oxidative stress.
GSTM1	• This gene encodes an isoform of glutathione S-transferase, an enzyme that conjugates glutathione to other organic structures. • A deletion variant, in which a large portion of the normal genetic code is missing, has been shown to encode a functionally inactive protein. • This allele has been observed in 50% of the population in screening studies (Zotova et al. 2004). • No research to date has examined the presence of this allele in relation to exercise-induced oxidative stress.
P22 PHOX	• Gene encodes the antioxidant a subunit of Nicotinamide adenine dinucleotide phosphate (NAPDH) oxidase, which is an enzyme in white blood cells (specifically macrophages) that produces free radicals (superoxide). • The C242T single-nucleotide polymorphism variant leads to the substitution of histidine to tyrosine on an amino acid residue in the encoded subunit, which reduces NAPDH oxidase activity (production of fewer free radicals). • The NADPH oxidase p22phox C242T polymorphism does not alter lymphocyte DNA damage or exercise performance at rest, immediately after exercise, or during recovery (Paik et al. 2009).
SOD2	• Gene encodes the antioxidant enzyme manganese superoxide dismutase. • One reported polymorphism leads to the substitution of alanine for valine at amino acid 16 (Platz 2009). • Persons with the alanine enzyme variant (or alanine allele) are more susceptible to oxidative stress and are at greater risk for developing cancer (Platz 2009). • No research to date has examined the presence of this allele in relation to exercise-induced oxidative stress.

this concept, athletes who possess variant genes that encode antioxidants that operate at a relative disadvantage compared to athletes that encode "optimal" antioxidants may benefit from dietary antioxidant supplementation. Furthermore, athlete carriers of polymorphisms that encode suboptimal vitamin/mineral transporters (not listed in Table 5.3) may also physiologically benefit from increased micronutrient intakes. However, geneticists are only beginning to examine the association between these polymorphisms and their effects on exercise-induced oxidative stress (Paik et al. 2009).

5.5 CONCLUSIONS

In summary, researchers have determined that diet-induced vitamin or mineral deficiencies in athletes reduce endurance capacity, impair immune cell function during prolonged exercise, exacerbate muscle protein breakdown beyond what is normally incurred through strenuous training, and lead to the whole-body accumulation of noxious free radicals during exercise; the last may have long-term health consequences (i.e., vascular damage, cognitive function, cancer development, etc.) if vitamin deficiency is severe and prolonged. Furthermore, vitamin and mineral deficiencies are highly prevalent in many athletes due to insufficient intakes coupled with increased physical activity levels, and this phenomenon is of even greater concern to athletes who attempt to optimize body composition through caloric restriction (Lukaski 2004).

Therefore and in summary, the primary recommendation to all athletes is to consume a well-balanced diet concomitant with a daily multivitamin/mineral supplement with the intent of preventing micronutrient deficiencies. The points discussed next summarize other vitamin and mineral recommendations discussed in this chapter. In addition, a hypothetical model with a typical daily supplement regimen is presented in Figure 5.7 and is briefly outlined in the text for a typical endurance athlete.

5.5.1 B VITAMINS AND MINERALS

As evidenced by the findings of Belko et al. (1983), endurance athletes should increase certain vitamin and mineral intakes by as much as 100% (or two times) the RDI to optimize his or her micronutrient status. These vitamins include all of the B vitamins, and minerals including calcium, chromium, magnesium, phosphate, and zinc. However, it should be noted that these intakes are obtainable with a well-balanced diet in addition to a daily multivitamin/mineral supplement.

5.5.2 ANTIOXIDANTS

Consuming high doses of antioxidants (i.e., vitamin A, β-carotene, vitamin C, vitamin E, selenium) does not improve and, in some instances, impairs endurance performance as well as the molecular adaptations to endurance exercise (Ristow et al. 2009). Based on these research findings, it is advisable that athletes concerned with aerobic performance do not consume copious amounts (i.e., five to ten times [or more] the current RDI) of these substances. However, athletes who are undergoing acute, extreme exercise stress (i.e., road cyclists or ultramarathoners participating in

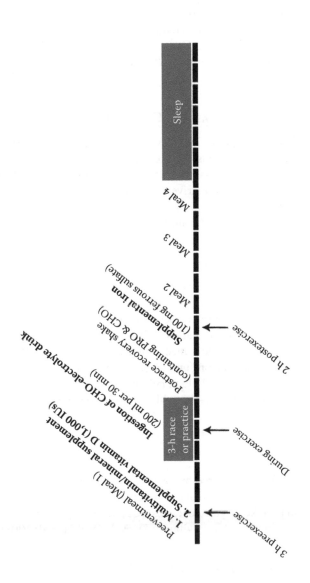

FIGURE 5.7 A typical daily vitamin/mineral supplementation schematic for endurance athletes. Note that no research to date has unequivocally demonstrated that vitamin/mineral timing around exercise optimizes vitamin/mineral status or enhances recovery, albeit it may be advantageous for endurance athletes to consume supplemental iron within a six-hour postexercise window due to high red blood cell turnover following exercise.

multiday events) have experienced a reduction in excessive muscle damage from the daily prophylactic supplementation of antioxidant concoctions up to four weeks prior to and throughout the event. Such formulations have included (1) 150 milligrams per day of vitamin C, 24 milligrams per day of vitamin E, and 4.8 milligrams per day of β-carotene; (2) 200 milligrams per day of vitamin C and 266 milligrams per day of vitamin E; (3) 400 milligrams per day of vitamin E; and (4) 266 milligrams per day of vitamin E, 1 gram per day of vitamin C, and 90 micrograms per day of selenium. Again, these intakes are obtainable with a well-balanced diet in addition to a daily multivitamin/mineral supplement.

5.5.3 ELECTROLYTES (SODIUM, POTASSIUM, CHLORIDE)

Blood sodium chloride loss and potassium elevations are primary concerns for athletes partaking in endurance events lasting greater than two hours in hot and cold climates (sweat rates have been estimated to range from 400 to 500 milliliters per hour). To remedy this, athletes should strive to consume 200 to 250 milliliters of a carbohydrate-electrolyte beverage (that contains sodium and other discussed electrolytes) per 30 minutes for prolonged endurance activities in all climates.

5.5.4 IRON

In general, researchers have reported that up to 60% of endurance athletes are tissue iron depleted (Hunding et al. 1981). Supplementing with 100 to 200 milligrams per day ferrous sulfate may optimize endurance performance, as these dosages have been found to restore blood hemoglobin and markers of tissue iron status and improve performance markers in iron-deficient endurance athletes (Hinton et al. 2000; Hunding et al. 1981). Further, consuming an iron supplement within six hours of a prolonged endurance event may enhance new red blood cell and hemoglobin formation due to the fact that red blood cell turnover has been shown to be elevated within this time frame (Smith et al. 1995).

5.5.5 VITAMIN D

Contrary to the current RDI and spurred by the rising concern about vitamin D deficiencies in athletes, it is recommended that endurance athletes supplement with 1,000 to 2,000 IU per day and partake in safe sun exposure up to 30 minutes per day for two to three days per week to increase blood vitamin D levels (Willis et al. 2008).

5.5.6 ULTRAENDURANCE AND STRENGTH/POWER ATHLETES

For those athletes who regularly partake in extreme endurance competitions (e.g., > 100-mile runs, 24-hour runs, expedition races, cross-country rides, extreme temperature or condition races, etc.), it may be advantageous for these individuals to consume supplemental antioxidants (i.e., 200 milligrams of vitamin C and 200 to 300 milligrams of vitamin E with or without selenium) on a daily basis up to four weeks prior to and during the event. Strength and power athletes are generally advised to consume a daily multivitamin/mineral; however, the intermittent nature and often short duration of activity allows for more opportunities to feed both fluids and food, which will likely contain some combination of required micronutrients.

5.6   WEB SITES PROVIDING SCIENCE-BASED INFORMATION ON MICRONUTRIENTS

- Nutrition Data: http://www.nutritiondata.com. Athletes can find general nutrition information on a wide variety of foods and analysis tools that allow users to determine how various foods affect their health.
- Medline Plus: http://www.nlm.nih.gov/medlineplus/vitamins.html. This Web site is a service of the U.S. National Library of Medicine as well as the National Institutes of Health; it provides a comprehensive database on information regarding vitamins, including the latest news, scientific journal articles, and current research studies.
- Linus Pauling Institute Micronutrient Information Center: http://lpi.oregon-state.edu/infocenter/. This Web site is a source for scientifically accurate information regarding the physiological roles of vitamins, minerals, and other nutrients.

6 Preexercise Nutrient Timing in Endurance Activity

Elizabeth M. Broad, Leonidas G. Karagounis, and John A. Hawley

CONTENTS

6.1 INTRODUCTION AND BACKGROUND

The importance of carbohydrate as a substrate for skeletal muscle during exercise has been known since the turn of the twentieth century. At this time, evidence was provided to show that both carbohydrate and fat contributed as energy sources for the muscle during submaximal aerobic exercise, but as exercise intensity increased, carbohydrate-based fuels (i.e., muscle and liver glycogen, blood glucose, lactate) predominated. A series of experiments undertaken in the 1920s provided perhaps the first information on the interaction of diet and exercise on substrate metabolism and exercise capacity. The results from these studies confirmed that carbohydrate and fat were oxidized by the muscle during submaximal exercise; that an individual's preceding diet influenced muscle metabolism both at rest in the postabsorptive state and during subsequent exercise. Further, with an increase in the relative intensity of exercise, there was a shift from utilization of fat as a fuel source toward carbohydrate-based fuels, and that individuals have a low tolerance for exercise when the diet preceding exercise is low in carbohydrate (i.e., high in fat). Classic work from researchers in Scandinavia in the 1930s further described how diet, training, and exercise intensity/duration affected carbohydrate and fat utilization. The findings from these early pioneering studies were instrumental in underpinning our current understanding of muscle fuel metabolism and laid the foundation for many of the modern-day studies of exercise-nutrient interactions (Kiens and Hawley 2011).

The introduction of the percutaneous needle biopsy technique in the 1960s (Bergstrom et al. 1967) saw the beginning of the "classic period" of exercise biochemistry that commenced in the late 1960s and progressed through the mid-1980s. As direct measures of muscle carbohydrate stores (i.e., muscle glycogen) were now possible, the emphasis shifted from measures of whole-body substrate oxidation (through respiratory exchange values determined from pulmonary gas exchange) and blood glucose concentrations toward endogenous carbohydrate as a fuel source during exercise. Among many of the experimental findings at this time was the seminal observation that there was an increased exercise endurance capacity when subjects were fed a carbohydrate-rich diet in the days preceding competition, and that carbohydrate feedings during exercise could postpone the development of fatigue and prolong endurance capacity. This chapter focuses on the various diet and exercise training strategies that are known to promote carbohydrate availability before and during exercise and to what extent such nutrient-exercise interactions have an impact on exercise performance in humans.

6.2   MUSCLE AND LIVER GLYCOGEN STORES IN HUMANS

Endogenous carbohydrate reserves are limited, and muscle and liver glycogen depletion often coincide with fatigue during both endurance events and many team sports. Accordingly, diet-exercise strategies to maximize these fuel depots are of paramount importance to the performance of many sporting activities. Carbohydrates are compounds having a ratio of one carbon atom to water ($C:H_2O$). As discussed in more detail in Chapter 2, the most common form of dietary carbohydrates are the monosaccharides, that is, glucose, fructose, and galactose. Of these, glucose is the principle currency for carbohydrate metabolism. Glucose is stored in polymer form and ranges in molecular weight from 50,000 to several million. In humans, glucose is stored as glycogen, and the branch-like structure of glycogen affords many terminal glucose sites that can be rapidly degraded during exercise to provide energy. The energy oxidation equivalent for the terminal oxidation of glucose to CO_2 and H_2O is 5.1 kilocalories per liter of consumed oxygen.

The endogenous sources of carbohydrate are muscle and liver glycogen, blood glucose and blood, muscle and liver lactate. The glycogen content of skeletal muscle of untrained individuals consuming a mixed diet is typically 80 millimoles per kilogram (mmol/kg) of muscle wet weight. For individuals involved in regular strenuous endurance training, muscle glycogen content is somewhat higher at approximately 125 millimoles per kilogram of muscle wet weight (Hawley, Schabort, et al. 1997) (Figure 6.1). After several days of a high-carbohydrate (eight to ten grams of carbohydrate per kilogram of body mass) diet and a decrease in training, muscle glycogen

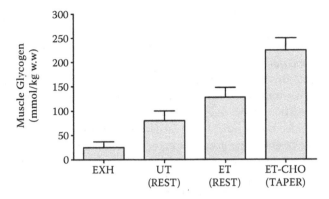

FIGURE 6.1 Muscle glycogen stores as a function of training status and diet-exercise manipulations. EXH = exercise-induced exhaustion; UT = untrained; ET = exercise trained; CHO = carbohydrate. (Data are from Hawley, J.A., E.J. Schabort, T.D. Noakes, and S.C. Dennis. 1997. Carbohydrate-loading and exercise performance: An update. *Sports Med* 24(2):73–81.)

content can be elevated to values greater than 200 millimoles per kilogram of muscle wet weight. Glycogen is stored in tissue with two to three grams of water per gram of glycogen (Olsson and Saltin 1970), which reduces the effective energy value of this substrate as an energy source and practically speaking results in a typical 2–3% increase in body mass of an athlete after several days of "carbohydrate loading." Accordingly, the extra mass to be carried by an athlete (i.e., during overground running) must be balanced against the likely benefit to performance before adopting such strategies.

In addition to skeletal muscle reserves, about 100 grams of glycogen are stored in the liver; liver glycogen can be hydrolyzed back to glucose and transported via the bloodstream to working muscle for oxidation. The major source of carbohydrate outside the muscle is found in the liver, which with an average weight of approximately 1.2 kilograms, contains about 100 grams of glycogen. As with muscle glycogen, the content of the liver glycogen pool can range widely depending on training status and diet. Liver glycogenolysis and the subsequent release of glucose into the systemic circulation consist of an essential mechanism for maintaining blood glucose concentrations during prolonged exercise.

6.3   PREEXERCISE NUTRIENT TIMING

6.3.1   THE WEEK PRIOR TO COMPETITION: CARBOHYDRATE LOADING STRATEGIES

In the late 1960s, Swedish investigators first described a novel exercise-diet regimen to "supercompensate" muscle glycogen stores. In an ingenious study (as side note, this was conducted on the study creators), Bergstrom and Hultman (1966) described an extreme protocol that involved glycogen-depleting exercise until exhaustion followed by a period (three days) of restricted carbohydrate intake and subsequent (two to three days) intake of large quantities of dietary carbohydrate. The extremes of exercise and diet elevated muscle glycogen stores to exceptionally high levels; a phenomenon that was localized to only those muscles involved in the exercise-induced depletion. This diet-exercise regimen prolonged exercise time to exhaustion at a fixed, submaximal work rate compared to when the same subjects ingested their habitual or a low-carbohydrate diet in the days before undertaking the prescribed exercise task (Bergstrom et al. 1967). Since this pioneering investigation, Sherman and colleagues (1981) have proposed a less-extreme exercise-diet program that does not require an athlete to exercise to exhaustion in the days prior to competition or subject them to extreme diet practices. Indeed, it is now widely accepted that several days of increased carbohydrate intake (eight to ten grams of carbohydrate per kilogram of body mass) in association with a reduction in exercise volume (not necessarily intensity) will supercompensate muscle glycogen stores to levels comparable with the classical loading protocol conducted by Bergstrom and Hultman (1966) (Figure 6.2).

There is some evidence that well-trained endurance athletes who consume a high-carbohydrate diet (>6 grams of carbohydrate per kilogram of body mass) on a day-to-day basis may not have the same capacity to increase their muscle glycogen content as untrained individuals (Hawley, Schabort, et al. 1997; Rauch et al. 1995). However, it should be noted that trained individuals can supercompensate their muscle (and presumably liver) glycogen stores on a daily basis when consuming a moderate- to high-carbohydrate diet. For review, see the work of Hawley, Schabort, et al. (1997). Indeed, Costill et al. (1981) have previously reported that muscle glycogen stores were not significantly different when trained runners ingested 525 or 650 grams of carbohydrate per day. These results suggest that muscle glycogen content

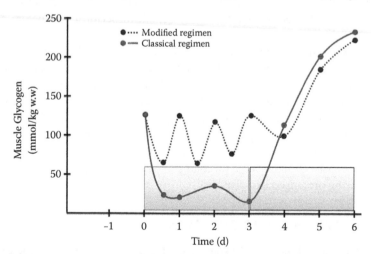

FIGURE 6.2 The effect of exercise-diet manipulation on muscle glycogen storage. The "classical" protocol was extreme and involved glycogen-depleting exercise until exhaustion followed by a three-day period of restricted carbohydrate intake and a subsequent two to three days while ingesting large quantities of dietary carbohydrate (Bergstrom and Hultman 1966). Subsequently, a less-extreme exercise-diet program was proposed by Sherman et al. (1981) that did not require an athlete to exercise to exhaustion in the days prior to competition or subject the athlete to extreme dietary practices (Sherman et al. 1981). The two exercise-diet regimens resulted in similar preexercise muscle glycogen stores.

may plateau in trained athletes when large amounts (approximately 600 grams of carbohydrate per day or > 8 grams of carbohydrate per kilogram of body mass) of carbohydrates are consumed.

With regard to the effects of carbohydrate loading on performance, it is well accepted that increasing muscle and liver glycogen stores in the week prior to an event/competition lasting longer than 90 minutes will postpone fatigue and enhance performance (Hawley, Schabort, et al. 1997). During this type and duration of exercise, exhaustion usually coincides with critically low (25 millimoles per kilogram of muscle wet weight) muscle glycogen content, suggesting the supply of energy from glycogen utilization cannot be replaced by increased oxidation of blood glucose. Glycogen supercompensation improves endurance performance in which a set distance is covered as quickly as possible (i.e., a time trial). In such exercise, high-carbohydrate diets have been reported to improve performance by 2–3%. However, there appears to be little advantage of elevating preexercise glycogen stores on a single bout of exercise lasting 60 to 90 minutes or strenuous exercise of short duration (i.e., five to ten minutes). In such cases, substantial amounts of glycogen remain in the working muscles after exercise.

6.3.2 THE DAY PRIOR TO COMPETITION

The 24-hour period immediately prior to competition is important for fine-tuning nutritional preparation. However, unless an athlete is specifically carbohydrate loading, it does not require any difference in approach than a normal training day would. Considering most individuals will undertake only light training (or rest) the day before an important competition or match, the focus during this time is to optimize muscle glycogen stores by maintaining an adequate carbohydrate intake (approximately seven grams of carbohydrate per kilogram of body mass), optimize hydration levels, and consume foods or beverages that ensure minimal gastrointestinal disturbance. Normalization of glycogen stores (in the absence of muscle damage) can be achieved within a 24-hour period (Burke et al. 1995), although this requires a consistent and continued food and fluid intake over that period, rather than focusing on the nutritional composition of one single meal the night before competition. For some individuals, this may also require a reprioritization of food components (for example, reducing protein or fat intake to allow a higher carbohydrate intake or increasing total energy intake) to ensure glycogen stores are optimized in this time period before competition.

6.3.3 IMMEDIATE PRECOMPETITION FEEDING STRATEGIES

The decision regarding consumption of carbohydrate prior to endurance exercise may depend on the goals of the exercise session. In the case of competition, where the goal is usually related to optimal performance, the evidence strongly supports consuming a preevent meal consisting predominantly of carbohydrate as it may reduce the rate of glycogen utilization during the event (Tsintzas and Williams 1998). For regular training, the goals may vary; hence, the preexercise feeding strategy may require modification. For example, if the training session is a lower-intensity session aiming to increase total mileage and stimulate greater fat utilization, the choice may be not to consume carbohydrate preexercise due to the suppression of lipolysis by insulin (Coyle et al. 1985). In this situation, the focus may be more on the consumption of nutrients during exercise. The goals of the immediate precompetition feeding can be summarized by the following:

1. Continue to contribute to muscle glycogen stores if they have not been fully restored since the last exercise session.
2. Optimize blood glucose concentrations and restore liver glycogen content (especially when the competition or training session is undertaken first thing in the morning after an overnight fast).
3. Achieve gut comfort: minimize hunger during the event, but also avoid sensations of fullness, bloating, or urgency.
4. Ensure euhydration and prime the gut with a fluid bolus to optimize fluid absorption during exercise.
5. Enable the athlete to feel comfortable and confident by including familiar foods and practice regimens.

There are no succinct rules for precompetition eating, but rather a range of guidelines that require adaptation by each individual to ensure all the goals are met. The importance of this meal or snack will also depend in part on the duration of the event (i.e., less important as a fuel source for events lasting less than 60 minutes than for events lasting > 90 minutes) and whether any during-competition feeding and fluid intake strategies will occur (i.e., of lesser importance if a source of carbohydrate or fluid can be consumed during the event). Certainly, it is well recognized that feeding carbohydrate prior to endurance exercise compared to starting the event in a fasted state will increase the likelihood of a superior performance (Chryssanthopoulos and Williams 1997; Flynn et al. 1989; Rollo and Williams 2010; Sherman et al. 1989).

6.3.4   Preexercise Nutrient Intake: Timing—What Do We Know?

Perhaps somewhat surprisingly, relatively few studies have systematically compared the effects of different timings of food/fluid intake before exercise on endurance exercise performance. Indeed, one of the earliest studies of preexercise feeding reported that the ingestion of 75 grams of glucose 30 minutes prior to exercise *impaired* performance (time to exhaustion at 80% of VO_2Max [maximum oxygen consumption]) compared to exercising in the fasted state or consuming a liquid meal with mixed nutrient composition (Foster et al. 1979). The results from that study received widespread publicity, and athletes were effectively warned against consuming carbohydrate in the hour before exercise in fear of the resultant hypoglycemia at the commencement of exercise and impairment of exercise tolerance/capacity. However, subsequent research on the timing of the preexercise meal revealed that the results from that study (Foster et al. 1979) had been overplayed. For example, in subsequent investigations it has consistently been shown that the initial fall in blood glucose concentrations at the start of exercise was temporary and short-lived and did not have a negative impact on performance in endurance exercise in the vast majority of individuals. Indeed, a review of the literature has noted that this early study is the only study in which performance was negatively impacted by the preexercise carbohydrate feeding. Thus, all subsequent investigations in which carbohydrate was fed within the hour before endurance exercise found either no effect or an improvement in performance (Hawley and Burke 1997).

Most researchers have investigated the impact of carbohydrate ingestion within a 75-minute period preexercise. Moseley and colleagues (2003) compared the ingestion of 75 grams of glucose with 500 milliliters of water taken 15, 45, or 75 minutes prior to exercising for approximately one hour (20-minute cycle preload followed by a time trial). Despite substantial differences in insulin and blood glucose concentrations, particularly in the first 10 minutes of exercise, no performance difference was observed between treatments. In a similar study, Lancaster et al. found no difference in performance and no functionally relevant difference in immune parameters when comparing 75 grams of carbohydrate consumed 15 or 75 minutes before exercise (Lancaster et al. 2003). Smith et al. (2002) found nonstatistically significant improvements in 4,000-meter swimming performance (improvements ranged from 24 seconds to 5 minutes in 8 of 10 subjects) when 5 milliliters per kilogram of body mass of a 10% glucose solution (mean absolute carbohydrate intake was 38 grams) was given 5 or 35 minutes prior to exercise when compared to placebo ingestion.

There is evidence that feeding on carbohydrate further from the start of exercise (e.g., four hours prior) can result in higher muscle glycogen stores at the commencement of exercise compared to commencing exercise in the fasted state (Coyle et al. 1985). Interestingly, no studies have considered whether there is a difference in endurance performance when timing of carbohydrate feeding was within 75 minutes compared to several hours before exercise. Maffucci and McMurray (2000) compared feeding 40 kilojoules per kilogram (approximately 82 grams of carbohydrate) three or six hours before exercise and found improved performance with the three- compared to the six-hour feeding protocol. However, the conclusions are complicated because the three-hour feeding protocol actually had a meal at six hours, then another meal at three hours before exercise (similar nutritional composition each time), whereas the six-hour feeding provided a single meal only, and a relatively short exercise period (37 minutes total). Flynn and investigators (1989) compared feeding 3.5 grams of carbohydrate per kilogram of body mass four or eight hours before a 120-minute exercise bout (105-minute steady state with 15-minute time trial) and found no difference in performance between the two trials.

There do remain some individuals who experience hypoglycemia in the first 10 to 20 minutes of exercise following consumption of carbohydrate in the last hour before exercise commencement (Kuipers et al. 1999). Some of these individuals may experience hypoglycemic symptoms and potentially impaired performance as a result, thus highlighting the need to individualize the preexercise feeding strategy to optimize performance. In such circumstances, the athlete should trial having a carbohydrate meal or snack with a lower glycemic index further away from the start of exercise (two to three hours) and may require a larger amount of carbohydrate. Manipulation of the warmup to include some high-intensity sprints to stimulate hepatic glucose output or consuming carbohydrate during the event may also be advisable.

6.3.5 Is the Glycemic Index of a Preevent Meal Important?

One way of manipulating the delivery rate of carbohydrate to the bloodstream, and hence a surrogate for altering the timing of feeding, is altering the glycemic index of the carbohydrate ingested. One of the first studies to determine the effect of the glycemic index of carbohydrate consumed preexercise revealed that a dose of carbohydrate with a high glycemic index consumed one hour before exercise reduced exercise performance compared to food with a low glycemic index (Thomas et al. 1991). The results of that study were the stimulus for further research in this area. While it is generally accepted that consuming a preexercise meal with a lower glycemic index results in a more favorable metabolic profile during exercise (Moore et al. 2010; Wu et al. 2003), many investigations have failed to assess the impact of this on performance. The outcomes of those studies that have measured performance are mixed, from improved performance following meals with a low glycemic index (DeMarco et al. 1999; Kirwan et al. 2001; Moore et al. 2010), to no difference in performance (Febbraio et al. 2000; Febbraio and Stewart 1996; Thomas et al. 1994), or even to reduced performance (Sparks et al. 1998) compared to a meal with a high glycemic index. The variations in outcomes could partly be due to the timing, type, or amount of carbohydrate consumed or the selection of performance or outcome parameters. Regardless, Donaldson et al. (2010) have recommended encouraging athletes to follow standard recommendations for carbohydrate consumption preexercise and let practical issues and individual athlete experience dictate the use of options with a high or low glycemic index.

6.3.6 Should the Preexercise Meal Contain Fat or Protein?

Surprisingly, there is minimal research published regarding the potential use of high-fat or high-protein preexercise meals on performance. Rowlands and Hopkins (2002) found no difference in 50-kilometer time trial performance following a 110-minute exercise preload when comparing a high-fat, high-protein, and high-carbohydrate meal consumed 90 minutes prior to the exercise bout, despite substantial differences in substrate oxidation and blood glucose concentrations between trials. Interestingly, these differences remained despite the athletes being fed a 6% carbohydrate-electrolyte solution throughout both the steady state and time trial. Similarly, both Okano et al. (1996) and Whitley et al. (1998) found no difference in performance when isoenergetic high-fat versus high-carbohydrate meals were consumed four hours prior to prolonged (90- to 120-minute) steady-state exercise followed by a time trial. In contrast to the Rowlands and Hopkins study, Whitley et al. found no difference in substrate metabolism during the steady-state exercise component despite the fact that the meals had induced different hormone, blood glucose, and plasma free fatty acid profiles during exercise. Similarly, Okano et al. found the substrate utilization differences induced by the preexercise meals were only present in the first 40 minutes of steady-state exercise. The only study in which performance during endurance exercise was found to be improved by prior ingestion of a high-fat meal (90% of energy, compared with high-carbohydrate meal) had followed the meal with an infusion of heparin to increase fat utilization (Pitsiladis et al. 1999)—a factor that would not be practical in the field.

Considering the potential impact on gastrointestinal comfort of high-fat foods, it is unnecessary to include fat in the preexercise meal or snack other than for taste.

6.3.7   How Much Carbohydrate?

There is little research regarding the optimal amount of carbohydrate that should be consumed immediately prior to endurance exercise. Sherman et al. (1991) compared 1.1 and 2.2 grams of carbohydrate per kilogram of body mass in a liquid meal consumed one hour before exercise and found no difference in performance between the two conditions. Similarly, in another trial in which isocaloric meals were consumed four hours preexercise, there was no difference in performance between 45 and 156 grams of carbohydrate (Sherman et al. 1989). Lancaster et al. (2003) not only found no difference in cycling time trial performance when comparing 25 to 200 grams of carbohydrate consumed 45 minutes before exercise, but also found no difference in immune responses to the exercise bout. Perhaps surprisingly, they also found no difference in performance or immune response to the placebo condition. In contrast, Cramp et al. (2004) observed a 3% faster performance in a mountain bike trial when three grams of carbohydrate per kilogram of body mass were consumed three hours prior to exercise compared to one gram of carbohydrate per kilogram of body mass, along with altering the pacing strategy of the cyclists. Overall, the greater influences on the amount of carbohydrate consumed before exercise may be gastrointestinal comfort, timing of ingestion, or mode of exercise rather than performance per se.

6.3.8   Is the Preexercise Meal Required If Athletes Consume Carbohydrate during Exercise?

Several studies have combined carbohydrate feeding preexercise with the consumption of carbohydrate during exercise (predominantly in the form of a carbohydrate-electrolyte solution). These studies have generally continued to show enhancement of performance above fasting or no carbohydrate during exercise. In this respect, two studies reported greater enhancement of performance by combining the preexercise meal with during-exercise carbohydrate intake compared to just consuming carbohydrate pre- or during exercise, respectively (Chryssanthopoulos and Williams 1997; Flynn et al. 1989). However, this additive effect may be dependent on the duration of the event, as more recently Rollo and Williams (2010) have shown no further improvement in performance during a one-hour run when a carbohydrate-electrolyte solution was consumed before and during the run compared to consuming a high-carbohydrate preexercise meal three hours before the run alone. Nevertheless, the consumption of carbohydrate in the immediate preexercise period remains beneficial for endurance performance.

6.4   SUMMARY AND GUIDELINES FOR PREEVENT FEEDING

In the week prior to a major competition lasting 90 minutes or longer, athletes should consume a high-carbohydrate intake (eight to ten grams of carbohydrate per kilogram of body mass) in association with a reduction in exercise volume (not necessarily intensity). Such a diet-exercise regimen will supercompensate muscle (and presumably liver) glycogen stores and enhance performance. There is strong evidence to recommend that athletes consume meals and snacks rich in carbohydrate within the 24-hour period prior to an important endurance exercise task or team sport lasting longer than 90 minutes. There is good evidence that consuming meals and snacks rich in carbohydrate within the 24-hour period prior to endurance exercise enhances performance. However, to date, no systematic assessment of the ideal timing of the immediate preexercise meal has been undertaken. Of course, numerous variables could influence such an analyses, including the glycemic index of the foods and fluids to be consumed, the fat and protein content of such food and fluids, the total amount of carbohydrate, whether the meal is liquid or solid, and whether the athlete is consuming carbohydrate during the exercise bout or event. Given that such variables would make it difficult to make "general recommendations" to athletes across a variety of sporting situations, it may well be that individual food preferences and gastrointestinal comfort would override the scientific outcomes in many instances. Perhaps what is more important is to guide athletes toward developing their own personal prerace and preexercise feeding plan, to practice it, to make alterations if required, then to systematically use this plan leading up to competition or training. For example, a beginning guideline would be as follows:

1. Consume a larger meal three to four hours before exercise.
2. Consume a smaller snack two hours before or liquid snack 30 to 60 minutes before exercise.
3. Choose a carbohydrate-based food/fluid with minimal fat (<5 grams) and fiber (<3 grams) content and a low-to-moderate protein content (<15 grams).

Foods should be low in fat and fiber to minimize the risk of gastrointestinal upset. Both fat and fiber can slow the rate of digestion and absorption of food. The choice of time of feeding and volume consumed will depend on a number of factors, including the time at which the event commences, type of event (e.g., running compared to cycling), and optimal gastrointestinal comfort and should be tested well in advance.

6.5   EXAMPLES OF USEFUL PREEXERCISE MEALS OR SNACKS

While Chapter 13 is dedicated to providing more detailed guidelines regarding types of foods, amounts of foods, and when to eat them for a select group of athletes, a brief list of meals that contain a high-carbohydrate content are provided here and could be used as considerations for preexercise meals several hours before or in the preexercise period.

- Breakfast cereal, skim milk, fresh or canned fruit
- Toast and baked beans or eggs
- Toast, bagel, English muffin, and jam or honey
- Pancakes with maple syrup

- Fruit and low-fat yogurt
- Creamed rice
- Rolls or sandwiches (low-fat fillings, not too much salad)
- Pasta with low-fat sauce
- Low-fat smoothie
- Porridge
- A liquid meal supplement may be preferable in individuals who suffer from known gastrointestinal issues or nerves prior to competition.

7 Macronutrient Intake during Endurance Activity to Optimize Performance

Michael J. Saunders and Nicholas D. Luden

CONTENTS

7.1 INTRODUCTION

Competitive endurance sport activities place significant metabolic demands on the body. For example, the energetic requirements during sustained endurance exercise may exceed 600 to 1,000 calories per hour in highly trained women and men. Providing for these caloric needs, and managing the associated disruptions in metabolic homeostasis, is essential for optimal performance and recovery from prolonged, heavy exercise. This chapter, specifically, focuses on the role of nutrition during exercise to influence metabolism and optimize performance for endurance athletes. For this purpose, endurance exercise is defined as any activity of approximately one-hour duration or longer (generally less than four hours), performed at moderate-to-vigorous intensities (approximately 50–85% VO_2Max

[maximum oxygen consumption]). Our scope is limited to the influences of energy-providing nutrients (carbohydrate, protein, and fat) consumed during exercise and particularly how deviations in temporal administration may influence resulting performance, recovery, and so on. Due to the universal role the macronutrients have on various physiological processes, similarities between pre-, during-, and postexercise recommendations are expected and unavoidable. However, it is our contention, as with many of the contributors of this book, that each individual athlete and sporting scenario are different, and for this reason, strategies from one area may not apply for one athlete but will apply for another. In addition, macronutrient consumption during endurance exercise is usually accompanied by water/electrolyte intake, as athletes consume much of their caloric intake during exercise from sports beverages, which deliver these constituents simultaneously. Thus, readers are referred to reviews from other sources regarding fluid and electrolyte intake during endurance exercise (Noakes 1993; Rodriguez et al. 2009a; Sawka et al. 2007; Shirreffs 2009).

7.1.1 Substrate Utilization during Endurance Exercise

The relative contributions of carbohydrate, fat, and protein to skeletal muscular energy requirements are influenced by various factors; the most important with respect to this chapter are the intensity and duration of exercise (discussed further in this chapter) as well as the nutrient intake of the athlete. As shown in Figure 7.1, during low-intensity exercise (approximately 25% VO$_2$Max) in the fasted state, the

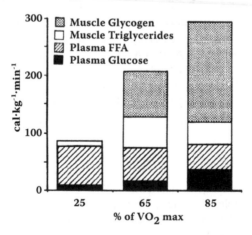

FIGURE 7.1 Maximal contribution to energy expenditure derived from glucose and free fatty acids taken up from blood and minimal contribution of muscle triglyceride and glycogen stores after 30 minutes of exercise expressed as a function of exercise intensity. Total amount of energy (kcal) available from plasma does change in relation to exercise intensity. FFA = free fatty acids. (From Romijn, J.A., E.F. Coyle, L.S. Sidossis, A. Gastaldelli, J.F. Horowitz, E. Endert, and R.R. Wolfe. Regulation of Endogenous Fat and Carbohydrate Metabolism in Relation to Exercise Intensity and Duration. *Am J Physiol* 265(3 Pt 1):E380–91, 1993. Used with permission.)

vast majority of energy is provided from fat oxidation, predominantly in the form of plasma-free fatty acids derived from lipolysis of peripheral adipocytes. At this intensity, carbohydrate provides a relatively small amount of energy, almost exclusively from blood glucose (Romijn et al. 1993). Proportionally, protein contributes very little to energy demands during endurance exercise (Lemon and Mullin 1980; Rennie et al. 2006). Most studies examining substrate utilization during exercise assume that protein metabolism is negligible and constant throughout exercise. Thus, contribution of protein to energy metabolism is not discussed further in this section. However, greater detail regarding protein metabolism is provided in the subsequent section regarding protein intake during exercise.

At moderate exercise intensities (60–70% VO_2Max), total fat oxidation increases via significant contributions from plasma-free fatty acids and intramuscular triglycerides. In addition, carbohydrate utilization rises considerably, particularly from muscle glycogen stores. At higher intensities (>80% VO_2Max), the proportional contribution of carbohydrate to total energy production increases further due largely to reductions in fat oxidation and increases in both blood glucose and (especially) muscle glycogen utilization (Romijn et al. 1993).

Substrate utilization is also influenced by exercise duration (Figure 7.2). At moderate exercise intensities, plasma free fatty acid utilization increases over time. The contribution of muscle glycogen to total energy production decreases progressively throughout exercise as levels of this substrate are reduced over time. Blood glucose utilization increases in the later stages of prolonged exercise to maintain high rates of carbohydrate oxidation necessary to sustain energy demands. Blood glucose levels are maintained during exercise largely through endogenous glucose production (via glycogenolysis and gluconeogenesis) in the liver and, to a lesser extent, gluconeogenesis in the kidney (Gerich 2010; Wasserman 2009). However, liver glycogen stores can be depleted during prolonged exercise, resulting in decreased blood glucose levels, ultimately limiting contributions of carbohydrate to total energy production (Coyle et al. 1986).

7.2   CARBOHYDRATE INTAKE DURING ENDURANCE EXERCISE

7.2.1   HISTORICAL PERSPECTIVE

The importance of carbohydrate for endurance exercise has been investigated for more than a century. Prior to 1900, scientists had observed that carbohydrate utilization increased during exercise (Chaveau 1896), and that dietary intake could influence the proportional utilization of carbohydrates and fats (Zuntz and Loeb 1894). The hypothesis that carbohydrate intake *during exercise* may improve endurance performance dates to at least the 1920s (Krogh and Lindhard 1920; Levine et al. 1924). For example, it was observed that blood glucose levels were related to the physical condition of runners following completion of the Boston Marathon, and it was suggested that carbohydrate intake "would be of considerable benefit in preventing the hypoglycemia accompanying development of the symptoms of exhaustion" (Levine et al. 1924). Subsequently, Dill and associates (1932) reported that ingestion of glucose by a dog during prolonged exercise resulted in a threefold increase in

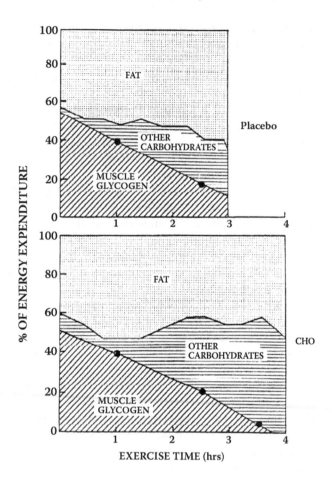

FIGURE 7.2 Summary of estimated percentage of energy expenditure derived from oxidation of muscle glycogen, carbohydrate sources other than muscle glycogen, and fats. Contribution of muscle glycogen was calculated from rate of decline in glycogen within vastus lateralis with assumption that a total of 10 kilograms of muscle were active and using glycogen at an average similar to that of the vastus lateralis. Total carbohydrate and fat oxidation were calculated from O_2 uptake and respiratory exchange ratio, whereas percentage of energy derived from carbohydrate other than muscle glycogen is displayed as difference between total carbohydrate oxidation and muscle glycogen oxidation. Rate of glycogen utilization averaged over 0- to 2-hour, 2- to 3-hour, and 3- to 4-hour periods of exercise are plotted at midpoint of respective periods (i.e., 1, 2.5, and 3.5 hours, respectively). CHO = carbohydrates. (Data from Coyle, E.F., A.R. Coggan, M.K. Hemmert, and J.L. Ivy. Muscle Glycogen Utilization during Prolonged Strenuous Exercise When Fed Carbohydrate. *J Appl Physiol* 61(1):165–72, 1986. Used with permission.)

work capacity. They concluded that a limiting factor for endurance capacity was "the quantity of easily available fuel" from carbohydrates.

It is not clear why carbohydrate intake during prolonged exercise did not become more widely investigated in the period following these early studies. However, in an excellent review of this topic, Coggan and Coyle (1991) note that blood glucose maintenance in humans was generally assumed to be important for central nervous system function, rather than fuel for skeletal muscle. As a result, it was believed that carbohydrate intake during exercise would only improve performance in athletes suffering from symptoms of neuroglycopenia. Studies conducted in the 1960s identified muscle glycogen as the primary source of carbohydrate fuel for prolonged exercise (Bergstrom and Hultman 1967; Corsi et al. 1969) and its significant influence on endurance performance (Bergstrom et al. 1967; Hermansen et al. 1967). However, these studies also advanced the concept that blood glucose was a negligible contributor to muscular energy demands during exercise (Coggan and Coyle 1991). It was believed that exogenous glucose was not oxidized at high rates (Costill et al. 1973), and that carbohydrate slowed the gastric emptying of fluid during exercise (Coyle et al. 1978). Thus, sports nutrition guidelines as late as the early 1980s suggested there were "limited benefits" to carbohydrate intake during exercise (without hypoglycemia), and drinks with low-carbohydrate concentrations were recommended, especially in conditions under which dehydration or hyperthermia was a concern (Costill and Miller 1980).

Since the early 1980s, the effects of carbohydrate intake during endurance exercise have been extensively investigated. It is now known that blood glucose is an important contributor to energy supplied during prolonged exercise, and that carbohydrate ingested during exercise is oxidized at relatively high rates. Thus, exogenous carbohydrate is an important supplemental fuel for exercise, as well as potentially sparing liver and muscle glycogen stores. Although it should be acknowledged that there are numerous studies indicating an absence of ergogenic effects with carbohydrate ingestion (i.e., Cole et al. 1993; Davis et al. 1988; Felig et al. 1982; Flynn et al. 1987; Millard-Stafford et al. 1990; Williams et al. 1990), many studies have shown that carbohydrate intake can improve exercise capacity and endurance performance under certain exercise conditions. Positive effects on performance have been noted most consistently during prolonged (>2 hours) exercise in cyclists (Coyle et al. 1983, 1986; Fielding et al. 1985; Mitchell et al. 1989) and runners (Millard-Stafford et al. 1992; Tsintzas, Williams, Boobis, et al. 1996). In addition, carbohydrate may improve performance in shorter (approximately one-hour) exercise protocols (Below et al. 1995; Jeukendrup et al. 1997), including those designed to simulate sports of varying intensity, such as tennis (Vergauwen et al. 1998), soccer (Ali et al. 2007; Currell et al. 2009; Ostojic and Mazic 2002), and basketball (Winnick et al. 2005).

7.2.2 Effects of Carbohydrate on Metabolism and Performance

As described, carbohydrate intake during exercise significantly alters substrate metabolism compared to exercise while fasted. Coyle and colleagues (1986) observed that declines in blood glucose during prolonged cycling at approximately 70% VO_2Max were prevented by carbohydrate consumption during exercise. With carbohydrate ingestion, oxidation was maintained at high rates throughout exercise (see Figure 7.2), and endurance capacity was 33% longer than in a placebo trial. Numerous studies have reported similar findings as well as the concept that carbohydrate intake during exercise can improve endurance by maintaining high rates of carbohydrate oxidation throughout the later stages of exercise (Coggan and Coyle 1987; Coyle et al. 1983; Jeukendrup et al. 1999; Neufer et al. 1987).

In addition to maintaining euglycemia, carbohydrate ingestion during exercise may attenuate hepatic glucose output; which may be completely suppressed with very high levels of carbohydrate ingestion (Jeukendrup et al. 1999). This could spare liver glycogen, which may be beneficial for maintaining blood glucose levels (and high rates of carbohydrate oxidation) if ingested carbohydrate is unable to sustain euglycemia late in exercise (Jeukendrup 2004).

The influence of carbohydrate intake during exercise on muscle glycogen utilization is a topic of continued debate. A majority of studies have reported no effect of carbohydrate ingestion on muscle glycogen utilization rates during exercise, especially during prolonged constant-intensity cycling (Bosch et al. 1994; Coyle et al. 1986; Flynn et al. 1987; Hargreaves and Briggs 1988; McConell et al. 2000; Mitchell et al. 1989). However, some studies have reported glycogen sparing with carbohydrate intake during running (Nicholas et al. 1999; Tsintzas et al. 1995; Tsintzas, Williams, Wilson, et al. 1996), perhaps due to a greater degree of hyperglycemia and hyperinsulinemia that may occur when carbohydrate is ingested during running (Tsintzas and Williams 1998). Glycogen sparing has also been reported during variable-intensity exercise (Nicholas et al. 1999; Yaspelkis et al. 1993). Although this could be indicative of a reduced rate of glycogen utilization when fed carbohydrate, it could also be the result of more glycogen resynthesis during the periods of low-intensity exercise in the presence of carbohydrate (Kuipers et al. 1986, 1987).

A few recent studies have challenged the prevailing view that carbohydrate ingestion does not spare muscle glycogen during continuous, moderate-intensity cycling. Stellingwerff and associates reported significant reductions in muscle glycogen utilization during the first hour of cycling (approximately 63% VO_2Max) when fed carbohydrate, resulting in significant muscle glycogen sparing in both type I and type II muscle fibers after three hours of exercise (Stellingwerff, Boon, et al. 2007). Although previous fiber-type-specific studies had reported glycogen sparing in type I fibers only (Tsintzas et al. 1995; Tsintzas, Williams, Boobis, et al. 1996), this apparent discrepancy is likely explained by longer exercise durations, which favor increased recruitment of type II muscle fibers as the type I fibers become depleted (Gollnick et al. 1974). This observation may also explain findings from De Bock and colleagues (2007), who report that carbohydrate intake spared muscle glycogen in type II muscle fibers (but not type I) following two hours of constant-load cycling at 75% VO_2Max. It is plausible that carbohydrate ingestion spared muscle glycogen in type I fibers during the early stages of exercise, but these fibers were depleted to similar levels when individuals were fasted by the end of exercise. Thus, early-exercise muscle glycogen sparing from the more heavily recruited type I fibers might have postponed additional recruitment of type II fibers, permitting greater contributions from these fibers later in exercise (De Bock et al. 2007). In summary, the scientific literature is presently equivocal regarding the effects of carbohydrate intake on muscle glycogen utilization during exercise. The considerable variations between existing studies could potentially be explained by differences in methodology (i.e., techniques used to assess muscle glycogen, use of fiber-specific glycogen analyses, time course of glycogen assessments); exercise conditions (exercise mode, duration, intensity, training status of subjects, preexercise nutrition); and the timing and amounts of carbohydrate provided during exercise. These issues require further examination to fully elucidate the effects of carbohydrate intake on muscle glycogen utilization.

7.2.3   CENTRAL EFFECTS OF CARBOHYDRATE AND PERFORMANCE

As discussed, carbohydrate intake during exercise can improve endurance performance by increasing carbohydrate availability for the later stages of prolonged exercise via increased oxidation of exogenous carbohydrate, sparing of liver or muscle glycogen stores, or possibly a combination of these effects. Carbohydrate intake has also been reported to improve performance during high-intensity endurance events (>75% VO_2Max) lasting approximately one hour (Below et al. 1995; Carter, Jeukendrup, and Jones 2004; Chambers et al. 2009; Jeukendrup et al. 1997; Rollo et al. 2009; Rollo and Williams 2010). However, ingested carbohydrate has little impact on muscle metabolism at these intensities (Jeukendrup et al. 1997; McConell et al. 2000), so performance enhancement under these conditions is probably independent of the aforementioned metabolic effects of carbohydrate.

Carbohydrate ingestion during exercise can improve psychological constructs such as perceived effort and affect (i.e., relative feelings of pleasure-displeasure) and could directly influence high-intensity performance by reducing inhibition of central motor drive to the working muscles (Backhouse et al. 2007; Backhouse et al. 2005; Davis 2000). Carter and associates examined the effects of carbohydrate intake during high-intensity cycling of approximately one hour in two related studies. In the first, cyclists received carbohydrate via intravenous infusion (thus bypassing the digestive tract) and observed no improvement in simulated 40-kilometer time trial performance (Carter, Jeukendrup, Mann, et al. 2004). In the second study, time trial performance was improved by a carbohydrate mouth rinse, which was not swallowed (Carter, Jeukendrup, and Jones 2004). These findings sparked considerable interest in this topic, and the positive effects of carbohydrate mouth rinsing have been supported by some (Chambers et al. 2009; Pottier et al. 2010; Rollo et al. 2008, 2009), but not all (Beelen et al. 2009; Rollo and Williams 2010; Whitham and McKinney 2007), subsequent studies. Particularly notable was a study by Chambers and associates (2009), who, using functional magnetic resonance imaging, determined that mouth rinsing of glucose or maltodextrin activated regions of the brain related to reward and motor control, supporting the hypothesis that stimulation of oral carbohydrate receptors may produce performance benefits via effects on the central nervous system. These findings suggest that the act of consuming regular doses of carbohydrate (i.e., at aid stations in distance running events) could hypothetically provide performance benefits, even if only small amounts are actually digested. However, it is significant that studies reporting improved performance of exercise lasting approximately one hour in duration with carbohydrate ingestion or mouth rinsing have generally performed testing in a fasted or postabsorptive state. In studies conducted following a standardized meal (two to three hours prior to exercise), no differences were observed between carbohydrate and placebo trials (Beelen et al. 2009; Rollo and Williams 2010). This finding could be related to observations that activation of certain brain regions may be reduced when carbohydrate is ingested in a postprandial state (Haase et al. 2009). Thus, further study is required to elucidate the specific conditions in which carbohydrate ingestion or mouth rinsing may be beneficial during vigorous exercise of approximately one-hour duration.

7.2.4 Carbohydrate Amount, Timing, and Type

Current guidelines from various sport/nutrition associations (American College of Sports Medicine, American Dietetic Association, Dieticians of Canada, International Society of Sports Nutrition) recommend that endurance athletes consume approximately 30 to 60 grams of carbohydrate per hour during exercise (Kreider et al. 2010; Rodriguez et al. 2009a, 2009b). Performance benefits with carbohydrate intake have been reported with as little as 16 to 22 grams of carbohydrate per hour (Fielding et al. 1985; Maughan et al. 1996), and there is surprisingly little evidence to suggest a strong dose-response effect above this amount (Flynn et al. 1987; Galloway et al. 2001; Mitchell et al. 1988, 1989). However, as described elsewhere, this may be at least partially related to difficulties assessing small differences in performance between repeated endurance trials (Jeukendrup 2004). Therefore, the recommended amounts reflect the carbohydrate intake rates utilized by a majority of studies reporting positive effects on performance. In addition, they conceptually represent levels that are high enough to influence the potential mechanisms discussed previously while promoting acceptable gastrointestinal tolerance.

A primary rationale for ingesting carbohydrate at relatively high rates is to maximize the contribution of exogenous carbohydrate to energy production during exercise. As discussed in a topical review (Jeukendrup and Jentjens 2000), oxidation of exogenous carbohydrate is initiated within 5 minutes of the initial feeding, rises throughout the first 75 to 90 minutes of exercise, and plateaus at high rates until exercise termination. It is recommended that carbohydrate feedings begin early in exercise to achieve high rates of exogenous oxidation as quickly as possible, and the total amount of ingested carbohydrate should be adequate to maintain high oxidation rates for the entire duration of exercise (Jeukendrup and Jentjens 2000). From a practical standpoint, this is most easily accomplished via regular feedings throughout exercise as large boluses of carbohydrate/fluid may be associated with gastrointestinal discomfort (Leiper 2001). Logically, this "early-and-often" timing strategy should maximize the potential sparing of both hepatic and muscle glycogen stores, as well as take full advantage of the aforementioned "central" benefits of carbohydrate ingestion, which might be more pronounced early in exercise (Rollo et al. 2008). Collectively, this may explain why McConell and colleagues (1996) observed that carbohydrate fed at regular intervals throughout exercise (but not when provided in a single late-exercise feeding) produced significant performance improvements over a placebo.

Exogenous carbohydrate utilization may be affected by a variety of factors, including the intensity of exercise and the amount, timing, and type of carbohydrate ingested (Jeukendrup 2008). Maximal oxidation rates of ingested glucose, maltodextrins (glucose polymers), sucrose, and maltose are similarly high (approximately 60 grams of carbohydrate per hour), while fructose and galactose are oxidized at considerably lower rates (approximately 30 grams of carbohydrate per hour) (Jeukendrup

2008). It is worth noting that fructose ingestion is also associated with lower blood glucose and insulin responses in comparison to glucose, as well as poorer gastrointestinal tolerance and ergogenic effectiveness (Bjorkman et al. 1984; Maughan et al. 1989; Murray et al. 1989). Thus, fructose is not considered an ideal choice as the primary source of exogenous carbohydrate during endurance exercise.

Exogenous carbohydrate oxidation rises with increasing consumption, with maximal oxidation achieved at intake rates of approximately 60 to 70 grams of carbohydrate per hour (approximately 1 gram of carbohydrate per minute). Consuming higher levels of any single form of carbohydrate does not increase exogenous oxidation and is more likely to result in gastrointestinal distress (Jeukendrup and Jentjens 2000). This provides a rationale for the upper limit of approximately 60 grams of carbohydrate per hour recommended in most current sports nutrition guidelines (Kreider et al. 2010; Rodriguez et al. 2009b).

Intestinal absorption is an important factor influencing maximal oxidation of carbohydrate as glucose transporters may become saturated at high ingestion rates (greater than one gram of carbohydrate per minute) (Jeukendrup and Jentjens 2000). However, while glucose is primarily absorbed from the intestine by the sodium-dependent glucose transporter 1 (SGT1), fructose is absorbed by a sodium-independent facilitated transport mechanism (GLUT5, glucose transporter 5) (Leiper 2001). Because they are transported by noncompetitive pathways, combining glucose (or maltodextrins) with fructose (or sucrose) may increase intestinal absorption and result in peak exogenous carbohydrate oxidation rates that are significantly higher than any single carbohydrate source. Indeed, when carbohydrate sources are combined and fed at high rates (2.4 grams of carbohydrate per minute), carbohydrate oxidation rates as high as 1.75 grams of carbohydrate per minute have been reported, as shown in Figure 7.3 (Jentjens and Jeukendrup 2005; Jentjens, Moseley, et al. 2004; Jentjens, Venables, et al. 2004; Wallis et al. 2005) (Figure 7.3).

The implications of these findings are intriguing as increased exogenous carbohydrate oxidation might influence exercise performance via previously described mechanisms. Jeukendrup and associates (2006) reported higher exogenous carbohydrate utilization when a combination of glucose (1.0 gram of glucose per minute) and fructose (0.5 grams of fructose per minute) was ingested in comparison to identical amounts of glucose ingestion (1.5 grams of glucose per minute), and this was accompanied by lower ratings of perceived exertion and higher self-selected cycling cadence in the later stages of prolonged exercise. No measures of performance were made in this study. Similarly, Rowlands and colleagues observed that adding fructose (0.5 grams of fructose per minute) to glucose (0.6 grams of glucose per minute) reduced perceptions of muscle tiredness, physical exertion, and fatigue; however, they reported no clear effect on sprint performance following two hours of cycling (Rowlands, Thorburn, et al. 2008). Currell and Jeukendrup (2008) were the first to directly observe a performance benefit with a high combination of glucose and fructose intake, using a protocol consisting of two hours of moderate-intensity cycling followed by a time trial of approximately one hour. Consumption of 1.8 grams per minute of glucose plus fructose improved power output and performance times by 8% when compared to glucose ingestion of the same amount and 19% versus a placebo trial (Currell and Jeukendrup 2008).

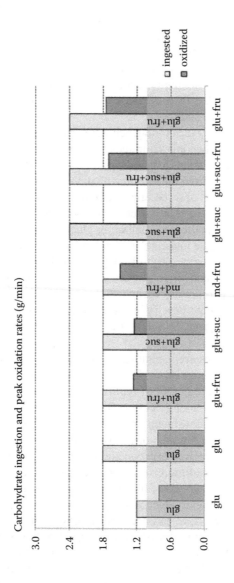

FIGURE 7.3 Oxidation of ingested carbohydrate. This figure is compiled from a number of studies investigating the oxidation of ingested carbohydrate during exercise. The bars on the left indicate the amount of carbohydrate ingested (grams of carbohydrate per minute), and the bars on the right indicate the exogenous carbohydrate oxidation rate. The shaded area shows the maximum range of oxidation rates that can be expected from a single carbohydrate with a maximum oxidation rate of about one gram of carbohydrate per minute. When multiple transportable carbohydrates are ingested at high rates, the oxidation rates can easily exceed one gram per minute, and the highest oxidation rates were found with a mixture of glucose and fructose (1.75 grams of carbohydrate per minute). fru = fructose; glu = glucose; suc = sucrose. (From Jeukendrup, A.E. Carbohydrate Feeding during Exercise. *Eur J Sport Sci* 8(2):77–86, 2008. Used with permission.)

While these findings provide initial evidence that multiple transportable carbohydrates may augment performance, a variety of practical implications of high carbohydrate intake remains that require further study. For example, most commercial sports beverages are formulated to be relatively dilute (approximately 4–8% carbohydrate), which allows them to accommodate for various physiological and psychological factors, such as prevention of dehydration, influences on gastric emptying, thirst perception, flavor, palatability, and so on (see Passe 2001 and Leiper 2001 for reviews of these issues with specific reference to sports beverages). Thus, ingesting currently recommended amounts of carbohydrate (30 to 60 grams of carbohydrate per hour) requires approximately 600 to 1,200 milliliters per hour of most sports beverages; 90 grams of carbohydrate per hour would require approximately 1,200 to more than 2,500 milliliters per hour. While these intake levels are possible in some instances (i.e., during cycling in hot conditions), they are probably not practical or desirable for many athletes. This is particularly true in runners (Lambert et al. 2008; Peters et al. 1999) and during exercise in cool temperatures, for which high fluid intakes may exceed sweat rates (Rehrer 2001). However, it was shown that high rates of ingestion of glucose plus fructose (>1.5 grams of carbohydrate per minute) from concentrated carbohydrate gels (Pfeiffer et al. 2010a) or bars (Pfeiffer et al. 2010b) produced similar exogenous oxidation rates as isocaloric beverages containing a combination of glucose and fructose. Furthermore, carbohydrate ingested in solid or semisolid forms has similar effects on performance compared to carbohydrate beverages (Hargreaves et al. 1984; Lugo et al. 1993; Murdoch et al. 1993). Thus, consuming carbohydrate gels and energy bars may be a desirable way for athletes to maximize their carbohydrate intake when high levels of fluid intake are not feasible or desirable.

A primary concern of athletes consuming large amounts of fluid or carbohydrate is the risk of gastrointestinal discomfort. Gastrointestinal problems are common during endurance sports (Jeukendrup et al. 2000; Peters, van Schelven, et al. 1993) and have been associated with carbohydrate intake during exercise (Brouns and Beckers 1993). In addition, highly concentrated carbohydrate solutions may limit gastric emptying rates (Coyle et al. 1978; Vist and Maughan 1995). However, it is possible that the utilization of multiple transportable carbohydrates may positively influence these factors. For example, ingestion of glucose plus fructose has been associated with greater "oxidation efficiency" (reflecting less carbohydrate remaining in the gastrointestinal tract) than isocaloric amounts of glucose (Jentjens, Moseley, et al. 2004; Jeukendrup et al. 2006; Rowlands, Thorburn, et al. 2008). In addition, enhanced gastric emptying and fluid delivery have been reported with glucose-plus-fructose intake (Jeukendrup and Moseley 2008). As a result, lower frequencies of severe gastrointestinal symptoms (i.e., bloating, urge to vomit) have been reported with ingestion of glucose plus fructose versus glucose alone (Jentjens, Moseley, et al. 2004), and generally good gastrointestinal tolerance has been reported with highly concentrated intakes (1.8 grams per minute) of glucose-plus-fructose gels during endurance exercise (Pfeiffer et al. 2009, 2010a).

It has been suggested that the optimal carbohydrate intake rate for endurance athletes is that which maximizes exogenous oxidation without causing gastrointestinal discomfort (Jeukendrup 2008). The previous information provides a theoretical framework regarding the physiological potential for maximizing exogenous oxidation rates. However, because individual responses to large intakes of fluid or carbohydrate appear to be highly variable, it is recommended that athletes experiment with their own maximal tolerable carbohydrate intake. Development of personal strategies requires a trial-and-error approach and must be tailored to the demands of the specific athletic endeavor (Jeukendrup 2008). Thus, individualized guidelines for a given event should logically include the consideration of a variety of factors, including

1. Exercise mode: Gastrointestinal symptoms are usually more severe in weight-bearing activities such as running versus cycling (Peters et al. 1999).
2. Exercise intensity and duration: Gastrointestinal tolerance or gastric emptying may be impaired when exercise is performed at higher intensities (Costill and Saltin 1974; Leiper 2001) or when exercise is prolonged (Jeukendrup et al. 2000; Peters et al. 1999).
3. Fluid/carbohydrate availability: Intake of fluid or carbohydrate may be limited by portability, access at aid stations, or sport-specific rules (i.e., halftime breaks in some team sports). In some instances, the specific carbohydrate sources available to the athlete may be restricted to those provided by event organizers.
4. Environmental conditions: Gastrointestinal discomfort may be more prevalent during prolonged exercise in the heat, perhaps related to hypohydration and hyperthermia (Neufer et al. 1989; Rehrer et al. 1994). In addition, more dilute carbohydrate solutions may be appropriate in hot/humid conditions to allow adequate fluid intake for rehydration, even if it does result in adequate delivery of carbohydrate.

As demonstrated, the development of specific guidelines to optimize potential physiological benefits of carbohydrate intake while managing individualized levels of gastrointestinal tolerance are complex. It is also worth noting that the gastrointestinal tract is highly adaptable, and individuals can probably alter their tolerances to fluid and carbohydrate intake (Brouns and Beckers 1993; Rehrer 2001). Thus, athletes participating in events in which high exogenous carbohydrate oxidation appears advantageous could potentially benefit from "training" themselves to increase their maximal tolerable carbohydrate intake rate (Rehrer 2001).

7.2.5 SUMMARY: CARBOHYDRATE INTAKE DURING ENDURANCE EXERCISE

Carbohydrate ingestion during endurance exercise elicits a variety of positive metabolic effects: Exogenous carbohydrate is oxidized at relatively high rates, euglycemia is maintained, and liver or muscle glycogen stores can potentially be spared. Carbohydrate intake may also attenuate central fatigue during exercise. Thus, there is a strong rationale for ingesting carbohydrate to enhance endurance performance during activities of approximately one hour or longer. Guidelines from most sports nutrition groups recommend 30 to 60 grams of carbohydrate per hour, primarily from carbohydrate sources that are oxidized at high rates (i.e., glucose, maltodextrins, etc.). Recent evidence suggests that adding fructose or sucrose to glucose/maltodextrins will increase peak exogenous carbohydrate utilization and oxidation efficiency beyond that of individual carbohydrate sources, which may have positive implications for gastrointestinal tolerance and performance. Specific recommendations for carbohydrate intake must be tailored to the specific demands or conditions of the event and the personal tolerances of the individual athlete.

7.3 FAT INTAKE DURING ENDURANCE EXERCISE

The ability of macronutrient intake to modify energy-yielding substrate utilization and physical performance is fundamental to endurance exercise and sport (Christensen and Hanson 1939; Krogh and Lindhard 1920; Zuntz and Loeb 1894). Carbohydrates have been emphasized in this context, and deservedly so. As described in this chapter, endogenous carbohydrates are quantitatively finite, and gluconeogenesis alone is unable to provide enough glucose for heavily working skeletal muscle. Fatigue during prolonged exercise is commonly associated with a diminished quantity of muscle and liver glycogen (Bergstrom et al. 1967; Hermansen et al. 1967) and in some instances hypoglycemia. For these reasons, carbohydrate intake during exercise is recommended as a means to enhance carbohydrate availability as well as to conserve endogenous carbohydrate stores.

The potential advantage of fat ingestion during exercise is less conspicuous than those of carbohydrates because the energy potential of fat stores (Horowitz and Klein 2000) far exceeds the energetic demand imposed by any endurance activity (Westerterp et al. 1986). However, fat feedings both prior to and during endurance exercise have been shown to promote fat oxidation (Costill et al. 1977; Vukovich et al. 1993). Due to the finite capacity of endogenous carbohydrates and the biological limits of exogenous carbohydrate oxidation, the notion that nutritional manipulation could preserve carbohydrates by replacing them with energy from fat is attractive. This is of keen interest to endurance athletes, as carbohydrate sparing could theoretically improve performance, as described previously. Unfortunately, fat ingestion during exercise is associated with gastrointestinal discomfort (Angus et al. 2000; Goedecke et al. 2005; Jeukendrup et al. 1998). Moreover, there is little evidence to support the performance benefits of fat supplementation during exercise.

7.3.1 Metabolic and Performance Implications of Fat Intake

Respiratory exchange data indicate that fat is increasingly relied on for adenosine triphosphate (ATP) formation as fixed-intensity exercise progresses in duration, with decreasing contributions from carbohydrates (Romijn et al. 1993). Further, a core adaptation to repeated bouts of endurance exercise is the improved ability to mobilize and oxidize fat, again diminishing the reliance on carbohydrates (Holloszy 1973). Thus, carbohydrate and fat metabolism are intimately interdependent, a concept proposed by Randle et al. in 1963. The influences of fat-promoting interventions on carbohydrate metabolism during exercise were initially studied in the 1970s. In a key investigation, rats were tube-fed corn oil, injected with heparin to further stimulate lipolysis, and then exercised for 30 minutes (Rennie et al. 1976). The authors elicited high free fatty acid levels and found that rats that were fed fat had a greater abundance of muscle and liver glycogen following exercise relative to a control group. The same research group subsequently showed that rats with elevated free fatty acids and slower rates of glycogen use (elicited via a similar protocol) were able to run approximately one hour longer than control rats (Hickson et al. 1977). Initial research in humans reported similar physiological responses to the aforementioned rat studies. Skeletal muscle glycogen use was reduced 40% during 30 minutes of running exercise preceded by a high-fat feeding (approximately five hours prior to exercise) and heparin infusion (Costill et al. 1977). However, the external validity of these results is limited as heparin infusion is not a feasible practice for athletes. Under more practical conditions (no heparin and smaller dose of fat), fat feedings appear to stimulate a less-marked metabolic response (Massicotte et al. 1992).

Endurance exercise affords the opportunity to ingest multiple, relatively small doses of fat over a prolonged period of time. Thus, it may be hypothetically possible for athletes to adequately consume high enough amounts of fat to promote an ergogenic response regarding alterations in substrate metabolism. However, most conventional sources of triglycerides are comprised of long-chain (≥14 carbons) fatty acids. Long-chain fatty acids and their incorporation into triglycerides are characterized by relatively slow oxidation rates following ingestion due to their reassembly into chylomicrons and subsequent transport to systemic circulation via the lymphatic system (Binnert et al. 1996). Thus, temporal limitations prevent long-chain triglycerides from playing a significant role in energy metabolism during typical endurance exercise (<4 hours). Conversely, medium-chain (eight to ten carbons) triglycerides are readily available for oxidative metabolism due to rapid entry into the portal circulation and carnitine–independent transportability into mitochondria (Bach and Babayan 1982; Decombaz et al. 1983). Therefore, the most promising and practical strategy to improve performance with a fat-promoting intervention is to provide multiple doses of medium-chain triglycerides throughout endurance exercise.

Since the mid-1990s, at least nine separate investigations have studied fuel metabolism and exercise performance in response to "fat" feedings during exercise (Angus et al. 2000; Goedecke et al. 2005; Jeukendrup et al. 1995, 1996, 1998; Thorburn et al. 2006, 2007; Van Zyl et al. 1996; Vistisen et al. 2003). Jeukendrup et al. (1995) examined metabolic influences of ingesting relatively small amounts of medium-chain triglycerides (ten grams per hour) during three hours of cycling, in isolation and in combination with carbohydrates. Performance was not assessed, but approximately 75% of exogenous medium-chain triglycerides were oxidized in the second hour of exercise when coingested with carbohydrates (approximately 7% of the total energy expended during exercise), compared to only 33% when taken alone. However, medium-chain triglycerides were oxidized in the place of endogenous fat, rather than endogenous carbohydrates. This finding was confirmed in a subsequent study by the same authors, who concluded that approximately 10 grams per hour of medium-chain triglyceride ingestion were an inadequate stimulus to alter whole-body substrate utilization patterns (Jeukendrup et al. 1996).

Van Zyl and colleagues (1996) examined the effects of such higher doses of medium-chain triglycerides ingested during exercise. Medium-chain triglycerides were provided in an 85-gram dose (three times the previously reported maximum tolerable dose) and were administered during two hours of fixed-intensity cycling and a subsequent 40-kilometer time trial. Endogenous carbohydrate utilization was reduced, and 40-kilometer time trial performance was enhanced by 3%. The authors cited carbohydrate sparing as the probable mechanism for the gains observed with medium-chain triglyceride plus carbohydrate. Although gastrointestinal comfort was not monitored, the performance results imply that any discomfort that may have been experienced during the trials were inconsequential. At least three comparable examinations have attempted to replicate the performance results of Van Zyl et al. with a medium-chain triglyceride dose of at least 85 grams (along with carbohydrates). Performance measures included a high-intensity time trial (Jeukendrup et al. 1998), a 4.5-hour ultraendurance session with intermittent sprints followed by a 200-kilojoule time trial (Goedecke et al. 2005), and a simulated 100-kilometer time trial (Angus et al. 2000). In each of these instances, performance was unaltered, and moderate-to-severe gastrointestinal discomfort was reported. Because gastrointestinal distress may interfere with performance gains in response to large doses of fat, efforts have been made to devise formulas that enhance nutrient delivery while easing gastrointestinal strain, such as specifically structured triglycerides (long-chain plus medium-chain hybrid triglycerides) (Vistisen et al. 2003) and fat adaptation interventions (Thorburn et al., 2006, 2007). However, even those that have successfully reduced gastrointestinal distress failed to replicate the performance gains documented by Van Zyl et al. (Thorburn et al. 2006).

7.3.2 SUMMARY: FAT INTAKE DURING ENDURANCE EXERCISE

Early animal and human data obtained using fat and heparin infusions yielded exciting preliminary results regarding fat ingestion and performance. However, fat-feeding studies conducted under more practical conditions have consistently caused gastrointestinal discomfort and have failed to generate reliable performance benefits. At this point, the collective literature cautions against ingesting fat (or one of its derivatives) during exercise. A better understanding of individual differences in tolerance, the influence of preexercise diet, and the possible usefulness of fat and carbohydrate coingestion during ultraendurance exercise are required to determine if this recommendation should be generalized to all endurance athletes and settings.

7.4 PROTEIN/AMINO ACID INTAKE DURING ENDURANCE EXERCISE

Proteins and their amino acid constituents are used in a variety of metabolic and biochemical processes at rest and during exercise, including full oxidation to carbon dioxide for ATP resynthesis, Krebs cycle anaplerosis, and gluconeogenesis, among others (Dohm 1986). Nutritional considerations during exercise naturally revolve around energy provision due to the marked rise in the demand for ATP during skeletal muscle work. Appreciation for protein as an energy-yielding molecule has changed considerably 150 years ago. The classic viewpoint, largely propagated by von Liebig (1840), was that protein is the primary fuel for contracting skeletal muscle. That position was maintained until Fick and Wislicenus (1866) performed a paradigm-shifting experiment in which they measured urinary nitrogen during and following a mountain ascent lasting more than eight hours. Based on estimates of work and mechanical efficiency, their nitrogen computations led others to conclude that "the best materials for the production, both of internal and external work, are non-nitrogenous material" (Frankland (1866) as discussed by Carpenter et al. (1997)). Remarkably, our current understanding of amino acid oxidation during exercise does not substantially deviate from the perspective of Fick and Wislicenus. It is generally agreed that amino acids play a relatively small role in energy metabolism; estimates range from less than 5–10%), or slightly more in conditions of diminishing carbohydrate reserves (e.g., prolonged exercise) (Lemon and Mullin 1980; Rennie et al. 2006). Due to the small absolute quantity of amino acids used during exercise and our ability to at least partially replenish the free amino acid pool (intra- and extracellular) through the catabolism of intact proteins and de novo amino acid synthesis (Dohm 1986), acute exercise even of extended duration does not appear to alter whole-body protein/nitrogen balance on a scale that would necessitate protein consumption. As such, research into the potential benefits of amino acid/protein ingestion during endurance exercise was virtually nonexistent until the early 1990s.

7.4.1 BRANCHED-CHAIN AMINO ACIDS

Newsholme and colleagues were among the first to suggest that amino acid or protein taken *during* exercise may be of ergogenic value (Blomstrand, Hassmen, Ekblom, et al. 1991). Their rationale for conducting human-based performance studies was not related to the aforementioned aspects of energy metabolism; rather, they were based on reports that central nervous system fatigue may develop from a tryptophan-induced increase in brain 5-hydroxytryptamine, a substance known to induce drowsiness and fatigue (Young 1986). The ratio of free tryptophan:BCAAs (branched-chain amino acids; leucine, isoleucine, and valine) may influence the rate of tryptophan transport across the blood-brain barrier due to competitive transport mechanisms. High tryptophan:BCAA ratios can occur during prolonged exercise due to decreasing BCAA levels (presumably from their oxidation) and an increase in free tryptophan, caused by elevated free fatty acids displacing albumin-bound tryptophan (Blomstrand et al. 1988). The investigators tested the hypothesis that BCAA provision would alter this ratio in a manner advantageous to performance and found that BCAAs conferred benefits to "slower," but not "faster," Stockholm Marathon participants (Blomstrand, Hassmen, Ekblom, et al. 1991). They speculated that faster runners may be more resistant to central and peripheral fatigue, making them less likely to benefit from amino acids. Notwithstanding the design limitations inherent in using a marathon model, the results were intriguing.

Blomstrand et al. (1997) later examined the physiological and ergogenic effects of adding seven grams of BCAA to a carbohydrate beverage during 60 minutes of cycling followed by a 20-minute performance session. Subjects performed more work in the carbohydrate and carbohydrate-BCAA trials compared to a placebo trial, with no distinction between the two carbohydrate trials. These results, along with similar findings from other investigators utilizing longer-duration performance protocols (>2 hours), refute the notion that BCAA ingestion can alleviate central fatigue, even when the tryptophan:BCAA ratio is maintained (Madsen et al. 1996; van Hall et al. 1995; Watson et al. 2004). Furthermore, amino acid ingestion may result in elevated levels of ammonia (MacLean and Graham 1993; MacLean et al. 1994), which has been implicated as a source of fatigue (Banister and Cameron 1990; Nybo et al. 2005; Secher et al. 2008).

7.4.2 INDIVIDUAL AMINO ACIDS

Individual amino acids such as tyrosine and alanine have also been tested for their effects on metabolism and endurance performance (Chinevere et al. 2002; Klein et al. 2009), although few studies have been completed to date. Tyrosine is the amino acid precursor for the excitatory substance dopamine, and tyrosine provision has been shown to increase brain dopamine levels in rats (Chaouloff et al. 1987). However, Chinevere et al. (2002) found that aliquots of tyrosine ingested during 90 minutes of cycling had no impact on time trial performance compared to placebo, carbohydrate-only, or carbohydrate-plus-tyrosine treatments. Alanine has also been investigated for its potential ergogenic properties, primarily because of its availability as an energy substrate for skeletal muscle and its role as a gluconeogenic precursor. Korach-Andre et al. (2002) reported that 68% of exogenous alanine (51 of 73 grams) was decarboxylated during three hours of cycling, which accounted for 10% of total energy expenditure, in addition to the approximately 5% derived from endogenous protein sources. Despite the extent to which exogenous alanine may be utilized, 75 grams of alanine delivered before and during 45 minutes of cycling did not influence performance during a subsequent 15-minute performance trial (Klein et al. 2009). However, the 60-minute protocol was probably too brief to detect performance differences that would emanate from modifications to energy substrate metabolism. Similar rates of alanine ingestion have not been investigated during protocols of longer duration.

7.4.3 INTACT PROTEINS AND PROTEIN HYDROLYSATES

Scientists did not directly examine the performance-related influences of adding protein to conventional carbohydrate supplements until recently (Ivy et al. 2003). At least 10 investigations have since examined the performance effects of coingesting carbohydrate and protein during prolonged exercise (>1 hour) (Breen et al. 2010; Ivy et al. 2003; Martinez-Lagunas et al. 2010; Osterberg et al. 2008; Romano-Ely et al. 2006; Saunders et al. 2004, 2007, 2009; Valentine et al. 2008; van Essen and Gibala 2006). Some of these studies have reported ergogenic effects from the inclusion of protein (Ivy et al. 2003; Saunders et al. 2004, 2007, 2009), while others have reported no discernable differences in performance between carbohydrate and carbohydrate plus protein (Breen et al. 2010; Martinez-Lagunas et al. 2010; Osterberg et al. 2008; Romano-Ely et al. 2006; Valentine et al. 2008; van Essen and Gibala 2006).

The discrepant findings among these studies may be related, at least partially, to differences in carbohydrate doses. In studies that administered carbohydrates at levels below those that elicit maximum exogenous carbohydrate oxidation rates, the addition of protein to matched-carbohydrate formulas (37 to 47 grams of carbohydrate per hour) extended time to exhaustion by 13–37% (Ivy et al. 2003; Saunders et al. 2004, 2007). Similar time-to-exhaustion outcomes have been reported in studies in which some carbohydrate calories were replaced isocalorically with protein (Romano-Ely et al. 2006) or when carbohydrate plus protein provided slightly fewer calories than carbohydrate (Martinez-Lagunas et al. 2010). Although improved "endurance" is of obvious interest to endurance athletes, fatigue resistance does not necessarily translate to proportional improvements in time trial performance, a measure of greater external validity. Surprisingly, the effects of adding protein calories to moderate doses of carbohydrate during time trial performances have yet to be examined. Nonetheless, protein added to moderate doses of carbohydrate may provide some ergogenic effects for endurance athletes, and protein substituted for carbohydrate calories may "replace" ergogenic effects potentially provided by additional carbohydrate calories. However, it is not possible from these studies to determine if protein provides a calorically independent benefit versus carbohydrate.

When studies have compared carbohydrate and carbohydrate-plus-protein beverages delivered at rates of approximately 60 grams of carbohydrate per hour or greater, most investigators have reported no differences in time trial performance (Breen et al. 2010; Osterberg et al. 2008; van Essen and Gibala 2006) or cycling endurance (Valentine et al. 2008), although one study reported a 3% improvement in late-exercise performance with carbohydrate plus protein (Saunders et al. 2009). In addition, one recent study reported a small (<1%) decrement in performance with carbohydrate-plus-protein feedings (approximately 66 grams of carbohydrate plus 18 grams of protein per hour) during high-intensity exercise (six-kilometer time trial following 45 minutes of variable-intensity cycling) (Toone and Betts 2010). However, this study may not be directly comparable to other investigations due to potentially different metabolic responses and gastrointestinal tolerances to carbohydrate-plus-protein ingestion at such high exercise intensities. Thus, the prevailing view at present is that coingestion of carbohydrate and protein does not confer ergogenic effects beyond the maximal benefits obtained when carbohydrate is provided at rates that elicit maximal exogenous oxidation.

A limitation in the literature on this topic is the lack of mechanistic evidence to explain reported protein-related improvements in endurance performance. The original rationale for experimenting with protein during prolonged exercise was that protein may potentiate the insulin response to carbohydrate ingestion (Ivy et al. 2003), similar to what had been shown at rest (Spiller et al. 1987; van Loon, Saris, Verhagen, et al. 2000). Elevated insulin could theoretically shift carbohydrate reliance away from glycogen, thereby delaying the onset of fatigue. However, carbohydrate-plus-protein ingestion has been shown to increase time to fatigue by 37%, without significant changes in insulin responses compared to carbohydrate (Ivy et al. 2003). Other candidate mechanisms could hypothetically include influences on protein oxidation (glycogen sparing) (Colombani et al. 1999; Koopman et al. 2004), Krebs cycle anaplerosis (Wagenmakers et al. 1990), and central fatigue (Blomstrand, Hassmen, Ekblom, et al. 1991; Blomstrand, Hassmen, and Newsholme 1991). However, none of these potential mechanisms has been directly examined in studies reporting improved performance with protein. In addition, the effect of ingestion of carbohydrate plus protein during exercise on muscle metabolism was examined during 90 minutes of cycling at 70% VO_2Max. Ingestion of carbohydrate plus protein produced no detectable differences versus a carbohydrate-only beverage in absolute muscle glycogen utilization or the concentration of Krebs cycle intermediates (citrate and malate) (Cermak et al. 2009), providing evidence against these potential mechanisms. Presently, no studies have provided an adequate mechanistic explanation for performance benefits with carbohydrate plus protein, and further investigation is required to establish the specific role of protein ingestion on endurance exercise metabolism and performance.

7.4.4 SUMMARY: INGESTION OF PROTEIN/AMINO ACIDS DURING ENDURANCE EXERCISE

As described previously, carbohydrate is a critical component of sports formulas designed to promote endurance performance. There also appears to be evidence to support the coingestion of carbohydrate and protein, especially when protein is added to moderate doses of carbohydrate. However, there remain too many unanswered questions to provide comprehensive recommendations regarding the consumption of protein during endurance exercise. Most notably, a majority of studies indicate that protein does not promote ergogenic effects that are greater than maximal benefits derived from high-carbohydrate doses. If subsequent investigations support the prevailing view that ingestion of carbohydrate plus protein provides equal performance benefits versus optimal carbohydrate doses, additional functional benefits must be more clearly established to widely recommend that endurance athletes replace small amounts of carbohydrate calories with protein. There is minimal evidence at present to suggest performance detriments from this approach during prolonged exercise; however, the addition of protein could potentially aid in the recovery process following heavy exercise. For example, numerous studies have reported that ingestion of carbohydrate plus protein *following* exercise improves indicators of postexercise recovery, such as enhanced performance in subsequent exercise, as shown in some (Berardi et al. 2008; Rowlands, Rossler, et al. 2008), but not all, investigations (Berardi et al. 2006; Betts et al. 2005; Millard-Stafford et al. 2005). Few studies have examined the effects of ingestion of carbohydrate plus protein consumed only *during exercise* on postexercise recovery (Breen et al. 2010; Valentine et al. 2008). Valentine et al. reported that postexercise markers of sarcolemmal disruption (myoglobin and creatine kinase) were reduced and muscle function (leg extension repetitions) improved with carbohydrate plus protein, compared to isocaloric and isocarbohydrate beverages. However, Breen and colleagues observed no significant influences of carbohydrate plus protein on similar markers of postexercise recovery versus carbohydrate.

Although more evidence regarding efficacy and physiological mechanisms is required before broad recommendations can be provided, it is our position that there are potential benefits to consuming carbohydrate plus protein during endurance exercise and minimal potential disadvantages to this approach. Logically, athletic endeavors that combine the demands of high levels of performance and rapid recovery may benefit the most from ingestion of carbohydrate plus protein, but further evidence is required to support this concept. As discussed previously, development of strategies for nutrient intake during exercise requires a trial-and-error approach and must be tailored to the individual athlete and the specific demands of the athletic endeavor. Individual athletes should therefore test the efficacy of protein intake in this approach.

8 Postexercise Nutrient Timing in Endurance Activity

Kyle Sunderland and Chad M. Kerksick

CONTENTS

8.1 INTRODUCTION

The recovery process following endurance activity is heavily dependent on restoration of glycogen stores. Rapid recovery of glycogen stores is essential to those athletes participating in multiple activities within a 24-hour time period (i.e., swimming, track and field, tournament-style play for basketball/soccer, etc.). Many factors exist that determine the rate of glycogen synthesis following endurance activity, such as the level of glycogen depletion that occurred during exercise, the time frame of carbohydrate ingestion, amount of carbohydrate ingested, and the type of carbohydrate ingested. Research has also discussed the idea of combining carbohydrate intake with protein to maximize glycogen stores and synthesis rate. Even more recently, caffeine has been introduced as a possible supplement to synergistically act with carbohydrate to aid in glycogen synthesis rates, while other nutrients exist that may provide additional benefit. Following endurance activity is the altered state of immune function whereby the body is susceptible to various types of infections. For this reason, other micronutrients have been suggested to protect the body following endurance activity to bolster the immune function of the body.

8.2 POSTEXERCISE GLYCOGEN SYNTHESIS

In an effort to equate all muscle glycogen concentrations across all studies discussed throughout this chapter, muscle glycogen concentrations are reported in millimoles of glucosyl units per kilogram of dry muscle weight (mmol/kg dry weight) unless otherwise stated. Therefore, muscle glycogen concentrations in studies that reported muscle glycogen content in millimoles glucosyl units/kilogram wet weight were multiplied by 4.28 to account for the water weight of the muscle (van Hall et al. 2000). Note the relevance as units presented in Chapter 6 utilized the wet weight calculations. Resting muscle glycogen levels are typically in excess of 500 millimoles/kilogram dry weight (Sherman et al. 1981). Exhaustive endurance activity can decrease glycogen levels to less than 30 millimoles/kilogram dry weight (Casey et al. 1995). Postexercise synthesis rates can range from 5 to 50 millimoles/kilogram dry weight/hour depending on factors that are discussed further in this section. These rates mean that it can take as little as 5 hours and as long as 40 hours to replenish most of the muscle glycogen stores following exhaustive endurance activity. This divergent range of recovery time elucidates the importance of the appropriate nutritional intake and timing central to the purpose of this chapter.

Glycogen synthesis occurs in two phases: a rapid and a slow phase. The rapid phase occurs in the first 60 minutes of recovery and occurs without the presence of insulin; therefore, it is termed the insulin-independent phase. This phase is characterized by an increase in translocation of glucose transporters to the plasma membrane of the muscle. This rapid phase is said to occur only if glycogen is sufficiently depleted by exercise (<50 millimoles/kilogram dry weight) and carbohydrate is consumed immediately following cessation of exercise. A possible mechanism for the rapid phase of glycogen synthesis is the increased activity of glycogen synthase following exercise. In this respect, when muscle glycogen levels are diminished, such as following strenuous endurance activities, glycogen synthase activity has been shown to increase (Price et al. 2000). In fact it has been suggested that glycogen depletion may be a more potent stimulator of glycogen synthase than insulin or muscle contraction (Nielsen et al. 2001). The slow phase of glycogen synthesis is characterized by a marked increase in insulin sensitivity inside the muscle. Studies have suggested the exercise-induced increases in insulin sensitivity of the muscle can last upward of 48 hours postexercise (Cartee et al. 1989). It is not known exactly the mechanism for this increase in muscle insulin sensitivity, although it may come from a combination of glycogen concentration, serum factor(s), adenosine monophosphate (AMP)-activated protein kinase (AMPK) and insulin-signaling molecules (Jentjens and Jeukendrup 2003).

8.2.1 CARBOHYDRATES

While the molecular mechanisms linking carbohydrate availability with increases in intramuscular insulin sensitivity with or without exercise need additional understanding, processes associated with restoration of muscle and liver glycogen stores, replacement of fluid and electrolytes lost in sweat, protein synthesis for repair and adaptation, and responses of the immune and antioxidant systems to help the athlete stay healthy are better understood. Many of these processes are highly dependent on the provision of nutrients in the hours after an exercise bout.

To enhance the rate of recovery, athletes are advised to consume carbohydrate as soon as possible after the completion of a workout or event. There is a potential for higher rates of muscle glycogen storage during the first two to four hours after exercise, but even in the face of carbohydrate intake, the rate and extent of glycogen recovery decline after two to four hours (Ivy, Katz, et al. 1988). In fact, it was primarily this finding that is attributed by many to be the genesis of nutrient timing and created the idea of a "window of opportunity" for glycogen storage during the early period of postexercise recovery. This study found that when carbohydrate ingestion was delayed by just two hours, the rate of glycogen synthesis decreased by approximately 50% (Figure 8.1) (Ivy, Katz, et al. 1988). However, it has been suggested that the true value of postexercise carbohydrate intake comes more from the provision of a substrate that promotes recovery of lost muscle and liver glycogen rather than a few hours of moderately enhanced glycogen synthesis (Burke et al. 2004). The outcome of delaying carbohydrate intake means that there will be very low rates of glycogen restoration until feeding occurs. Any delay is important when there are only four to eight hours between exercise sessions, but it may have less impact over a longer recovery period, as long as sufficient carbohydrate is consumed (Burke et al. 2004). Evidence suggests that maximal glycogen storage during the first four hours after exercise can readily be achieved by a pattern of small but frequent meals that provide a total carbohydrate intake of approximately 1 gram of carbohydrate per kilogram of body mass per hour (likely 70 to 85 grams of carbohydrate per hour) (Burke et al. 2004).

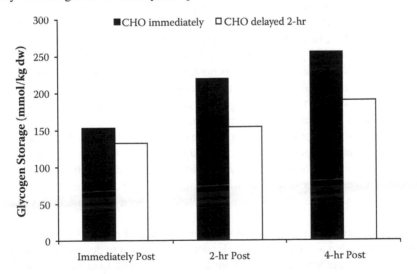

FIGURE 8.1 Glycogen storage following exhaustive exercise with carbohydrate ingestion immediately post (filled bars) or after two hours of rest (open bars). CHO = carbohydrate. (Adapted from Ivy, J.L., A.L. Katz, C.L. Cutler, W.M. Sherman, and E.F. Coyle. Muscle Glycogen Synthesis after Exercise: Effect of Time of Carbohydrate Ingestion. *J Appl Physiol* 64(4):1480–85, 1988.)

It should be noted, however, that athletes who need to recover quickly from endurance exercise must ask themselves which macronutrient will promote their fastest recovery. The rate of glycogen storage by the muscle when carbohydrate is provided following exercise has been found to be between 20 and 50 millimoles/kilogram of dry muscle weight per hour; however, when carbohydrate is not provided, the rate of storage is decreased to 7 to 12 millimoles/kilogram of dry muscle weight per hour. In 1981, Costill et al. were the first to investigate the role of dietary carbohydrate in recovery from exercise and how it impacts the recovery of glycogen. They reported that a high-carbohydrate diet (70% carbohydrate) following exhaustive exercise caused a greater increase in muscle glycogen stores 24 hours postexercise than a low-carbohydrate diet (20% carbohydrate) or a "mixed-carbohydrate" diet (50% carbohydrate). For example, the high-carbohydrate diet condition increased muscle glycogen by 127%, while the mixed-carbohydrate diet caused a 50% increase, but the low-carbohydrate diet only increased muscle glycogen by 6% when measured again 24 hours after exercise (Costill et al. 1981). As a result, the importance of delivering high levels of carbohydrate after stressful exercise (including prolonged, moderate-intensity, and shorter, more intense exercise) is critically important to ensure optimal recovery of glycogen stores. In 1988, the same laboratory studied the effects of following a low-carbohydrate diet that provided carbohydrate in an amount equivalent to 50% of their estimated exercise energy expenditure or a diet that matched carbohydrate intake with exercise energy expenditure for several days in highly trained runners. While both diets were being consumed, changes in muscle glycogen content, running economy, and ratings of perceived exertion were measured (Kirwan et al. 1988). Muscle glycogen content was higher at all measured points when more carbohydrate was ingested in the diet. In addition and after only three days, running economy decreased when running at both low and high intensities (Kirwan et al. 1988). Finally, Parkin et al. (1997) reported that delaying carbohydrate intake (1.75 grams of carbohydrate per kilogram of body mass per hour) by 2 hours had no effect on muscle glycogen stores 8 or 24 hours postexercise when compared to immediately taking carbohydrate following exercise. While these findings seemingly refute the other study previously mentioned regarding the timing of carbohydrate, the amount of carbohydrate ingested was much different.

As a result, these studies show that as long as adequate carbohydrate is consumed, muscle glycogen is replenished effectively and can even be increased above baseline levels within 24 hours. If, however, rapid replenishment of glycogen is needed, immediate ingestion (or at least within two hours) of carbohydrate is recommended to maximally stimulate replenishment of muscle glycogen (Figure 8.1) (Ivy, Katz, et al. 1988).

As can be seen, the need for carbohydrate is evident if recovery of muscle glycogen is required, but a number of investigations have sought to determine exactly how much carbohydrate was required. Blom et al. (1987) examined the effects of consuming three different amounts of glucose on glycogen synthesis following exhaustive interval cycling. The subjects ingested 0.18 (low dose), 0.35 (moderate dose), or 0.70 (high dose) grams of glucose per kilogram of body mass per hour after exercise. The glycogen synthesis rate for the low-glucose group was approximately nine millimoles/kilogram of dry muscle weight per hour. The rate of glycogen resynthesis was more than doubled (approximately 25 millimoles/kilogram of dry muscle weight per hour) when a moderate amount of glucose was provided; the high dose of glucose did not stimulate any further increase in the rate of glycogen resynthesis. These findings led the authors to hypothesize that there is a "leveling off" effect of glycogen resynthesis at a carbohydrate intake somewhere between 0.35 and 0.70 grams of carbohydrate per kilogram of body mass per hour. An additional study reported similar outcomes after carbohydrate intakes between 0.75 and 1.50 grams of carbohydrate per kilogram of body mass per hour found similar rates (approximately 22 millimoles/kilogram of dry muscle weight per hour) of glycogen synthesis (Ivy, Lee, et al. 1988). Finally, van Loon et al. (van Loon, Saris, Kruijshoop, et al. 2000) reported that ingestion of 1.2 grams of carbohydrate per kilogram of body mass per hour (typically 85 to 100 grams of carbohydrate per hour) resulted in glycogen synthesis rates of approximately 45 millimoles/kilogram of dry muscle weight per hour, an exceptionally fast rate of glycogen resynthesis. In accordance, other studies have supported this outcome that aggressive and rapid regimens of carbohydrate intake (more than one gram of carbohydrate per kilogram of body mass per hour) result in exceptionally high rates of glycogen resynthesis (Hickner et al. 1997; van Hall et al. 2000). As a result, it seems prudent to suggest that a carbohydrate intake of at least one gram of carbohydrate per kilogram of body mass per hour is needed to ensure maximal rates of glycogen synthesis.

In addition to the timing, amount, and frequency of carbohydrate intake, the type of carbohydrate ingested has been suggested to have an impact on recovery of glycogen stores. Blom et al. (1987) were among the first to establish that fructose, a low-glycemic carbohydrate, when ingested postexercise does not replenish glycogen stores as effectively as glucose or sucrose, both high-glycemic forms of carbohydrate. In 1993, Burke et al. (1993) studied the effects of glycemic index on muscle glycogen levels 24 hours after a bout of glycogen-depleting exercise. A key, practical consideration for this research study was that prior to this study, no study had utilized meals consisting of either high-glycemic or low-glycemic carbohydrates and instead had focused on studying single-carbohydrate sources of varying glycemic indexes, such as fructose, glucose, sucrose, and the like. The authors reported that when subjects consumed meals with a high glycemic index, significantly greater glycogen storage 24 hours following exhaustive exercise occurred in comparison to when meals with a low glycemic index were consumed. It is therefore suggested that following endurance activity a beverage or meal containing glucose or sucrose (or some form of carbohydrate with a high glycemic index that also comprises the majority of carbohydrates found within the food source) is preferential over carbohydrate sources with a low glycemic index (such as fructose) to adequately replenish glycogen stores.

Last, additional studies have investigated the impact of ingesting different forms of carbohydrate. On a first look, liquid forms of carbohydrate are known to empty from the stomach at a quicker rate when compared to solid forms of carbohydrate (Rehrer et al. 1994). Keizer and colleagues (1987) initially reported similar glycogen synthesis rates between liquid and solid forms of carbohydrate (24.8 and 24.6 millimoles/kilogram of dry muscle weight per hour, respectively). Careful interpretation of these data should be considered as the solid meal actually contained greater amounts of carbohydrate than the liquid meal, in addition to other differences in the composition of meals in this study, which likely confounded their results.

In light of this, Reed et al. (1989) performed a more controlled study in which subjects ingested 0.75 grams of carbohydrate per kilogram of body mass per hour in either liquid or solid form immediately following and two hours after exercise. They concluded that glycogen synthesis rates were similar between the liquid (21.8 millimoles of glycogen per kilogram of dry muscle weight per hour) and solid forms (23.5 millimoles of glycogen per kilogram of dry muscle weight per hour) of carbohydrate.

Another important factor to consider is the impact of gastric emptying and how this could affect glycogen synthesis and performance. To address this point, the authors (Reed et al. 1989) also included a group of subjects who received a glucose infusion. When glucose was infused (0.75 grams of glucose per kilogram of body mass per hour), the glycogen synthesis rate was 24.0 millimoles/kilogram of dry muscle weight per hour, which was not different from glycogen synthesis rates when either solid or liquid forms of carbohydrate were ingested (Reed et al. 1989). Therefore, the authors determined that gastric emptying rates of carbohydrate did not hinder glycogen storage postexercise. Consequently, it seems that the form of carbohydrate (solid or liquid) or the gastric emptying ability of the carbohydrate do not have an impact on the ability of muscle to replenish lost muscle glycogen during the postexercise period.

In summary, carbohydrate is a critical fuel substrate that drives the resynthesis of glycogen after exercise. In most scenarios, athletes do not have an immediate need to recover, and in these situations, maximal recovery is easily achieved with an adequate amount of carbohydrate (more than eight grams of carbohydrate per kilogram of body mass per day) in the diet, irrespective of the timing with which these nutrients are ingested. However, when athletes have an immediate need to recover, optimal timing can facilitate faster (and thus more complete) recovery of muscle glycogen. In these scenarios, athletes are recommended to ingest 1.2 to 1.5 grams of carbohydrate per kilogram of body mass per hour immediately after exercise and again at least every hour for four to six hours after exercise.

8.2.2 CARBOHYDRATES AND PROTEIN

Lately, the concept of adding protein to carbohydrate feedings following endurance exercise to increase glycogen synthesis has garnered interest. The physiological mechanism behind this approach involves the ability of certain proteins and amino acids to increase plasma insulin levels above those of carbohydrate alone. For example, Zawadzki et al. (1992) were the first to investigate the effects of adding protein to a carbohydrate supplement following exercise. Immediately and two hours following a two-hour exercise bout, subjects ingested (1) 112 grams of carbohydrate, (2) 40.7 grams of protein, or (3) the combination of carbohydrate and protein. When provided in combination, glycogen synthesis rates were 38% greater than those achieved with carbohydrate alone. While seemingly impressive results, it was impossible to determine if the greater rate of glycogen resynthesis was due to the added protein or if they were a result of greater energy availability because no isocaloric dose of carbohydrate was compared to the combined carbohydrate and protein group, a key limitation of interpreting the outcomes of this study. A later study by Ivy et al. (2002), however, supported the initial findings of Zawadzki et al. using an isocaloric carbohydrate group. In this study, protein addition (0.37 grams of protein per kilogram of body mass) to carbohydrate (1.03 grams of carbohydrate per kilogram and body mass) resulted in significantly higher glycogen restoration following four hours of recovery from an exhaustive cycling bout when compared to an isocaloric carbohydrate dose (1.45 grams of carbohydrate per kilogram body mass).

In opposition, Tarnopolsky et al. (1997) reported that a carbohydrate intake of one gram of carbohydrate per kilogram of body mass per hour following exercise resulted in similar glycogen synthesis rates as those achieved by an isocaloric combination of carbohydrate (0.75 grams of carbohydrate per kilogram of body mass), protein (0.1 grams of protein per kilogram of body mass) and fat (0.02 grams of fat per kilogram of body mass). Van Hall et al. (2000) reported similar rates of glycogen resynthesis occurred when a combination of carbohydrate (one gram of carbohydrate per kilogram of body mass per hour) plus protein (0.3 grams of protein per kilogram of body mass per hour) or carbohydrate by itself (one gram of carbohydrate per kilogram of body mass per hour) were ingested every 15 minutes following exercise. Collectively, the results provide consistent evidence that when carbohydrates are ingested in high enough amounts (at least one gram of carbohydrate per kilogram of body mass per hour) at regular intervals (at least every 60 minutes), protein addition does not appear to positively influence rates of glycogen resynthesis. Alternatively, athletes should consider their ability to regularly ingest this quantity of carbohydrates at regular intervals, a point reinforced by Jentjens and Jeukendrup (2003):

> It should be noted that from a practical point of view, it might not be possible for an athlete to consume such large amounts of carbohydrate (i.e., 1.2 grams of carbohydrate per kilogram of body mass per hour). Alternatively, athletes may want to consume a moderate carbohydrate intake (0.8 grams of carbohydrate per kilogram of body mass per hour) in combination with some protein and/or amino acids, because this practice has been shown to result in similar muscle glycogen synthesis rates to the ingestion of a large amount of carbohydrate only (1.2 grams of carbohydrate per kilogram of body mass per hour).

8.2.3 OTHER NUTRIENTS THAT AID GLYCOGEN SYNTHESIS

Even with the high rates of glycogen synthesis found with sole ingestion of carbohydrates and the practicality of a carbohydrate and protein combination, athletes often will take other nutrients following endurance exercise in an attempt to aid their recovery. One of these nutrients, creatine monohydrate, has been investigated for its ability to impact levels of muscle glycogen following exhaustive exercise. In 1996, Low et al. examined the effects of muscle cell swelling on glycogen synthesis. In their examination, they used harvested skeletal muscle cells from rats and exposed them to solutions of different osmotic potentials, thereby changing the volume of each cell. Their results indicate that glycogen synthesis increased by 75% with a 78% increase in muscle cell volume. In addition, when cell volume was decreased by 30%, glycogen synthesis was also decreased by 31%. Furthermore, these changes were found to be independent of changes in glucose uptake (Low et al. 1996), providing consistent in vitro evidence that changes in cell volume may have an impact on changes in glycogen synthesis.

Robinson et al. (1999) were the first to report that creatine supplementation could augment human muscle glycogen content. They investigated the impact of simultaneous ingestion of creatine monohydrate and carbohydrate following exercise on changes in muscle creatine levels. When creatine monohydrate and carbohydrates were coingested, muscle creatine levels increased by 14% and 23% in exercised and nonexercised legs, respectively (Robinson et al. 1999). Secondary to these results, muscle glycogen content was increased by 23% following five days of creatine monohydrate plus high-carbohydrate feedings after exhaustive exercise when compared to ingesting high amounts of just carbohydrates. The authors credited this increase in glycogen to the increases in intracellular volume as a result of creatine monohydrate supplementation; however, no measurements of body water were made, and this finding requires further investigation.

Nelson and colleagues (2001) followed this study by investigating the effect of prior creatine monohydrate supplementation on a glycogen supercompensation strategy. They subjected their participants to a one-legged exhaustive exercise bout followed by a three-day high-carbohydrate diet, which resulted in a 41% increase in muscle glycogen. The subjects then supplemented for five days with creatine monohydrate (20 grams per day), followed by an exhaustive exercise bout. Following this exercise bout, the subjects again ingested a high-carbohydrate diet for three days. During the second carbohydrate-loading period, a 53% increase in muscle glycogen occurred, which was 16% more total glycogen than the glycogen content achieved during the initial carbohydrate-loading period (Nelson et al. 2001).

Evidence has also shown the possibility of caffeine enhancing muscle glycogen synthesis following exhaustive exercise. Caffeine has long been known to improve performance when taken prior to and during endurance activity; however, until recently, it was thought that it would impede glycogen synthesis. Caffeine ingestion in small doses (one to three milligrams caffeine per kilogram of body mass) before and during an exhaustive exercise bout was not shown to be detrimental to postexercise glycogen synthesis (Battram et al. 2004). Although this study was not conducted on postexercise intake of caffeine, the subjects were given approximately 1 gram of carbohydrate per kilogram of body mass per hour (75 grams of carbohydrate) immediately after exercise and every hour for four hours, which resulted in glycogen levels returning to baseline five hours after exercise with no difference in glycogen synthesis rates seen when caffeine was ingested instead of placebo. This study concluded that although caffeine has been shown to have negative effects on insulin-mediated glucose disposal in the resting state, exercise induces other factors (i.e., insulin-independent mechanisms, low levels of glycogen postexercise, etc.) that drive glycogen synthesis, which appears to override previously mentioned negative effects.

While Battram et al. (2004) revealed that caffeine ingestion before and during endurance exercise did not impair postexercise glycogen synthesis, Pedersen et al. in 2008 reported that postexercise consumption of caffeine could improve glycogen synthesis. Pedersen and colleagues utilized postexercise carbohydrate intake of one gram of carbohydrate per kilogram of body mass per hour and combined

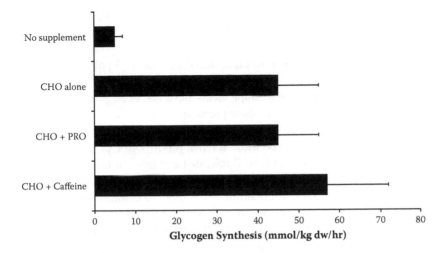

FIGURE 8.2 Average glycogen synthesis rates following endurance activity with different nutritional supplements. CHO = carbohydrate; PRO = protein.

this ingestion with two separate caffeine feedings (immediately postexercise and two hours postexercise) of four milligrams of caffeine per kilogram of body mass. During the recovery period, placebo ingestion resulted in glycogen synthesis rates that were very similar to normal rates following carbohydrate intake (38 millimoles/kilogram of dry muscle weight per hour). Interestingly, caffeine ingestion with carbohydrate resulted not only in improved glycogen synthesis rates over the four-hour recovery period, one of the highest reported glycogen synthesis rates for human subjects following oral supplementation, and the rate of glycogen resynthesis was 57.7 millimoles/kilogram of dry muscle weight per hour (Figure 8.2).

8.3 IMMUNE FUNCTION

The immune system is negatively affected by heavy exertion, such as prolonged, intense, endurance activity. Epidemiological studies conducted on runners following a marathon or ultramarathon have indicated on multiple occasions that such activity will increase an athlete's chance of upper respiratory infections (Nieman et al. 1990; Peters, Goetzsche, et al. 1993; Peters et al. 1996). Interestingly and almost paradoxically, regular, chronic endurance training is suggested to either have little to no effect on the immune system or may actually strengthen the immune system (Nieman 2008). For this reason, an acute depression in immune function after strenuous exercise, sometimes referred to as the "open window," is the most likely culprit for the increase in upper respiratory tract infections. Depending on the immune marker measured, this open window may last between 3 and 72 hours, and although transient in nature, this depression is thought to provide an opportunity for pathogens to gain a foothold within the body and increase the risk for infection (Nieman 2008). Following a marathon race, numerous cytokines increase to very high levels, including interleukin (IL) 6, IL-8, IL-10, IL-1ra, IL-1β, and tumor necrosis factor alpha

(TNF-α) (Nieman et al. 2001). Furthermore, cytokine increases have been shown to be positively correlated with markers of muscle damage and inflammation (Nieman et al. 2005). In humans, many nutritional interventions attempting to attenuate this immunity dysfunction have been studied, including zinc, N-3 polyunsaturated fatty acids, plant sterols, antioxidants, glutamine, and bovine colostrum (Nieman 2008). While many of these nutritional supplements have not been proven successful in closing the open window, a few do show promise.

Curcumin is derived from the popular Indian spice turmeric and, along with the other two curcuminoids, is responsible for the yellow color of turmeric. Clinical trials have shown that curcumin is well tolerated and poses minimal side effects in doses up to eight grams per day (Johnson and Mukhtar 2007). Curcumin has also been shown to have similar anti-inflammatory activity as common nonsteroidal anti-inflammatory drugs (NSAIDs), but favorably without the adverse side effects shown by these medications (Ammon and Wahl 1991). In a study performed on laboratory mice, chronic curcumin supplementation improved recovery of performance activities following a muscle-damaging bout of exercise and decreased levels of inflammatory cytokines in comparison to placebo (Davis et al. 2007). In this study, curcumin supplementation increased time-to-exhaustion trials by at least 100% performed both 48 and 72 hours following the muscle-damaging exercise bout. Following the muscle-damaging bout, placebo-fed mice decreased their voluntary activity for three days, while the curcumin-fed mice had no decrease in voluntary activity. Finally, curcumin feeding blunted any increase in muscle damage and inflammatory markers (creatine kinase, IL-1β, IL-6, TNF-α). However, until additional studies in humans are completed, the findings from this research should be interpreted cautiously.

Quercetin is quickly becoming another popular sports supplement for endurance athletes due to its antioxidant effects and its ability to affect mitochondrial biogenesis. A study conducted in 2007 revealed that trained cyclists ingesting 1,000 milligrams per day of quercetin had a significantly decreased incidence of upper respiratory tract infections than those cyclists consuming placebo (Nieman et al. 2007). Several measures of immune function, however, were not impacted; therefore, it was postulated that quercetin may decrease upper respiratory tract infections via direct anti-pathogenic pathways. In addition to decreased upper respiratory tract infections, quercetin supplementation has been shown to improve 30-kilometer cycling time trial performance by 3.1% (MacRae and Mefferd 2006). These improvements could be due to the effects of quercetin on mitochondrial biogenesis, which has been shown in mice to improve maximal endurance capacity (Davis et al. 2009), although this is merely speculative at this point until additional research is completed.

Similar to glycogen recovery, it appears the best option in supplementation for improving immune function following endurance activity is carbohydrates. Stress hormones (i.e., cortisol, growth hormone, norepinephrine) have been linked with immune function, and low blood glucose levels have been shown to increase these hormone levels during times of prolonged intense exercise (Nieman 1998). Also, carbohydrate, along with glutamine, is a significant fuel source for lymphocytes and monocytes, which play major roles in immune function. Ideally, athletes can increase their carbohydrate intake during prolonged exercise to maintain their blood glucose levels, which will help to avoid detrimental increases in stress hormones. However, if blood glucose is not maintained during exercise, it becomes extremely important for an athlete to consume carbohydrates following any prolonged exercise bout, which will rapidly increase blood glucose levels, blunt increases in catabolic hormones, and help to minimize inflammation and risk for upper respiratory tract infections. In this respect, carbohydrate ingestion amounts sufficient for glycogen recovery will also be appropriate to support immune system function and therefore will help to aid recovery following prolonged endurance activity.

8.4   FLUID AND ELECTROLYTE REPLACEMENT

Following endurance activity, replacing the fluid and electrolytes that an athlete loses is essential. Sweat rates during endurance activities can range depending on the athlete; those that are "light sweaters" can lose as little as 300 milliliters of sweat per hour, whereas those classified as "heavy sweaters" can lose in excess of two liters per hour (Maughan 1991). The aggressiveness of fluid replacement is dependent on how quickly an athlete must recover, similar to glycogen recovery. In most cases following endurance activity, an athlete will have ample time (≥24 hours) to recover; therefore, fluid replacement can be accomplished with normal meals and snacks accompanied by plenty of plain water. If this approach is taken, then it is recommended that meals and snacks contain sufficient sodium to replace what is lost from sweat. On the rare occasion that an endurance activity is followed by a short period of rest, then a more aggressive rehydration approach is needed and can be aided by sodium-laden sports drinks and snacks. If, however, subsequent endurance activities were to be performed in a hypohydrated state, performance would most certainly be negatively impacted. It is commonly reported that body weight decreases as little as 2% have a negative impact on performance (Sawka et al. 2007). Shirreffs and Maughan (1998) showed that a 2% decrease in body weight caused by dehydration can cause an individual to lose 1.5 grams of sodium, 300 milligrams of potassium, and 2 grams of chloride. The concentration of sodium in sweat can range greatly, from 20 millimoles/liter to 110 millimoles/liter (Kirby and Convertino 1986; Shirreffs and Maughan 1998). This sodium concentration means that heavy sweaters in combination with a high-sodium concentration in the sweat could lose in excess of five grams of sodium per hour. When put into the context that most sports drinks only contain 100 to 200 milligrams of sodium per 12 fluid ounces, it would require a fairly high amount of sports drinks to be ingested (approximately 300 fluid ounces) to replace all of the sodium lost during a single hour of activity. For this reason, salt tablets and pinches of salt added to drinks are often recommended in these specialized situations.

It is currently suggested by the American College of Sports Medicine that "individuals needing rapid and complete recovery from excessive dehydration should drink approximately 1.5 liters of fluid for each kilogram of body weight lost" (Sawka et al. 2007). However, if this fluid intake is plain water, then this will only cause an increase in urine production and not appropriately rehydrate the individual (Shirreffs et al. 1996). Appropriately formulated sports drinks provide fluid, optimal amounts of carbohydrates, and sodium. Including higher amounts of sodium in a postendurance activity drink not only will aid in replacing the sodium lost as

sweat but also will increase water retention by the body and increase thirst, resulting in greater fluid intake.

In another study by Shirreffs et al. (1996), two groups of subjects consumed four
different volumes of fluid postexercise (50%, 100%, 150%, and 200% body weight
lost) on four separate occasions. One group consumed a 23 millimoles/liter sodium
solution, and the other consumed a 61 millimoles/liter solution. In each of these
groups, urine output was increased with increasing fluid intake; however, the group
consuming the sodium solution with 61 millimoles/liter excreted less urine during
each visit. This indicates that a higher sodium content helps the body to retain more
water when compared to ingesting a solution with a lower sodium concentration
(Shirreffs et al. 1996). In addition, a positive fluid balance six hours after exercise
was achieved only when the higher concentration of sodium was ingested in amounts
equivalent to 150% and 200% of body weight lost. Consequently, consuming a volume equivalent to 200% of an individual's body weight lost will not properly rehydrate that individual unless the beverage consumed contains a high concentration of
sodium (Figure 8.3). However, one must keep in mind that the sodium concentrations used in this study are equivalent to 265 milligrams and 700 milligrams in a
500-milliliter serving, respectively. These concentrations are much higher than are
typically seen in the average sports drink on grocery store shelves today but nonetheless support the notion that adequate sodium ingestion is an important consideration
to promote optimal hydration.

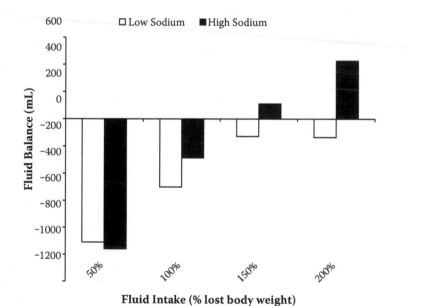

FIGURE 8.3 Fluid balance six hours postexercise following ingestion of beverages with
low- and high-sodium concentrations. (Adapted from Shirreffs, S.M., A.J. Taylor, J. Leiper,
and R. Maughan. Post-Exercise Rehydration in Man: Effects of Volume Consumed and Drink
Sodium Content. *Med Sci Sports Exercise* 28(10):1260–71, 1996.)

8.5 CURRENT RECOMMENDATIONS

The current literature on postexercise nutrient timing for endurance activity is expansive and sometimes conflicting. Many conclusions can be drawn from this extensive compilation of studies; however, based on the scientific literature, the following recommendations exist for postexercise nutrient timing for endurance activity (Figure 8.4):

- Timing of carbohydrate intake following endurance activity is of great importance if another bout of activity is required within 24 hours.
- Ingestion of 1.2 grams of carbohydrate per kilogram of body mass per hour is sufficient to recover glycogen storage if another bout of intense exercise will not take place within 24 hours.
- To aid with muscle recovery, 0.8 grams of carbohydrate per kilogram of body mass per hour in combination with 0.4 grams of protein per kilogram of body mass per hour would be more appropriate.
- The addition of caffeine (four milligrams of caffeine per kilogram of body mass every two hours) could increase glycogen synthesis to an even greater extent.
- The addition of curcumin and flavonoids, such as quercetin, has been shown to reduce the risk of upper respiratory tract infections following prolonged bouts of intense exercise and may be considered as effective training aids, while quercetin supplementation might aid in promoting greater adaptations to regular endurance training.
- Fluid replacement using a beverage containing a high-sodium concentration and a volume that provides at least 150% of lost body weight is required to maintain a positive fluid balance.

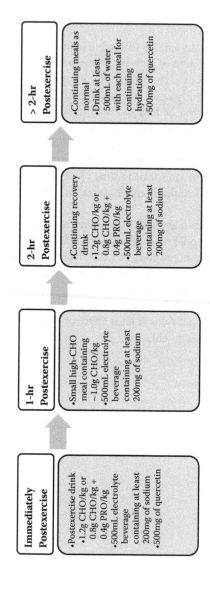

FIGURE 8.4 Recommendation for recovery nutrition following an endurance activity. CHO = carbohydrate; PRO = protein.

9 Early Timing Considerations for Resistance Activity

Chad M. Kerksick

CONTENTS

9.1 INTRODUCTION

The introduction of amino acids into the body, by either oral ingestion or infusion, rapidly increases muscle protein synthesis, while the impact on muscle protein breakdown is less robust (Biolo et al. 1997). In a somewhat similar fashion, acute bouts of resistance exercise while fasted also stimulate increases in muscle protein synthesis, but if no source of carbohydrate or protein is provided, the net balance of muscle protein will remain negative (muscle protein breakdown > muscle protein synthesis) (Phillips et al. 1997). This response occurs because of a rise in muscle protein breakdown that surpasses the rate of muscle protein synthesis (Biolo et al. 1995). When resistance training is completed and an amino acid source is ingested (or infused) in close temporal proximity, the net protein balance becomes positive (muscle protein synthesis > muscle protein breakdown) (Biolo et al. 1997; Tipton, Ferrando, et al. 1999). This research has led investigators to feverishly examine the impact of postexercise feeding to promote a positive balance of muscle protein, a topic outlined in Chapter 10 of this text.

Maintaining a positive balance of muscle protein is widely considered the ultimate objective of exercise training and nutrient feeding. The available research that has investigated nutrient timing-related considerations prior to beginning or while completing some form of resistive activity is limited, particularly when the available research is compared in magnitude to nutrient timing considerations associated with aerobic or endurance-style exercise. As outlined throughout Chapters 6, 7, and 8 of this book, a good deal of research exists examining timing considerations surrounding aerobic exercise. The same can be said regarding nutrient administration after completing a bout of resistive exercise (Chapter 10). Certainly, one of the primary interests and considerations for maximizing resistance training adaptations through concomitant adaptations to resistance exercise and some form of feeding is to enhance muscle hypertrophy and improve muscle quality. A great deal of appreciation, however, has developed for the impact of feeding on various clinical populations known to experience significant amounts of muscle wasting as well as decreases in the quality of their muscle tissue. In this respect, skeletal muscle is widely considered to play an important role in reducing risk for a number of metabolic as well as cardiovascular diseases, including diabetes, insulin resistance, osteoporosis, cardiovascular and heart disease, and aging (Wolfe 2006). For these reasons, any factor or combination of factors that increases the quantity and quality of skeletal muscle mass is likely to be clinically relevant. The purpose of this chapter is to outline the available literature that has examined the impact of ingesting some form of nutrients either before or throughout resistive activities.

9.2 PREEXERCISE

Although much less research has been conducted examining the impact of preexercise nutrient ingestion along with resistance exercise, it is almost paradoxical to highlight that one of the most widely discussed studies involving nutrient timing and resistance exercise concluded that ingestion of essential amino acids and carbohydrate immediately before resistance exercise resulted in higher levels of muscle protein synthesis when the exact same nutrients were ingested in a postexercise fashion (Tipton et al. 2001). Using a crossover study approach and stable isotope tracer analysis, Tipton and colleagues (2001) had participants ingest 35 grams of carbohydrates and 6 grams of essential amino acids immediately before and immediately after a single bout of lower-body resistance exercise. Blood and muscle levels of amino acids sharply increased in both conditions, but a greater delivery of amino acids was found to occur when the nutrients were ingested before exercise. A similar study was conducted a few years later that compared oral ingestion of 20 grams of whey protein immediately before and 20 grams of whey protein immediately after a single bout of resistance exercise (Tipton et al. 2007). Again, blood levels of amino acids increased in both conditions, and the overall balance of amino acids switched from negative to positive after whey protein ingestion at either time point. In this study, however, the net uptake of amino acids into the muscle was not different between preexercise and postexercise ingestion, suggesting that ingestion of whey protein immediately before and immediately after resistance exercise is responsible for similar changes in muscle protein synthesis. An important perspective to keep in mind is that both timing considerations significantly increased amino acid delivery and amino acid balance, suggesting that either nutrient timing consideration has the potential to increase muscle protein synthesis. However, it appears that when an intact protein source (whey protein) is ingested immediately before exercise that digestion of this protein source may limit amino acid availability (Tipton et al. 2007).

Most recently, Fujita et al. (2009) utilized a similar study design but employed analytical procedures to directly measure changes in muscle protein synthesis as opposed to the indirect approach used in previous studies. When these techniques were considered, no differences in the fractional synthesis rates of muscle protein synthesis were found when a combination of essential amino acids and carbohydrates was ingested immediately before or immediately after a single bout of resistance exercise, although both interventions resulted in significant increases from baseline (Fujita et al. 2009).

A detailed discussion of the technical differences that existed between all three studies outlined in this study is beyond the scope of this chapter. In summary, studies that have directly employed highly analytical procedures and compared the physiological differences between nutrient ingestion immediately before and immediately after resistance exercise at best provide conflicting results. Additional investigation is needed to clarify the independent effects of nutrient ingestion before versus after resistance exercise.

To examine the impact of ingesting a multinutrient supplement each day 30 minutes before seven days of heavy resistance training, Kraemer and colleagues (2007) had participants perform consecutive days of resistance training along with completing various performance measures and blood draws. When the supplement was ingested before exercise, markers of muscle damage were reduced in comparison to placebo ingestion, while also potentiating increases in anabolic hormones such as growth hormone, testosterone, and insulin-like growth factor 1, leading the authors to conclude that preexercise ingestion of a multinutrient supplement may exert favorable adaptations in recovery and anabolism (Kraemer et al. 2007).

Similarly, Shelmadine and colleagues (2009) had college-aged men resistance train for 28 days; groups ingested a maltodextrin placebo or a commercially available product containing creatine monohydrate, β-alanine, arginine, ketoisocaproate (KIC) and leucine 30 minutes before exercise. When the combination of nutrients was ingested, greater increases in upper-body strength occurred along with greater levels of myofibrillar protein and transcription factors associated with satellite cell activation. The authors concluded that over a 28-day period, preexercise (30 minutes prior) ingestion of a combination of nutrients known to stimulate positive adaptations to resistance training resulted in greater strength improvements and cellular markers of protein activity when compared to placebo ingestion (Shelmadine et al. 2009).

Finally, ingestion of a combination of protein and carbohydrate before (or after) a damaging bout of eccentric muscle contractions did not have an impact on recovery of lost muscle strength or invoke any favorable change in muscle damage markers. This suggests that timing (or even the administration in general) of protein and carbohydrates may not afford any positive impact on recovery from damaging exercise (White et al. 2008).

In summary, preexercise ingestion of nutrients may provide an opportunity to maximally deliver amino acids and other key nutrients to the muscle prior to exercise; however, outcomes from these studies have lacked consistency (Table 9.1). In addition, when other research not involving timing-related questions are considered, the delivery of amino acids and stimulation of muscle protein synthesis up to two hours prior to exercise (Witard et al. 2009) has been shown to exert similar positive effects as studies that provided an amino acid source after exercise (Biolo et al. 1997; Phillips et al. 2002). Thus, an argument can be made that muscle is as responsive and may be more responsive to nutrients ingested outside the postexercise window commonly reported (Ivy and Portman 2007; Kerksick et al. 2008).

TABLE 9.1

Summary of Studies that Provide Some Combination of Nutrients Before and After Resistance Training

Reference	Duration	Timing	Nutrition	Key Findings
			Preexercise vs. Postexercise Nutrient Administration	
Tipton et al. 2001	Acute bout	Immediately before or after exercise	6 g EAA and 35 g sucrose drink	Net muscle protein synthesis in response to drink consumed prior to resistance exercise was greater than that when drink was consumed after resistance exercise.
Tipton et al. 2007	Acute bout	Immediately before or after exercise	20 g whey protein	Timing of whey protein ingestion before or after resistance exercise did not affect extent of net muscle protein balance.
White et al. 2008	Acute bout	15 min before or after exercise	23 g whey protein + 75 g CHO	Timing of CHO/PRO supplement had no beneficial effect on markers of muscle damage.
Wilson et al. 2009	Acute bout	Immediately before or after exercise	3 g HMB	No acute or timing effects of HMB supplementation on markers of muscle damage.
			Preexercise and Postexercise Nutrient Administration	
Andersen et al. 2005	14 weeks	Immediately before and after exercise	25 g PRO vs. 25 g maltodextrin	Hypertrophy of type I and type II muscle fibers occurred only in the PRO condition.
Burk et al. 2009	8 weeks	Morning and immediately before exercise (TFR) or morning and 5 h after exercise (TDR)	70 g PRO (82% casein)	1 RM strength increases in bench press and squat were similar in TFR and TDR, and fat-free mass increased only in TDR.
Coburn et al. 2006	8 weeks	30 min prior to and after exercise	20 g whey PRO + 6.2 g leucine (SUP) vs. 26.2 g maltodextrin (PL) vs. nothing (CON)	Strength increases were greater in SUP condition when compared to PL and CON. Muscle CSA increases in SUP and PL were similar.

Cribb and Hayes 2006	10 weeks	Immediately before and after exercise (PRE-PO) or in the morning and late evening (MOR-EV)	1 g/kg/body weight of supplement containing PRO/Cr/glucose	PRE-PO timing resulted in greater increases in 1 RM strength in 2 of the 3 tested exercises, LBM, and increases in type II muscle fiber cross-sectional area when compared to MOR-EV.
Cribb, Williams, and Hayes 2007	10 weeks	Midmorning, after workout, and before sleep	1.5 g/kg/day of PRO, CHO-PRO, or CHO-PRO w/Cr	The CHO-PRO-Cr group increased LBM to a greater extent than PRO or CHO-PRO. CHO-PRO-Cr and PRO both decreased fat mass greater than CHO-PRO. The CHO-PRO-Cr group saw a greater increase in type II fiber CSA, which corresponded to a greater increase in overall strength.
Cribb, Williams, Stathis, et al. 2007	11 weeks	Midmorning, after workout, and before sleep	1.5 g/kg/day of WP, WP-Cr, CHO-Cr, or CHO	All groups increased LBM, with CHO-Cr being greater than CHO. CHO-Cr and WP-Cr increased muscle fiber CSA to a greater extent than CHO. CHO-Cr, WP-Cr, WP groups showed a greater increase in contractile protein content when compared to CHO, which corresponded to a greater increase in overall strength.
Hoffman et al. 2009	4 visits	Pre- and postworkout	42 g of PRO and BCAAs or 14.9 g of CHO	PRO supplementation allowed for more reps to be performed during the third and the fourth workout.
Hoffman et al. 2010	10 weeks	Pre- and postworkout or early morning and late night	42 g of PRO and BCAAs	Supplementation, irrespective of timing, can increase strength and power after training.
Verdijk, Jonkers, et al. 2009	12 weeks	Pre- and postworkout	Two servings of 10 g casein or PLA	Casein supplementation did not augment the effects of training on body composition or muscle fiber CSA.

g = gram; kg = kilogram; EAA = essential amino acid; CHO = carbohydrate; PRO = protein; HMB = β-hydroxy-β-methylbutyrate; h = hour; $1RM$ = one-repetition maximum; WP = whey protein; Cr = creatine; $BCAAs$ = branched-chain amino acids; CSA = cross-sectional area; LBM = lean body mass.

9.3   COMBINING PRE- AND POSTEXERCISE INGESTION

The combination of nutrient provision before *and* after resistance exercise was the first recommendation that involved some form of nutrient administration before or during consistent resistance exercise. In this study, Cribb and Hayes (2006) had participants supplement with protein and carbohydrates either immediately before and immediately after each workout or in the morning and evening (both times were at least five hours outside each workout) each day on nontraining days only (four days each week). Supplements were identical in each group and provided an estimated 32 grams protein, 34 grams carbohydrate, 0.4 grams fat, and 5.6 grams creatine monohydrate (Cribb and Hayes 2006). In a comprehensive analysis approach, greater whole-body (lean-body mass), cellular (cross-sectional area of type II fibers), and subcellular (contractile protein) levels of hypertrophy were found when the nutrients were provided in close proximity to the workouts (Cribb and Hayes 2006). While exceptional results were found, this does not necessarily mean that nutrients should be ingested before exercise as the study design could not rule out any potential impact of postexercise nutrient ingestion.

Providing additional clarity to this nutrient timing strategy, Hoffman and colleagues (2009) used a design that was similar to that of Cribb and Hayes (2006), but failed to replicate the initial findings. As before, two groups ingested nutrients either immediately before or immediately after exercise, but no changes in body composition were seen in either group. While strength increased in both supplementation groups, no differences in strength changes existed between these groups. On a closer look, it is likely that the greater resistance training background (collegiate football players) in this study may have had an impact on the changes reported. In this respect, Phillips and colleagues (1999) have shown previously that individuals with a greater training background present with reduced muscle protein turnover when compared to untrained individuals.

Finally, another factor to consider is the greater protein intake by the participants in the Hoffman et al. (2009) study, which can lead a person to conclude that timing surrounding resistance exercise may only be needed or exerts a meaningful impact when regular protein intake is low. Interestingly, a recent study used an approach that combined the two approaches investigated in the Cribb and Hayes (2006) and Hoffman et al. studies. Burk et al. (2009), over an eight-week period, had participants ingest supplements either in the morning (~10:00 a.m.) and evening (~10:00 p.m.) of exercising days or in the morning and immediately before exercise (~4:00 p.m.). The participants resistance trained for four days per week and ingested supplements only on training days. Daily administration of nutrition was identical between the groups and provided comparable amounts of protein, but the nutrition was relatively void of carbohydrate. When protein was not consumed in close proximity to the exercise bout, greater increases in lean mass resulted, providing additional results that conflict with the initial findings of Cribb and Hayes (Burk et al. 2009). Again, while the design from this study was not ideally suited to determine the impact of preexercise or during-exercise administration of nutrients, it does provide support that timing of nutrients surrounding bouts of resistance exercise sessions can alter phenotypic adaptations. An important note to consider for this study that may have had an impact on the outcomes was the source of protein utilized. Most studies commonly employ some form of whey protein; however, this study utilized casein protein. While this topic is discussed in much greater detail in Chapter 12 of this text, studies have nicely illustrated the distinct differences in digestion of whey and casein protein in an acute (Boirie et al. 1997; Dangin et al. 2001, 2003) as well as prolonged fashion (Phillips et al. 2009; Tang et al. 2009).

In addition to these studies that have directly measured some alteration of nutrient timing employed either before or during resistance exercise, a number of studies have utilized nutrient administration schemes that involve preexercise and postexercise administration of nutrients, commonly carbohydrate (Andersen et al. 2005; Coburn et al. 2006; Cribb et al. 2006; Hoffman et al. 2010); protein (Andersen et al. 2005; Coburn et al. 2006; Cribb et al. 2006; Cribb, Williams, Stathis, et al. 2007; Hoffman et al. 2010; Verdijk, Jonkers, et al. 2009); and sometimes these two macronutrients in combination with creatine monohydrate (Cribb and Hayes 2006; Cribb et al. 2006). Andersen and colleagues (2005) compared pre- and postresistance exercise administration of either carbohydrate or protein over 14 weeks and concluded that protein provided a slight advantage over carbohydrate regarding muscle function.

Hoffman et al. (2010) had 15 male strength and power athletes consume either 42 grams of protein or a similar amount of carbohydrate before and after a bout of heavy resistance training involving the squat, dead lift, and barbell exercises. They concluded that the addition of a protein supplement before and after a bout of heavy resistance aids in recovery 24 and 48 hours after the exercise bout.

Coburn and colleagues (2006) had 33 participants ingest a combination of protein (20 grams) and leucine (6.2 grams) or a carbohydrate placebo (26 grams) before and after resistance training sessions over an eight-week period. These authors reported that muscle hypertrophy was increased when any form of nutrition (carbohydrate or protein/leucine) was provided in comparison to a nonexercising control group, but there was no difference in hypertrophy between carbohydrate and protein ingestion.

Verdijk had 26 elderly men (72 ± 2 years) resistance train for 12 weeks while ingesting a small dose of protein (10 grams) before and after each resistance training session. No differences in skeletal muscle mass and strength were found when protein was ingested; however, recent findings suggest elderly individuals may have reduced sensitivity to protein and amino acids (Cuthbertson et al. 2005).

In addition, studies have been completed that have provided some combination of macronutrients (carbohydrate or protein) with and without creatine monohydrate (Cribb et al. 2006; Cribb, Williams, and Hayes 2007). One of these studies concluded that a combination of creatine monohydrate and carbohydrate, whey protein by itself, and a combination of creatine monohydrate and whey protein were responsible for the greatest increases in strength when provided before and after resistance training bouts over an 11-week period (Cribb, Williams, and Hayes 2007). A similar study by this research group over a 10-week period concluded that providing a combination of creatine monohydrate, carbohydrate, and protein provided greater improvements in maximal strength and a 40% greater increase in hypertrophy as measured by lean body mass, fiber cross-sectional area, and contractile protein. However, it should be noted that ingestion of just protein and a combination of protein and carbohydrate before and after resistance exercise also significantly increased strength and hypertrophy (Cribb, Williams, and Hayes 2007).

In summary, a number of studies are available that provide evidence that nutrient administration before and after resistance exercise sessions can improve adaptations to resistance training, such as strength and muscle hypertrophy. A limited number of these studies were designed, however, to fully ascertain whether the influence of nutrient timing plays a significant part. Regardless, it seems prudent to suggest to athletes interested in maximizing adaptations to resistance training that providing multiple boluses of nutrients may impart a favorable opportunity for the muscle to build more protein; this recommendation would also apply to the aged and other clinically relevant populations who suffer from muscle wasting and poor muscle quality.

9.4 DURING EXERCISE

Historically, ingestion of nutrients throughout a bout of resistance exercise has not been a popular or widely adopted practice. While no definitive answer exists to explain this discrepancy, a speculative attempt would suggest that any delay in published studies examining nutrient ingestion alongside resistance exercise took a backseat first to investigations involving nutrient ingestion during aerobic exercise. This combined with the popularity and explosion of interest in postresistance exercise nutrient administration are thought to be the primary reasons for the lack of available data. However, a few studies have appeared in recent years. Initial interest focused on the impact of blunting cortisol secretion as a result of ingesting a 6% carbohydrate solution throughout an acute bout of resistance exercise (Tarpenning et al. 2001). The authors discovered that when carbohydrate is ingested throughout resistance exercise, the exercise-induced release of cortisol was blunted (7% increase in cortisol) during and even after the exercise bout was completed. In comparison, cortisol secretion experienced a 99% increase when no nutrients were ingested throughout the same bout of resistance exercise (Tarpenning et al. 2001). Because of the well-accepted role of cortisol in increasing breakdown of muscle protein, this modulation of cortisol secretion was thought to influence protein turnover, resulting in a more favorable balance of anabolic and catabolic hormones (Goldberg 1969).

Bird and colleagues followed this initial study with two published papers from the same study that examined changes in myofibrillar protein breakdown (Bird et al. 2006c) and changes in serum concentrations of anabolic and catabolic hormones (Bird et al. 2006a). In this study, 32 untrained young men between the ages of 18 and 29 years performed a single bout of resistance consisting of three sets of 10 repetitions at 75% one-repetition maximum with one minute rest between sets. During the exercise bout, participants consumed either a 6% carbohydrate solution, a six-gram essential amino acid mixture, a combination of carbohydrate and essential amino acids, or a placebo. All solutions were approximately a total volume of 675 milliliters but were subsequently divided into 25 servings to be ingested every 15 minutes during the exercise bout. Blood samples were collected before exercise and every 15 minutes throughout the exercise bout and 15 as well as 30 minutes after completion of the exercise bout. When carbohydrate was ingested (groups ingesting carbohydrate only and carbohydrate plus essential amino acid), glucose and insulin concentrations were increased above baseline, while ingestion of just essential amino acids increased insulin during the postexercise period. Furthermore, the placebo group exhibited a 105% increase in cortisol, which corresponded with 56% greater urinary levels of 3-methyl-histidine, a marker of muscle protein break-down. Moreover, the groups ingesting essential amino acids only and carbohydrate only had decreased levels of muscle protein breakdown, but these differences only reached statistically significant levels (27% reduction in 3-methyl-histidine) when the two treatments were combined (groups ingesting carbohydrate only and carbohydrate plus essential amino acid) (Bird et al. 2006c).

A separate published study from this same investigation reported on changes in serum levels of growth hormone and testosterone and reported that, although pro-found impact was seen for insulin and cortisol levels, feeding throughout a bout of resistance exercise had no impact over growth hormone and testosterone changes (Bird et al. 2006a). A follow-up study by this same research group again had young participants ingest either a 6% carbohydrate solution, a six-gram mixture of essential amino acids, a combination of carbohydrate and essential amino acids, or a placebo solution (Bird et al. 2006b). All solutions were divided into small doses and ingested every 15 minutes throughout resistance exercise sessions. All participants followed a resistance training program for 12 weeks, completing two resistance exercise workouts per week. Blood samples were collected after 0, 4, 8, and 12 weeks of resistance training. In addition, urinary levels of 3-methyl-histidine and muscle fiber cross-sectional area were determined before and after the 12-week resistance training program. As exhibited during their single-bout data, cortisol increased in the placebo group after each phase of testing, while no such changes were displayed for the essential amino acid group. Either group that included carbohydrate (carbohydrate only and carbohydrate plus essential amino acid) significantly lowered cortisol levels. The combination of carbohydrate and essential amino acids (carbohydrate only and carbohydrate plus essential amino acid) caused a 26% reduction in urinary levels of 3-methyl-histidine; the placebo group increased by 52% after 12 weeks of resistance training. Also, muscle fiber cross-sectional area increased in all groups and all fiber types (I, IIa, IIb) after training, but the combination of carbohydrate and essential amino acids was responsible for the greatest gains in cross-sectional area (Bird et al. 2006b).

The results from these studies provide consistent evidence; however, caution should be used when interpreting their conclusions. For starters, a number of studies suggest that greater insulin levels do not necessarily translate into an inhibition of myofibrillar protein but do operate powerfully at the whole-body level. While a case could be made to suggest that protein throughout the body can be recycled and reincorporated into various tissue types, insulin appears to exert its most predominant anti-proteolytic function through lysosomal activity, as opposed to the ubiquitin proteolytic system, which is known to target myofibrillar proteins. In addition, kinetic analysis of protein balance using stable isotope tracers has revealed that protein synthesis can be increased in magnitude approximately 10- to 20-fold compared to the measured changes in protein breakdown (Biolo et al. 1997; Volpi et al. 2003). As a result, when interventions are employed, the augmentation (both magnitude and latency) of muscle protein synthesis is more important than alterations in muscle protein breakdown when endpoints of interest involve greater accretion of lean tissue. These comments are not to draw away from the positive outcomes reported by this research but, instead, are meant to augment the importance of considering both the synthetic and proteolytic considerations.

Last, another key factor to consider is the availability of amino acids as a function of increased blood flow that stems from completing the exercise bout. Bohe and colleagues (2003) nicely illustrated that muscle protein synthesis is driven largely, if not exclusively, by the extracellular concentration of amino acids. Therefore, because these study designs were not employed to identify any favorable impact of ingesting nutrients during a resistance exercise bout in comparison to other ingestion times, it cannot be ruled out that the favorable increases were simply a function of increased amino acid transport resulting in favorable metabolic and phenotypic adaptations, which may or may not have occurred if identical nutrients were ingested at other times.

9.5   SIGNIFICANCE AND FUTURE DIRECTIONS

Nutrient ingestion before or during resistance exercise is still largely underresearched, with a few notable studies available in each area. Unfortunately, none of these studies was designed to identify if the timing of nutrients was responsible for positive changes or whether the favorable changes were merely just because of increased nutrient availability and delivery because of increased blood flow. Surprisingly, the greatest number of studies employed a regimen of nutrient administration that provided some combination of protein and carbohydrates before and after each bout of resistance exercise. Initial studies using the approach suggested remarkable physiological changes (Cribb and Hayes 2006); however, recent studies have failed to universally support these initial findings, particularly if the individuals were highly trained and already consuming adequate protein (Hoffman et al. 2009). In addition, the popularity of preworkout formulations in the bodybuilding world has increased immensely without any concrete data showing that when the nutrients are ingested seemingly makes a difference. For these reasons, a wide number of well-controlled training studies need to be completed with specific interest in determining if timing makes any difference on the phenotypic outcomes associated with regularly performing resistance training.

10 Postexercise Nutrient Timing with Resistive Activities

Oliver C. Witard and Kevin D. Tipton

CONTENTS

10.1 INTRODUCTION

Postexercise nutrition plays an important role in optimization of recovery from exercise and adaptations to exercise training (Hawley et al. 2006). The early focus of exercise nutrition research was on restoration of glycogen stores following endurance exercise. Consequently, the timing of nutrient intake for optimization of recovery from endurance exercise has been extensively studied (Millard-Stafford et al. 2008). More recently, much attention has been given to nutrition for recovery from resistive activities, in particular for optimization of muscle anabolism. In recent years, the timing of nutrient intake in relation to resistance exercise has been intensively studied. Both longitudinal endpoint studies, and acute metabolic study designs have been utilized to examine the critical importance of nutrient timing for muscle hypertrophy. The focus of this research has been primarily on the timing of protein intake, with less emphasis on carbohydrate or fat intake.

This chapter examines and critically reviews the evidence regarding timing of nutrients—focused primarily on protein—intake in relation to resistive-type exercise primarily in humans. The importance of timing of nutrient intake for optimization of the anabolic response has begun to gain more attention in recent years. However, as pointed out, a paucity of information exists that has directly investigated the optimal timing of nutrient intake in relation to resistance exercise. For this reason, it will be shown that whereas timing of amino acid intake clearly has an impact on the metabolic response to exercise, the precise timing of nutrient ingestion in relation to resistance exercise for optimal anabolic adaptations may not be as firmly established as is often advocated. Many details of this response remain to be fully elucidated. This review perhaps has implications for many populations, including athletes and exercisers striving to increase muscle mass and strength and populations such as the elderly who wish to counteract or reduce the loss of muscle mass.

The importance that is placed on nutrient timing for the anabolic response to exercise seems to have gathered a great deal of momentum. The most prevalent opinion is that protein, perhaps along with carbohydrate, should be consumed in the immediate aftermath of exercise (Burd et al. 2010; Kerksick et al. 2008; Lemon et al. 2002; Little and Phillips 2009). The notion is that the anabolic response will be impaired, if not alleviated, if nutrients are not ingested within as few as 45 to 60 minutes following exercise (Ivy and Portman 2007). This time period has been coined the "anabolic window of opportunity" (Ivy and Portman 2007), and a great deal of attention has been given to this concept, in both scientific research and review articles (Burd, Tang, et al. 2009; Kerksick et al. 2008; Lemon et al. 2002; Little and Phillips 2009), as well as the lay literature (Ivy and Portman 2007), including numerous Web sites. As mentioned, the focus of this chapter is to critically evaluate the scientific evidence supporting this concept and not supporting it and to discuss other aspects of postexercise nutrient timing.

10.1.1 METHODOLOGICAL APPROACHES

A discussion of the study designs utilized for evaluation of nutrient timing in relation to exercise is important for making conclusions about this issue. The study design chosen, of course, will have basic assumptions and limitations that must be considered, and it is these factors that allow researchers to develop the conclusions from any study. Two basic study designs are typically utilized: longer endpoint studies, often referred to as "training" studies; and acute metabolic studies. The utility of longitudinal endpoint study designs is for the study of adaptations to regular, consistent training. Yet, transient metabolic (acute) response studies of individual exercise bouts result in the accumulation of new muscle proteins, which along with changes in activity and function of these proteins, over time is responsible for the phenotypic adaptations induced by training (Hawley et al. 2006). Thus, both longitudinal and acute studies may provide valuable information concerning the timing of nutrient intake with resistive exercise.

The metabolic basis for a change in muscle protein levels resulting in adaptations is net muscle protein balance, the difference between muscle protein synthesis and muscle protein breakdown, over a predetermined period of time. To accrue muscle proteins, the rate of muscle protein synthesis must exceed muscle protein breakdown, resulting in a positive muscle protein balance over a given period of time. Studies that have measured muscle protein balance acutely following resistance exercise have unequivocally found that, whereas muscle protein synthesis is markedly elevated, muscle protein balance remains negative in the absence of nutrient supply (Biolo et al. 1997; Phillips et al. 1997). Provision of an amino acid source combined with exercise is required to switch muscle protein balance from negative to positive (Biolo et al. 1997; Rasmussen et al. 2000; Tipton, Ferrando, et al. 1999). This switch is largely due to increases in muscle protein synthesis rather than changes in muscle protein breakdown (Biolo et al. 1997; Rennie and Tipton 2000). Thus, skeletal muscle hypertrophy, a common goal for populations involved in resistive-type activities, depends on the interaction between exercise and nutrition. This interactive effect seems to be influenced by the timing of nutrient intake relative to the exercise bout, thus influencing the accretion of muscle protein with training (Tipton and Witard 2007).

A critical assumption for acute metabolic studies to glean information regarding timing of nutrient intake is that measurement of the acute metabolic response to resistance exercise and nutrient timing predicts chronic adaptations that occur in response to strength training over a prolonged period of time, and certainly support exists for this contention. Previously, it has been demonstrated that acute changes in muscle protein balance, induced by the ingestion of essential amino acids following exercise, reflect those that occurred chronically over a 24-hour period (Tipton et al. 2003). Furthermore, short-term changes in muscle protein synthesis and muscle protein balance (Wilkinson et al. 2007) are qualitatively predictive of chronic adaptations (Hartman et al. 2007) to feeding with different protein sources following resistance exercise. There is no reason to believe that this relationship would not exist with reference to protein timing. Hence, studies (Fujita et al. 2008; Levenhagen et al. 2001; Rasmussen et al. 2000; Roy et al. 1997; Tipton et al. 2001, 2007) that have examined the impact of timing of protein intake in relation to exercise on acute changes in muscle protein metabolism may be used to predict adaptations to long-term training.

Whereas acute metabolic studies have predictive value, the importance of a longitudinal approach to address the importance of nutrient timing should not be underestimated. Longitudinal studies may be used to measure the adaptation that is important (e.g., increased muscle mass or strength) to the type of training that the athlete or exerciser deems important. On the other hand, training studies often reach equivocal, or even conflicting, conclusions regarding a nutritional intervention, such as timing of intake. The length of the training period for any given study may be weeks, months, or in theory, even years. Inherent difficulties controlling numerous extraneous variables, such as dietary intake, emotional issues, sleep patterns, and so on, have undoubtedly contributed to variable results, thus hindering a clear interpretation of longitudinal endpoint studies that attempt to address the importance of timing of protein intake (Tipton and Ferrando 2008). Whereas differences in adaptations to training may be more easily discerned with longer training periods, expense and increasing difficulty with control often limit the length of the training period that is possible for a study; for this reason, the number of these studies available is markedly reduced. Ultimately, the importance of nutrient timing for individuals involved in resistance training is determined by the resulting adaptations rather than a metabolic response per se, and more quantitative conclusions are possible if the studies are performed properly. Hence, the determination of long-term changes in muscle size, strength, and function in studies controlled as tightly as possible are important. Given appropriate interpretation of results considering the inherent limitations, these studies clearly provide critical information concerning the optimal timing of nutrient intake following resistive exercise. For these reasons, more of these studies are warranted at this time.

10.2   THE ANABOLIC WINDOW OF OPPORTUNITY

As mentioned, the consensus recommendation for maximization of the anabolic response to resistance exercise and protein intake is to ingest protein within close temporal proximity to the exercise (i.e., during the anabolic window of opportunity) (Ivy and Portman 2007; Lemon et al. 2002; Little and Phillips 2009). This recommendation is based on the results of several studies, both acute metabolic studies and longitudinal endpoint studies. Much of the support offered for this contention comes from studies in which greater lean tissue gains were found in subjects ingesting protein following exercise compared to those ingesting carbohydrate or a placebo (Andersen et al. 2005; Cribb, Williams, Stathis, et al. 2007; Hartman et al. 2007; Hulmi et al. 2009; Kerksick et al. 2006; Rankin et al. 2004; Willoughby et al. 2007). However, surprisingly few studies actually have compared changes in muscle mass and strength with ingestion of a protein-containing supplement in close proximity to exercise with ingestion at times other than close to exercise. Table 10.1 summarizes the existing data that directly compare the impact of nutrient timing on adaptations associated with resistance training.

Advocates of the importance of the anabolic window, both lay and scientific (Ivy and Portman 2007; Lemon et al. 2002), often cite an investigation by Levenhagen et al. (2001) as support for this notion. In this study, muscle protein balance was determined during recovery when a mixed macronutrient (ten grams protein, eight grams carbohydrate, and three grams fat) supplement was consumed either immediately or three hours after 60 minutes of moderate-intensity endurance exercise in recreationally trained adults. Net accretion of muscle protein was reported when nutrients were administered immediately postexercise; conversely, a net loss of muscle protein occurred when nutrients were given three hours after exercise. Indeed, muscle protein synthesis was increased more than threefold in the early versus late condition. Thus, these results seemingly support the importance of ingesting a protein-containing supplement immediately following exercise.

However, interpretation of these findings in the context of muscle growth is likely not as straightforward as first considered. First, the mode of exercise was cycling rather than resistance exercise, bringing into question the applicability if someone were to extrapolate these findings to a resistance training scenario. Whereas net muscle protein balance increased with immediate protein ingestion (Levenhagen et al. 2001), no distinction of protein type was made. It is clear that cycling exercise results in increased mitochondrial protein synthesis with no impact on myofibrillar proteins (Wilkinson et al. 2008). Thus, it is likely that the increase in the synthesis of mixed muscle proteins following cycling noted by Levenhagen et al. (2001) was primarily due to mitochondrial or sarcoplasmic proteins rather than the myofibrillar proteins responsible for increased size and strength. When essential amino acids are ingested one or three hours following resistance exercise, the response of mixed muscle protein synthesis and net muscle protein balance is identical (Rasmussen et al. 2000), suggesting that either time point is satisfactory to increase muscle protein synthesis and promote a positive muscle protein balance. However, it also remains that following resistive exercise, the type of exercise that stimulates myofibrillar protein synthesis (Wilkinson et al. 2008), the importance of immediately ingesting protein is lessened. When also considering the differential responses seen to occur with

TABLE 10.1

Overview of Studies that Directly Compared the Impact of Nutrient Timing on Adaptations Associated with Resistance Training

Reference	Participants	Training	Nutrients	Timing	Measurement	Main Findings
Esmarck et al. 2001	Elderly males	12-wk RT (3/wk)	MMN supplement (10 g protein, 7 g carbohydrate, 3 g fat)	Imm. post 2 h post	Muscle hypertrophy Dynamic strength Isokinetic strength	↑Imm. post, ↔2 h post ↑Imm. post (46%), ↑2 h post (36%) ↑Imm. post (15%), ↔2 h post
Candow, Chilibeck, et al. 2006	Elderly males	12-wk RT	Protein supplement (0.3 g·kg BM⁻¹·day⁻¹)	Imm. pre Imm. post	Lean tissue mass Muscle hypertrophy Strength	↔Imm. pre, ↔Imm. post ↔Imm. pre, ↔Imm. post ↔Imm. pre, ↔Imm. post
Cribb and Hayes 2006	Rec. trained bodybuilders	10-wk RT	MMN supplement (protein, creatine, glucose)	Imm. pre & post (PRE/POST) Morn. & eve. (MORN/EVE)	Lean body mass Muscle hypertrophy Strength	↑PRE/POST > ↑MORN/EVE ↑PRE/POST > ↑MORN/EVE ↑PRE/POST > ↑MORN/EVE
Hoffman et al. 2009	Trained power athletes	10-wk RT	Protein supplement	Imm. pre & post (PRE/POST) Morn. & eve. (MORN/EVE)	Strength Upper-limb power Lower-limb power	↑PRE/POST = ↑MORN/EVE ↑PRE/POST = ↑MORN/EVE ↑PRE/POST = ↑MORN/EVE
Burk et al. 2009	Young males	8-wk RT (crossover study design)	Protein supplement	Morn. & imm. post ex (TFR) Morn. & eve. (5 h postex; TDR)	Lean body mass Strength	↔TFR, ↑TDR ↑TFR = ↑TDR

$Rec. = recreationally; RT = resistance training; MMN = mixed macronutrient; BM = body mass; Imm. = immediately; Morn. = morning; Eve. = evening; TFR = time-focused regimen; TDR = time-divided regimen.$

ingestion of different protein sources (Moore, Tang, et al. 2009), it seems that both the mode of exercise and protein source should be considered in addition to or even in place of the timing of these nutrients.

Other acute metabolic data exist to suggest that other timing considerations may hold just as much importance as postexercise ingestion for optimizing the anabolic response of muscle. Certainly, postexercise feeding is not the only time consideration shown to optimize the interactive metabolic response to resistance exercise and an amino acid source. Both essential amino acids (Tipton et al. 2001) and whey protein (Tipton et al. 2007) ingestion prior to exercise result in superior or similar, respectively, anabolic responses compared to ingestion immediately following exercise. Moreover, the exercise-induced stimulation of muscle protein synthesis was similar when a protein-containing meal was ingested approximately two hours prior to exercise (Witard et al. 2009) compared to when an amino acid source is provided following exercise (Biolo et al. 1997; Phillips et al. 2002). This comparison is illustrated in Figure 10.1. Taken together, these results suggest that muscle is as responsive, if not more responsive, to nutrient ingestion during time periods outside the limits usually ascribed to the anabolic window (Ivy and Portman 2007) compared with a situation in which nutrition is provided within this window.

Recent data suggest that the anabolic window may extend to much more than merely the first hour or less following the exercise. The stimulation of muscle protein synthesis and muscle protein balance extends to at least 36 hours and up to 48 hours (Chesley et al. 1992) following resistance exercise (Phillips et al. 1997); recent data in this light suggest that it is indeed myofibrillar proteins that are responding (Burd et al. 2010). Thus, for people only to consider that an anabolic window of opportunity exists outside the often-reported one to three hours postexercise fails to consider these outcomes. This contention is supported by a report that protein ingestion 24 hours following resistance exercise resulted in a greater response of

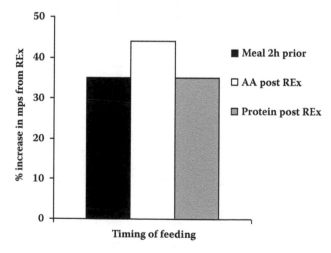

FIGURE 10.1   Additive effect of exercise on muscle protein synthesis when a source of protein is ingested prior to exercise compared with following exercise. AA = amino acids; REx = resistance exercise (Biolo et al. 1997; Phillips et al. 2002; Witard et al. 2009).

muscle protein synthesis than protein ingested with no exercise (Burd, Tang, et al. 2009). Whereas a direct comparison of the response of muscle protein synthesis or muscle protein balance to ingestion of protein immediately and 24 hours following exercise has yet to be made (thus the response could, in fact, be slightly greater immediately following exercise than 24 hours after), it is clear that the muscle is still responsive for up to, at least, 24 hours following exercise. The interaction of elevated blood amino acids from protein ingestion and resistance exercise is evident for at least 24 hours (Burd, Tang, et al. 2009). As a result, the importance of immediate postexercise ingestion of protein and other nutrients does not seem as critical as has been espoused (Ivy and Portman 2007; Lemon et al. 2002). The timing of amino acid or protein ingestion undoubtedly alters the metabolic response (Tipton and Witard 2007); however, much more work is necessary before definitive conclusions may be made about the optimal time of ingestion.

One of the longitudinal investigations that is often used to support immediate postexercise protein ingestion compared the changes in muscle size and strength in elderly volunteers with 12 weeks of resistance exercise training (Esmarck et al. 2001). Subjects were divided into two groups. One group ingested a protein-containing supplement immediately after exercise, and the other group waited two hours to ingest the supplement. The results were interesting, albeit somewhat puzzling. Muscle strength increases were greater in the immediate ingestion group and, in fact, were limited in the group ingesting the supplement two hours after exercise. Moreover, muscle hypertrophy was observed only in the immediate ingestion group. Interestingly, the hypertrophy measured with immediate ingestion of the protein supplement was similar to that reported in other resistance training studies with elderly volunteers and no particular supplementation or feeding intervention (Fiatarone et al. 1990; Frontera et al. 1988; Welle et al. 1996). Hence, the results of this study (Esmarck et al. 2001) suggest that immediate ingestion of protein does not offer any advantage over unsupervised nutrition with training—at least in the elderly. Thus, Esmarck et al. (2001) did not actually demonstrate any superior anabolic responses with immediate ingestion of protein during resistance training. Moreover, it should be noted that waiting two hours to ingest the protein actually inhibited the normal response to resistance exercise training (Esmarck et al. 2001). In fact, that group lost lean body mass—a very unusual situation with resistance exercise training—making these results quite puzzling and difficult to interpret. It should be emphasized that these results were noted in elderly (albeit healthy) volunteers and may not apply to younger weightlifters. Nevertheless, whereas it may be that immediate protein intake is important to preserve lean mass, this study does not support a superior anabolic response with immediate ingestion, as is so often stated.

Other longitudinal training studies may be used to provide support for the notion that optimal muscle and strength gains stem from ingestion of protein within close proximity to resistance exercise. Cribb and Hayes (2006) reported that during 10 weeks of resistance training, supplementation, including protein, immediately before and after each workout resulted in significantly greater improvements in maximal strength and hypertrophy compared with a matched group of young individuals who consumed isocaloric and isonitrogenous supplements in the morning and evenings (times not associated with the exercise bouts). The superior results were fairly comprehensive as they were demonstrated on whole-body (lean body mass), cellular (cross-sectional area of type II fibers) and subcellular (contractile protein) levels (Cribb and Hayes 2006). Thus, whereas these data support the notion that protein ingestion in close temporal proximity to exercise may provide optimal anabolic results, they do not necessarily support the notion that protein must be ingested immediately *following* exercise. Given the design of the study, there is no way to rule out that the preexercise ingestion played an important role. A possible role for preexercise amino acid and protein ingestion is supported by acute metabolic data (Tipton et al. 2001), a topic covered in greater detail in Chapter 9 of this text.

On the other hand, other recent studies do not support the necessity for protein ingestion in close temporal proximity to exercise for maximal muscle hypertrophy. Hoffman and colleagues (2009) used a design that was similar to that of Cribb and Hayes (2006) but did not replicate those results. While many aspects of this study were different, it is likely that the greater resistance training background (collegiate football players) of the participants in the Hoffman study may have had an impact on the adaptations achieved. In this respect, previous studies have shown that individuals with a greater training background had reduced muscle protein turnover in comparison to untrained individuals (Phillips et al. 1999). Another factor to explain the difference in results could be the greater protein intake reported by the Hoffman participants, suggesting that timing may be of no consequence if protein intake is achieved at higher levels. Furthermore, a recent investigation found a greater increase in lean body mass when protein was not consumed in close proximity (one dose in the morning and a second dose five hours after exercise) to resistance exercise than when consumed in close proximity (one dose in the morning and one dose immediately before exercise) over eight weeks of training (Burk et al. 2009). Of an important note, neither group immediately ingested nutrients postexercise, bringing into question whether postexercise timing is needed to facilitate greater training adaptations. While evidence does exist from the Esmarck study that postexercise ingestion may hinder adaptations, these results were challenging to explain at best and bring to light the need for more training style studies that specifically examine the role of timing on strength and hypertrophic adaptations after several weeks of resistance training.

Clearly, there is a great deal of equivocation in the results from studies investigating the importance of immediate postexercise ingestion of protein for gains in muscle. The reasons for this lack of certainty likely are multifactorial, and this is an extremely important consideration to consider and may have to do with the differences in study design between these studies. In the studies described, the subjects varied from completely untrained (Burk et al. 2009) to recreationally trained (Cribb and Hayes 2006) to very well trained (Hoffman et al. 2009). The impact of the training state of the subjects on the interactive response of muscle hypertrophy to resistance exercise and nutrition is unknown, but an acute metabolic study with no nutrition component suggested that subjects with a greater training background had reduced muscle protein turnover when compared to untrained individuals (Phillips et al. 1999). Furthermore, these studies used variable amounts of protein and other nutrients in the context of variable total protein and energy consumption, such that direct comparisons may not be possible. The dearth of studies directly assessing this question makes it all but impossible to make solid conclusions about the optimal

timing. Moreover, it appears that the optimal timing of protein or amino acid ingestion may differ depending on the type of amino acid source as well as concurrent
ingestion of other nutrients (Tipton and Witard 2007). Therefore, definitive conclusions cannot be made at this juncture, and approaches that are more systematic are
encouraged in the future.

It is considered that the accumulation of muscle, in particular myofibrillar, proteins in response to resistance exercise and protein ingestion may be similar to that
demonstrated for muscle glycogen. Specifically, research has indicated that with
various exercise and feeding combinations, the rate of muscle glycogen resynthesis
can be optimized over a short term, but when adequate amounts are provided, the
total accumulation of glycogen (or myofibrillar proteins in this example) is similar
(Keizer et al. 1987; Parkin et al. 1997). Indeed, it has been shown that an initial rate
of protein synthesis with immediate ingestion of protein is greater when no protein
is ingested, and that subsequent protein ingestion continues to stimulate protein synthesis (Rasmussen et al. 2000). After so many hours—provided all other nutrient
intake, particularly protein, and activity patterns are the same—the accumulation
of protein will be the same for both timing situations. A depiction of this scenario
as envisioned is provided in Figure 10.2. As seen in the figure, an arbitrarily chosen

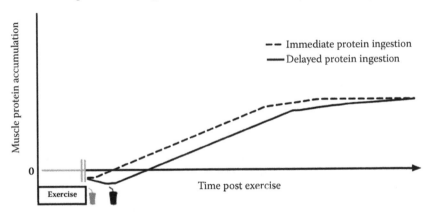

FIGURE 10.2 Proposed depiction of the accumulation of muscle, primarily myofibrillar,
proteins when protein is ingested immediately after (broken line) or postponed for a period
of time, such as two hours after (solid line) completion of a resistance exercise session. We
theorize that initial accumulation of protein rises steeply when protein is ingested immediately following exercise but plateaus as muscle protein synthesis and net muscle protein
balance are reduced. Since net muscle protein balance remains negative following exercise,
when protein ingestion is delayed, a small amount of muscle protein is lost until amino acids
from protein consumption become available to provide the interactive effect of exercise and
amino acids on muscle protein synthesis. However, the response of muscle protein synthesis
and net muscle protein balance is similar to immediate protein ingestion; thus, accumulation
of protein follows a similar pattern, albeit delayed by two hours. Assuming equivalent activity
patterns and nutrient, particularly protein, ingestion during the recovery period, there would
be little difference, at least of any physiological significance, in muscle protein accumulation
between immediate and delayed protein ingestion regimens. Instead, temporal diversities in
muscle protein accumulation may be achieved by varied timing approaches.

time point of approximately 48 hours is when protein accumulation is equivalent. Certainly, given the theoretical nature of this scenario, it is not known how this pattern would develop, especially when additional factors such as physical activity, or lack thereof, as well as energy and nutrient intake are considered. In this respect, more work is needed to determine how these factors influence the response of muscle growth to the timing of nutrient intake.

On the other hand, despite a relative lack of information, if we take a risk-benefit type of approach, some practical recommendations may be made. Despite the lack of clear evidence for unambiguous efficacy of immediate postexercise protein ingestion, it is probably a good recommendation to make for most individuals who desire increased muscle mass and strength with resistance training. The operative question regards which risks are associated with ingesting protein immediately following exercise. For the vast majority of individuals, there are no appreciable risks to that approach. Thus, it is unlikely to impair the response and could improve it, so why not consume protein in the first hour or two following resistance exercise? Most athletes and exercisers are quite likely to consume some protein, whether as part of a meal or as a postexercise supplement in the natural scheme of things in any case.

10.3   OTHER NUTRIENTS

While little direct information is available regarding the optimal timing of protein intake in relation to resistance exercise, if anything, there is even less regarding carbohydrate or fat intake. There is some, albeit minimal, information regarding carbohydrate intake following resistance exercise, but currently little to no information exists regarding the timing of fat ingestion following resistance exercise.

10.3.1   NET MUSCLE PROTEIN BALANCE

Any impact of carbohydrate intake on protein metabolism following resistance exercise is almost certainly mediated by insulin release. However, increased insulin has minimal, if any, impact on muscle protein synthesis following resistance exercise (Biolo et al. 1999). Thus, adding carbohydrate to protein ingestion following resistance exercise does not increase muscle protein synthesis (Koopman et al. 2007; Staples et al. 2010). However, there seems to be an impact on muscle protein breakdown (Biolo et al. 1999), thus improving muscle protein balance (Biolo et al. 1999; Borsheim et al. 2004; Miller et al. 2003). However, without an amino acid source postexercise, carbohydrate ingestion does not result in positive muscle protein balance (Borsheim et al. 2004; Miller et al. 2003; Tipton et al. 2001). Thus, the impact of postexercise carbohydrate ingestion on muscle hypertrophy during training would be minimal other than perhaps to supply needed energy.

To our knowledge, only one study has compared the response of muscle protein metabolism with different times of carbohydrate ingestion. In a nicely controlled study, Roy et al. (1997) provided carbohydrate either immediately and one hour following resistance exercise or at other times not associated with the exercise. Whereas there was no statistically significant difference in muscle protein synthesis, markers of whole-body (urinary urea nitrogen excretion) and myofibrillar protein breakdown (urinary 3-methyl histidine excretion) were reduced in the immediate postexercise ingestion trial (Roy et al. 1997). Thus, albeit with no direct measure, these data suggest that muscle protein balance is improved with immediate coingestion of carbohydrate. Therefore, as with protein, as long as carbohydrate intake immediately postexercise fits into the overall energy and macronutrient requirements of any individual's diet, it seems that carbohydrate intake would make sense for most athletes.

In addition to timing of postexercise carbohydrate ingestion in relation to exercise, the question of the timing of carbohydrate ingestion in relation to protein is potentially interesting. Examination of the muscle protein balance data following carbohydrate ingestion suggests that the response is somewhat delayed; that is, muscle protein balance does not seem to increase until approximately one hour after carbohydrate ingestion (Borsheim et al. 2004; Miller et al. 2003). Given that the response to amino acids is rapid (Fujita et al. 2008; Levenhagen et al. 2001; Rasmussen et al. 2000; Roy et al. 1997; Tipton et al. 2001, 2007), delaying amino acid ingestion for 60 minutes after carbohydrate ingestion would superimpose the responses, resulting in maximal positive muscle protein balance. However, when carbohydrate was provided one hour after resistance exercise and amino acids two hours after resistance exercise and compared to simultaneous ingestion at one hour after exercise, the overall response of muscle protein balance was not different (Witard, O.C., Cooke, T.L., Ferrando, A.A., Wolfe, R.R., and Tipton, K.D. 2004, unpublished data). Interestingly, from a physiological perspective, muscle protein balance initially (the first hour after amino acid ingestion) was slightly greater when carbohydrate and amino acid ingestion were separated, but over time the response evened out (Figure 10.3). Thus, whereas perhaps physiologically interesting, from a practical perspective, separation of carbohydrate and amino acid ingestion does not provide a superior anabolic response to concurrent ingestion.

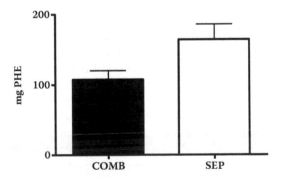

FIGURE 10.3 Anabolic response (amino acid uptake) to ingestion of carbohydrate and essential amino acids during recovery from resistance exercise measured over (a) a one-hour period following amino acid ingestion, and (b) a seven-hour (overall) period following exercise. COMB = carbohydrate and amino acids were ingested concurrently one hour following exercise. Thus, the one-hour measurement period began at one hour following exercise in this group. SEP = carbohydrate was ingested at one hour following exercise, and amino acids were ingested two hours following exercise. PHE = phenylalanine. Thus, the one-hour measurement in this group was from two to three hours following exercise.

10.3.2 GLYCOGEN RESYNTHESIS

In addition to the impact of carbohydrate intake on protein metabolism, glycogen resynthesis is an important issue to consider. It has been well recognized for many years that carbohydrate intake following intense endurance exercise is important for restoration of glycogen stores and maintenance of subsequent training intensity and performance (Ivy 1998). Similarly, there is a considerable reduction in muscle glycogen with resistance exercise, particularly in type II fibers (Pascoe et al. 1993; Roy and Tarnopolsky 1998). Thus, as with endurance exercise, ingestion of carbohydrates to enhance restoration of glycogen content in muscle is important. The rate of muscle glycogen synthesis is greater when carbohydrates are ingested soon after exercise compared to a placebo (Pascoe et al. 1993; Roy and Tarnopolsky 1998). However, as with protein ingestion and protein metabolism mentioned, few data exist showing the results of a comparison of immediate postexercise carbohydrate ingestion to ingestion at other time points. To date, only one study has examined this direct comparison. Roy and Tarnopolsky (1998) demonstrated that ingestion of carbohydrate, with or without fat and protein, resulted in superior rates of glycogen resynthesis when ingested immediately and at one hour after exercise compared to other times not related to the exercise (i.e., in the morning with breakfast). Six hours following exercise, glycogen was restored almost to preexercise levels. The rates of resynthesis were similar to those observed in similar circumstances following endurance exercise (Zawadzki et al. 1992). When glycogen levels are measured 24 hours following exercise—at least endurance exercise—the extent of muscle glycogen replenishment is similar whether carbohydrate administration is immediate or delayed, as long as the total amount of carbohydrate ingestion is similar (Keizer et al. 1987; Parkin et al. 1997). Thus, if the next workout is within a few hours of the previous resistance exercise bout, immediate carbohydrate is much more important than if the next exercise bout will occur within 24 or more hours.

The importance of carbohydrate ingestion for glycogen replenishment is not restricted to fuel use considerations. Recent evidence suggests that the molecular response to resistance exercise is related to muscle glycogen availability. The responses of translational (Akt/mammalian target of rapamycin (mTOR)) pathways (Creer et al. 2005) and transcriptional activity (Churchley et al. 2007) to resistance exercise are reduced when exercise commences with reduced muscle glycogen. Whereas no determinations of muscle protein synthesis or muscle protein balance were made in these studies, the results suggest that the anabolic response to the resistance exercise is reduced when glycogen levels are low at the beginning of exercise despite equivalent exercise bouts. Moreover, whereas the work was matched in the previously mentioned studies (Churchley et al. 2007; Creer et al. 2005), in a practical setting the ability to perform exercise will be reduced with low muscle glycogen (Churchley et al. 2007; Haff et al. 2003). Thus, muscle anabolism will be reduced due to lower work output and an inherent inability of the anabolic mechanisms to respond. Clearly, the importance of sufficient carbohydrate intake for resistance exercise is emphasized by these data.

10.4 SUMMARY

Timing of amino acid and protein intake markedly influences the response of net muscle protein balance to resistance exercise and hence muscle anabolism. Unfortunately, the optimal timing of nutrient ingestion is complex and remains to be fully elucidated. Determinants of the optimal timing are almost certainly multifactorial and likely depend on an intricate combination of protein type, content of the essential amino acids, and other nutrients ingested concurrently (Tipton and Witard 2007).

Thus, it remains that the often-reported anabolic window of opportunity may not be as prevalent as initially reported; that is, skeletal muscle remains responsive to nutrient ingestion for longer periods of time than initially thought following exercise. Indeed, several lines of evidence suggest that preexercise feeding may be more beneficial for muscle anabolism, but this topic is not without controversy. This said, from a purely practical standpoint, nutrient ingestion within one hour postexercise is likely to be a convenient time to ingest protein, and there certainly is no evidence that it will impede the anabolic response. For this reason, it is recommended due to its potential to yield improvements. It is unclear how important carbohydrate intake is for muscle anabolism. However, there is no reason to suggest it will hurt. Moreover, carbohydrate intake soon after exercise may be critical for restoration of muscle glycogen, particularly if a subsequent exercise bout will be undertaken within a few hours.

10.5 NUTRIENT TIMING GUIDELINES AFTER RESISTANCE EXERCISE

1. Immediate postexercise, protein and carbohydrate ingestion is recommended provided it fits within the overall energy and macronutrient requirements of the diet.
2. The sensitivity of skeletal muscle to protein remains elevated for up to 24 hours after resistance exercise, so a delay of one to two hours for ingestion of protein or carbohydrate is unlikely to inhibit the anabolic response.
3. Timing of protein and carbohydrate intake should be determined individually given the training and competitive demands of the athlete, as well as the overall energy, protein, and carbohydrate goals of the diet.

11 Industry, Innovation, and Nutrient Timing in Sports Nutrition

Robert Wildman and Mark Haub

CONTENTS

11.1 INTRODUCTION

Numerous nutritional factors have appeared in the marketplace over the last half century purported to enhance physical status or athletic performance. Among the many ingredients are creatine; β-hydroxy β-methylbutyric acid (HMB); carnitine; proteins; amino acids (e.g., leucine, glutamine, arginine, and ornithine); herbs (e.g., *Tribulus terristrus*, grape seed extract, ginseng); and minerals (e.g., zinc, magnesium, boron and chromium). Many of these ingredients have appeared in different forms (e.g., chelated compounds, organic components, etc.). While some of these nutritional factors have proven to be worthy of consideration for general dietary support in meeting the augmented needs of athletes and serious exercisers, additional concepts have emerged over the past decades that have helped to sculpt the strategy of their use and degree of efficacy. Nutrient timing, or more specifically the strategic consumption of specific nutrients and level in accordance to a training session or competition, has become one of those important concepts. As an example, with all other factors controlled, ingesting a protein supplement instead of dinner six hours after a resistance training session probably will not have a favorable impact on net protein balance as long as the level of total protein, calories, and other key nutrients are matched for the day. Meanwhile, an acute increase in net protein synthesis due to taking that same protein supplement immediately after a resistance training session versus not eating for several hours suggests that postexercise is a critical timing point with regard to net protein turnover, especially when protein accretion is considered incrementally over numerous training sessions (Tipton and Ferrando 2008). The concept of nutrient timing is valuable to endurance sports as well, and companies have been working feverishly over the past decade or so to investigate reformulations of their sport beverages to keep up with science and their competition to provide better and effective products for consuming athletes.

In more recent years, sport nutrition companies have sought to leverage nutrient timing in the marketing of products. This has bolstered the *when* component of the *who, what, when, why,* and *how much* approach to sport nutrition marketing. What is more, the concept of nutrient timing has augmented efforts to develop novel compounds as well as modify existing, established nutrients in sports nutrition. In this chapter, we consider some of the avenues taken by sport nutrition companies and review the support for some individual nutrients and combinations with regard to nutrient timing.

11.2   INDUSTRY OPPORTUNITIES FOR NUTRIENT TIMING INNOVATION

The idea of creating specific nutrient forms and formulations that can have an impact on the efficacy of nutrient timing is intriguing to sport nutrition companies for several reasons. First, it strengthens the marketability of products, which in turn can lead to a higher retail price. Second, it allows for the invention of new nutrient concepts or the reinvention of certain high-profile nutrients to market a *competitive advantage* or *point of differentiation* in an aggressive and crowded, yet highly lucrative, sport nutrition marketplace. *Nutrition Business Journal* reported that the total sales in the combined sport nutrition and weight loss industry was roughly $23 billion in 2010 and would continue to climb ("Sport Nutrition and Weight Loss Report" 2011). Of that, sales of sport nutrition supplements such as pills and powders contributed over 14%, with sport/energy beverages contributing roughly 57% (Figure 11.1). In general, there are several opportunities for innovation for sport nutrition companies with regard to nutrient timing. These include before (pre-), during (peri-, intra-), and after (post-) training or competition as summarized in Figure 11.2. As such, nutrients can be manipulated and combined with other ingredients to create novel delivery systems and marketing opportunities.

11.2.1   FAST NUTRIENTS

The stress of exercise training and competition is significant, and the perception of *timing is critical* is very real to athletes, serious weight trainers, and fitness

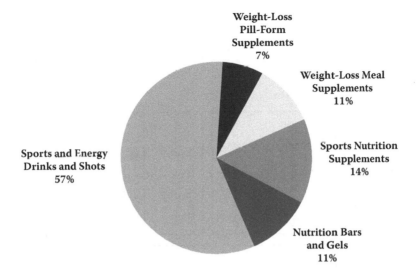

FIGURE 11.1 U.S. sports nutrition and weight loss sales by product category. From *Nutrition Business Journal Sport Nutrition & Weight Loss Report*, 2011.

enthusiasts. It simply makes sense to these individuals that nutrients brought into their body just before, during, or immediately after exercise can enhance performance, recovery, or adaptation. Sport brands such as Gatorade® and Accelerade® were founded on rapid delivery of nutrients either immediately before or during exercise and postexercise in more recent years. Target nutrients within the sport nutrition industry include energy substrates, primarily carbohydrate and certain amino acids, medium-chain triglycerides; support nutrients, including caffeine (and analog sources), creatine, branched-chain amino acids, glycerol, carnitine, arginine/citrulline, and electrolytes or "sweat mimetics"; the latter of which tend to be provided in a water matrix (hydrating fluid).

Athletes seek products that they can take immediately before (e.g., less than 30 minutes prior to) or during performance. Packages, magazine or Web ads, or product brochures and other sales pieces often provide an image of an individual drinking an RTD (ready-to-drink) energy beverage in the gym or a tight shot of a sweaty, muscular arm crushing a two-ounce drink purported to raise nitric oxide levels and increase blood flow to muscle. The goal is to create the perception that the product was having an immediate impact on performance, like lighting a short fuse or pumping high-octane fuel in the gas tank of a car. However, what the ads do not convey are some of the main considerations that have an impact on the timing, including how quickly and efficiently the product will be digested and its nutrients absorbed thus becoming available to working muscle or other parts of the body (e.g., central nervous system) that can have an impact on performance. Most water-soluble nutrients will be absorbed into the portal vein on their way to the liver prior to circulation and potential integration into tissue. Among the nutrients that are deemed as "fast" are certain carbohydrates and protein fractions as well as particular hydrolysates, which are discussed further in this chapter.

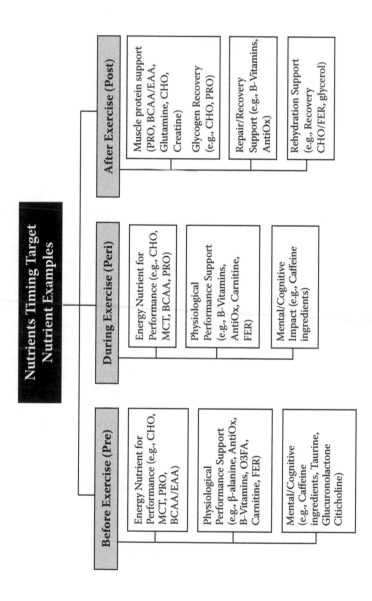

FIGURE 11.2 Examples of nutrient timing for target nutrients by industry. Note: Before Exercise = less than 60 minutes prior to exercise; During Exercise = onset/during training or competition; After Exercise = 30 to 60 minutes after completion or throughout the day after intense training or competition; CHO = carbohydrate; PRO = protein; BCAA = branched-chain amino acids; EAA = essential amino acids; AntiOx = antioxidants; O3FA = omega-3 fatty acids; MCT = medium-chain triglycerides; FER = fluid and electrolyte replacement.

11.2.2 Nutrient Forms

Several options exist for sport nutrition companies to consider with regard to nutrient form and how it applies to nutrient timing concepts. For instance, naturally occurring differences in form (e.g., glycated/aglycone forms), chelations, and molecular modifications via processing can have an impact on gastrointestinal transit rate, absorption rate and efficiency, or locations, as well as timing and level of bioavailability. Furthermore, manipulating nutrient form provides an opportunity to reinvent ingredients and possibly increase the retail price of a product that utilizes it as a "hero" ingredient. This has been the case with creatine and the amino acid leucine.

Manufacturers can combine nutrients with additional factors known to influence the speed of absorption of associated ingredients, which could also potentially influence its endpoint efficacy. For instance, some supplements contain extracts of black pepper (*Piper nigrum*) and long pepper (*Piper longum*) based on the recognized positive effect of key active compounds (e.g., piperine) on digestion/absorption time and bioavailability of certain compounds (Srinivasan 2007). One such product is FAST-C® which combines L-ascorbic acid (vitamin C) with Bioperine®, a commercialized black pepper and long pepper extract with a high content of piperine. Elsewhere, L-carnitine tartrate is produced by the Swiss company Lonza under the commercial name CarniPure®. Carnitine is a naturally occurring compound found in various tissues of the body and is linked to fat oxidation. Supplementation of L-carnitine L-tartrate at two grams daily was reported to have a positive impact on biochemical markers of purine metabolism (i.e., hypoxanthine, xanthine oxidase); free-radical formation (malondialdehyde); muscle tissue disruption (myoglobin, creatine kinase); and muscle soreness after physical exertion (Ho et al. 2010). Researchers have yet to demonstrate that acute ingestion of carnitine can have similar benefits on fat oxidation. What is more, time will tell if carnitine should be strategically consumed from a timing perspective (e.g., postexercise) and with specific levels/types of carbohydrate and protein for greater muscle integration and long-term benefit as one recent study suggests (Wall et al. 2011).

In addition, manufacturers can look to market naturally occurring metabolites, or precursors of key nutrients, that might be critical in short- or long-duration performance. One example is β-alanine, an amino acid that is not used in protein synthesis but is used as a precursor of carnosine, a key acid-buffering factor in skeletal muscle (Harris et al. 2006; Hill et al. 2007). At present, 400 to 800 milligrams of β-alanine are recommended several times daily to achieve a target dose approximating 3 grams daily to reduce the likelihood of symptoms of paresthesia, which are observed in some people when a single dose exceeds 800 milligrams. While this effect is currently employed by some bodybuilding brands to elicit a palpable or "tangible" effect before exercise, other athletes might find the experience unpleasant or distracting. Meanwhile, PowerBar® has a global exclusive license to a modified release β-alanine that is believed to lower paresthesia. At present, opportunities remain to better understand the strategic timing of ingestion of this ingredient and from different sources or in different forms or nutrient combinations. Some brands are applying β-alanine in a timing-based product. For instance, Pro Science FINISH™ by EAS® recommends taking this β-alanine-based product within 60 minutes of completing a training session.

In another example, α-ketoisocaproate (KIC) and HMB are leucine metabolites that have been reported to increase net protein turnover and fat-free mass development, with considerations being taken for the training status of the individual (Zanchi et al. 2011). Certainly, there is a lot of opportunity to better understand if strategic timing of ingestion is warranted even though these ingredients are viewed as daily supplements to be taken over several weeks. However, preliminary research suggests that while consumption of three grams of HMB immediately before or after a damaging exercise bout does not have an impact on performance, there are suggestions that it might reduce markers of cell damage, and nonsignificant trending of data also suggests that there might be a minor effect on the delayed onset of muscle soreness (Wilson et al. 2009). Further still, manufacturers can utilize modified raw ingredients that can alter aspects of digestion, intestinal transit, or absorption rate. Two examples are PeptoPro®, which is a casein hydrolysate, short-chain peptide delivery system, and Vitargo®, an enzymatically modified starch designed for faster digestion/absorption and muscle glycogen restoration.

11.2.3 PHASIC, TIME-RELEASED, OR LONG-ACTING NUTRIENT DELIVERY

The notion of a phasic, time-released, or long-acting approach formulation to have an impact on nutrient timing is rooted in the understanding that recovery and adaptation from an exercise training session or competitive bout can take several hours and up to a day or more depending on the type, intensity, and duration of the challenge as well as the level of training of the individual. For instance, it has been noted that the effects of a resistance training session on protein turnover can last for several hours and up to 24 hours (Chesley et al. 1992). Meanwhile, the complete recovery of muscle glycogen stores in muscle can take up to a full day as well if glycogen stores are reduced to nadir levels during exercise (Wildman et al. 2010).

Milk proteins are often separated into "fast" and "slow" proteins as well. Here, the faster proteins tend to be whey based, and the slower are casein based (Boirie et al. 1997). While classifying these protein fractions as such is not really that simple and many physiological factors can have an impact on this concept, the concept does make sense to athletes and bodybuilders and has proven to be very marketable. Some of the reasons for the acceptance of multiphase protein delivery are based on the perceived need to deliver amino acids to challenged muscle fibers as soon as possible after completing exercise. In addition, it is common knowledge among bodybuilders and serious weight trainers that net muscle protein turnover mechanics are influenced for several hours after a training session. As a testament, many articles in popular muscle magazines often point to the strategic combination of whey and casein proteins as part of an optimal nutrition profile training recovery for several hours postexercise.

Carbohydrates have also been classified based on speed of delivery, again establishing some fertile ground for marketing carbohydrate combinations in a timing sequence manner. Interestingly, the preliminary thinking was that simpler carbohydrates, in lieu of their size and form, would be absorbed more quickly. However, one of the key understandings in sport nutrition research over the past couple decades is that osmolality and digestability are critical factors that can dictate movement through the stomach

TABLE 11.1
Relative Properties of Different Carbohydrates

Carbohydrate Type	Molecular Size	Digestibility/ Absorption[a]	Glycemic Effect[b]	Insulinemic Effect[b]
Glucose (dextrose)	Very small	Fast	High	High
Fructose	Very small	Very slow	Very low	Very low
Sucrose	Very small	Moderate	Moderate	Moderate
Corn syrup	Medium	Fast	High	High
High-fructose corn syrup (HFCS)[c]	Medium	Moderate	Moderate	Moderate
Maltodextrin	Medium	Fast	High	High
Waxy maize starch (WMS)	Large	Slow	Low	Low
Vitargo®	Very large	Very fast	Very high	Very high
Amylose	Large	Very slow	Very low	Very low

[a] Assumes similar absorption rates of postdigestion glucose. Fructose will be absorbed by a slower process than glucose.
[b] Due to limitations in research data availability and industry information some of the values on this table are based on estimations. Also, these properties are based on independent effect. Properties can be modified when integrated into more complex food and supplement formulations.
[c] Assumes commonly used HFCS-55 (55% fructose).

to facilitate substrate exposure to various amylases and disaccharidases for compete digestion and monosaccharide absorption transport systems. Thus, researchers are beginning to understand that certain larger, higher molecular weight carbohydrates that have a lower osmolality can have similar and potentially faster monosaccharide (e.g., glucose) entry into circulation and delivery to muscle. Table 11.1 provides an overview of different carbohydrates used in sport nutrition products and their characteristics.

Sport nutrition companies have also looked to precursor molecules that might provide a timing advantage. An example would be to utilize the alanine precursor citrulline as a potential means of producing nitric oxide. While arginine remains the direct precursor of nitric oxide, it is subject to breakdown in the wall of the digestive tract as well as in serum via various arginases (Luiking et al. 2010). Citrulline, on the other hand, enjoys greater longevity and is used as a means to create a time-released nitric oxide system along with arginine and possibly other factors such as grapeseed extract, which also has some supporting evidence of impacting the nitric oxide system (Edirisinghe et al. 2008; Luiking et al. 2010). Or, manufacturers can utilize delivery systems known to deliver components in a time-delayed fashion. For instance, placing ingredients in the core of the coated tablet can slow their delivery. Meanwhile, some tablet and soft gel technologies have a two-layer design that allows for a time-released system.

11.3 MARKETING INNOVATION

Scientific breakthrough, secret weapons, and patented technologies are all important marketing concepts in the sport nutrition industry. The stakes are high, and the brand that is able to convince the consumer that it has the best science, cutting edge technology, and intellectual property that will result in the physical or performance outcome the consumer seeks will be successful. Thus, marketing messages and claims are a key consideration in industry innovation, and it is critical to clearly convey the points of difference as well as create consumer "buy-in" of the innovation in relation to the ergogenic properties of the product.

11.3.1 New Technology for Old Ingredients

Often, when a new blockbuster ingredient breaks into the market, either with or without proven efficacy, supply of the raw ingredient fails to meet demand as more companies look to apply it. As a result, the raw ingredient costs more, which in turn raises the product price tag for consumers. However, with time, supply becomes better able to meet demand, and the price of the raw ingredient decreases. When this happens, brands will lower the finished product price to gain market share.

Creatine monohydrate, arguably the most efficacious nutritional supplement ingredient for increasing fat-free mass and strength in novice weightlifters (Kreider 2003), provided a clear example of this. The retail price of creatine monohydrate supplements was higher in the mid-1990s and then decreased over the next decade as supply increased. New creatine forms and combination ingredient systems continue to pop up annually, including creatine ethyl ester, creatine malate (di- and tri- forms), creatine citrate, micronized creatine, and creatine orate; however, none has demonstrated a real advantage to creatine monohydrate based on cost and physiological efficacy (Spillane et al. 2009). Thermolife International LLC patented and released creatine nitrate, a new development that remains to be proven efficaceous by university researchers.

11.3.2 Product Programs/Kits

Many sport nutrition brands create product suites in which one or more specific products are to be consumed in conjunction with the different phases of a training session or competition. Certainly, this concept is not new within the bodybuilding community; however, in more recent years products have been named or taglines including terms such as "pre-" or "post-" have appeared on labels based on the recognition of such prefixes from magazine and Web site articles and talk at the gym. Some Web sites of retailers will even categorize products based on pre-, during, and postexercise. Gatorade has brought to market the G series, which includes Prime, Perform, and Recover, which specifically target pre-, during, and posttraining or competition timing. Meanwhile, EAS markets Pro Science Finish products that are to be consumed within 60 minutes of completing training, as mentioned previously.

11.3.3 Research Marketing

Marketing of sport nutrition products has endured eras during which it seemed that companies could make all types of claims with little to no applicable research to determine proof of efficacy for the consumer. Bar graphs and exaggerated graphics and photographs suggesting effects were common to packaging, as were statements in relation to patented or patent-pending ingredients or manufacturing technologies displayed on the principal display panel (front panel) and on the information panel or often inserted into the supplement facts panel or ingredients. Research and intellectual property (e.g., patents, proprietary blends) are very marketable, and companies use these tools in an attempt to create points of differentiation between their product and that of the competition.

In 1994, the U.S. federal government signed into law the Dietary Supplements Health and Education Act (DSHEA), which provided a set of guidelines for the supplement industry. By and large, DSHEA restricted the ability of the Food and Drug Administration (FDA) to exert authority over supplements as long as manufacturers made no claims that their products treated, prevented, or cured diseases. Thus, the sport nutrition industry has enjoyed a long run of making exaggerated or misleading claims regarding physical development or performance, and caveat emptor (Latin for "let the buyer beware") became the general rule for consumers. The FDA and Federal Trade Commission (FTC) have stepped in periodically and issued warning letters, levied lawsuits, and indeed did ban certain substances, such as ephedrine and androstenedione, from use in supplements in 2004.

Interestingly, the sport nutrition industry has demonstrated some degree of self-regulation over the past couple of decades, and there has been the emergence of ingredients and brands based on research trials that are setting the bar for the industry. Thus, the classic marketing strategy of showing pictures of muscular men in lab coats with a beaker of colored fluid, a clipboard, and swooning scantily clad women as lab techs has begun to give way to university-trained exercise scientists and properly designed human trials involving potentially ergogenic ingredients and finished products. For instance, EAS set the standard in the 1990s with several studies performed at universities and involving creatine monohydrate and HMB. MuscleTech and Pro Performance (GNC) and newer brands such as GENR8 and 8-Ball (FSI) have continued this tradition, and much of the research involves nutrient timing concepts.

Research validation of sport nutrition products is critical for the credibility of the industry in the consumer's mind and is now necessary as the FDA recently made more demands for substantiation of supplement claims made on packaging and other marketing pieces. In December 2008, the FDA released a Guidance for Industry on "Substantiation for Dietary Supplement Claims Made Under Section 403(r) (6) of the Federal Food, Drug, and Cosmetic Act" (FDA 2008). This communication states that the standards for substantiation are competent and reliable scientific evidence, which subsequently was defined in FTC case law as "tests, analyses, research, studies, or other evidence based on the expertise of professionals in the relevant area, that has been conducted and evaluated in an objective manner by persons qualified to do so, using procedures generally accepted in the profession to yield accurate and reliable results."

It was also noted that although there is no preestablished formula regarding how many or what type of studies are needed to substantiate a claim, the FDA will consider what the accepted norms are in the relevant research fields and consult experts from various disciplines. If there is an existing standard for substantiation developed by a government agency or other authoritative body, the FDA may accord some deference to that standard.

In determining whether the substantiation standard has been met with competent and reliable scientific evidence, the FDA (2009) recommends that supplement companies consider the following issues in their assessment (each of these issues is discussed further in this guidance):

1. The meaning of the claim(s) being made;
2. The relationship of the evidence to the claim;
3. The quality of the evidence; and
4. The totality of the evidence.

Basically, products need to be comprised of quality ingredients that are safe to consume. What is more, efficacy studies should involve people and in conditions, consumption levels, and so on that have direct application to real-world uses. Studies should minimize any confounding factors as well as include a placebo. Further still, double-blind evaluation is most ideal for removing bias on the part of the participants or researchers. Last, research needs to be published in peer-reviewed journals, subjected to the scrutiny of peer researchers and scientists, and be reproducible in other labs by unrelated researchers and without any conflicts of interest.

11.4   INNOVATIONS IN SPECIFIC NUTRIENTS

As discussed, there are many nutrient categories that sport nutrition companies can explore for developing finished products. These include protein, protein hydrolysates, amino acids or known metabolites, processed carbohydrates, nutrient chelates, and more. This section is a general overview of some types of nutrients or products that have demonstrated innovation and had research support.

11.4.1   Protein Innovations

Athletes continue to regard protein as one, if not the most, important energy nutrient, with good reason: Protein is the predominant nonwater component of muscle tissue, contributing more than 80% of the dry weight. Protein consumption is woven throughout their diet, and over the past decade or so the notion that protein timing is an important consideration has been in the spotlight along with protein needs, which are augmented for athletes and other people who train seriously (Tipton and Ferrando 2008). Further still, research performed on different protein sources (e.g., milk vs. soy) (Phillips et al. 2009; Wilkinson et al. 2007) and within the same protein type (Cribb et al. 2006) have suggested that all protein may not be the same with regard to potential impact on muscle tissue of athletes and exercisers.

During exercise, delivery of protein along with carbohydrate has been reported to provide potential benefit. For instance, in one study involving cyclists, the consumption of a carbohydrate and protein beverage (7.3% carbohydrate and 1.8% protein) and a carbohydrate-only (7.3%) beverage in two rides to exhaustion at 75% and 85% VO_2Peak separated by 12 to 15 hours resulted in improvements in performance (Saunders et al. 2004). The addition of the protein to the carbohydrate resulted in 29% improvements in endurance performance during a 75% VO_2Peak ride to voluntary exhaustion followed by a 40% improvement in the follow-up 85% VO_2Peak ride to exhaustion. In addition, peak postexercise plasma creatine phosphate kinase levels, indicative of muscle damage, were 83% lower after the trial of carbohydrate plus protein (Saunders et al. 2004). Of note, other studies have also reported a similar impact of protein (and in different delivery forms) in addition to carbohydrate on performance or muscle damage indices as well as the delayed onset of muscle soreness (Romano-Ely et al. 2006; Saunders et al. 2007). While the true mechanism behind the positive findings in these studies has been challenged as an added energy affect (Toone and Betts 2010; Valentine et al. 2008; van Essen and Gibala 2006), it would be hard to challenge that this does represent an industry attempt at formula innovation that in turn has led to a marketing platform.

During periods of perceived need, protein cannot get into circulation of athletes soon enough. However, many proteins are complex, three-dimensional structures that need to be denatured and digested. It has been long held that individual amino acids are the only absorbable form of protein. Part of this thinking was based on the discovery and understanding of individual amino acid transporters on the mucosal surface of the small intestine and cell membranes. Also, it is individual amino acids that are coded for in the genes that trillions of cells in the human body use as building blocks to construct protein. However, this concept was reshaped in the last quarter of the twentieth century based on our evolving understanding of alternative transport systems and processes such as pinocytosis. This helped drive innovation in protein delivery timing.

Capitalizing on this notion, DSM, a major ingredient supplier, produced a casein hydrolysate called PeptoPro®, which is greater than 60% dipeptides and tripeptides generated via a patented enzyme system. DSM contends that the dipeptides and tripeptides produced by this process are more readily absorbed, leading to faster delivery into circulation, thus getting to muscle and other tissues more quickly. In one exercise study, the combination of carbohydrate with PeptoPro improved cycling time trial performance versus straight carbohydrate alone (Saunders et al. 2009). Participants consumed 200 milliliters of carbohydrate (6%) or a combination of carbohydrate (6% or 60 grams per liter) and PeptoPro beverage (1.8% or 18 grams per liter) every five kilometers and 500 milliliters of beverage immediately postexercise. The researchers reported that late-exercise time trial performance was enhanced by the addition of PeptoPro as the cyclists were 1.6% faster in the final 20 kilometers, reducing their time by 43 seconds, and 2.5% faster in the last five-kilometer climb, reducing cycling time by 25 seconds. It was also of note that ingestion of carbohydrate plus PeptoPro prevented increases in plasma creatine kinase, a marker of muscle tissue damage, and the delayed onset of muscle soreness after exercise (Saunders et al. 2009). In a resistance training study, the addition of PeptoPro to carbohydrate (6% protein and 12% protein) led to greater insulin release and glucose disposal than solutions with protein only (6%) and protein (6%) plus 3% carbohydrate (Koopman et al. 2007). DSM has funded other research studies involving PeptoPro and aspects related to digestion/absorption or performance, making it one of the most researched branded ingredients available to sport nutrition companies (Beelen, Koopman, et al. 2008; Beelen, Tieland, et al. 2008; Kaastra et al. 2006; Verdijk, Jonkers, et al. 2009).

11.4.2 Carbohydrate Innovations

The need for carbohydrate is a foremost thought among athletes. Carbohydrate consumed hours before training or competition helps to maximize muscle glycogen stores, while carbohydrate during training or competition will help fuel working muscle as well as maintain blood glucose levels (Coyle 1992; Coyle et al. 1991). Glucose is the primary carbohydrate fuel for working muscle, and its contribution to total energy increases relative to exercise intensity and decreases with prolonged duration secondary to waning muscle glycogen (Romijn et al. 1993, 2000). Clearly, maximizing glycogen content before and after exercise training and competition is crucial for optimal performance in many sports. Carbohydrate consumption during exercise increases the availability of carbohydrate to working muscle fibers, which can have a positive influence on endurance performance as well as intermittent high-intensity performance, the latter of which could be applicable to sports such as football, ice hockey, and soccer (Kreider et al. 2010; Wildman et al. 2010).

While it was long believed that simpler carbohydrates, in lieu of less digestive requirements, would be absorbed quicker than larger starch molecules, recent research efforts have not supported this notion. Researchers have been testing larger, higher molecular weight carbohydrates in an attempt to hasten transit through the stomach and allow for faster digestion and absorption. In one such study, cyclists ingested one gram per kilogram of either glucose, resistant starch (70% amylose/30% amylopectin), 100% amylopectin (waxy maize), or a placebo in an 18.7% carbohydrate solution 30 minutes before a 90-minute ride at 66% VO_2Peak, which was followed by a 30-minute isokinetic performance trial (Goodpaster et al. 1996). Serum glucose and insulin levels were significantly higher 15 minutes after the cyclists ingested glucose compared to the other treatments. Likewise, after 30 minutes and just prior to exercise onset, serum insulin levels were still higher for the glucose treatment trial. When compared to placebo, carbohydrate oxidation was greater in the glucose, resistant starch, and amylopectin trials when compared to placebo, and performance was greater in the glucose and amylopectin trials. However, oxidation and performance did not differ between the different carbohydrate types.

Vitargo (Swecarb) is a starch molecule produced via a patented mild acid extraction process and marketed in the United States and other countries by GENR8. Preliminary research does support the hypothesis that glucose from Vitargo is more rapidly absorbed than other carbohydrate sources (Leiper et al. 2000; Piehl Aulin et al. 2000; Stephens et al. 2008). This effect is probably based on lower osmolality, high digestability, and rapid emptying into the small intestine from the stomach (Leiper et al. 2000). In one study, well-trained men endured glycogen-depleting exercise and then consumed 75 grams of Vitargo or a glucose/maltodextrin solution (low molecular weight, high osmolality) immediately after and at 30, 60, and 90 minutes postexercise (Piehl Aulin et al. 2000). It was reported that the high molecular weight, processed carbohydrate solution led to a 68% faster glycogen recovery within the first two hours of recovery. Elsewhere, eight healthy men were provided 100 grams of Vitargo or a glucose/maltodextrin solution after cycling to exhaustion at approximately 73% VO_2Peak (Stephens et al. 2008). Participants then rested for two hours before completing a 15-minute time trial. During the resting period, both blood glucose and insulin were significantly higher in the high molecular weight carbohydrate group as compared to the glucose/maltodextrin trial. In addition, work output for the high molecular weight carbohydrate group was significantly greater (average 10% higher) during a 15-minute time trial that began two hours after completion of the initial exhaustive exercise bout (Stephens et al. 2008).

11.4.3 Sport Drink Innovations

Nutrient delivery immediately before and during athletic performance can have an impact on performance and recovery (Kreider et al. 2010; Wildman et al. 2010). While Gatorade launched the sport drink industry about a half century ago with a fluid-and-electrolyte replacement containing a simple carbohydrate source, over the past couple decades some researchers have been focusing efforts on the addition of other nutrients, including protein, B vitamins, additional minerals, and other nutrients to sport drinks. Among the major players in the sport drink industry are Gatorade (Pepsi-Cola), Powerade (Coca-Cola), and Accelerade (Mott's). In addition, Cytomax (Cytosport), Amino Vital (Ajinomota), Heed (Hammer Nutrition), and Vitargo S2 (GENr8) are capturing respectable portions of the market share. Table 11.2 presents some of the key players and example products from their portfolios and comparative nutrient compositions. Perhaps in no other category of the sport nutrition market is finished product research so obvious. In fact, Gatorade built the Gatorade Sport Science Institute in 1988 as the physical structure where much of the research is conducted, analyzed, or shared with professionals and consumers (http://www.gssi-web.com/). Gatorade continues a steady stream of performance-based research in their facility as well as in more practical settings (J.W. Smith et al. 2010; Stover et al. 2006).

Another good example was the first widely available sport drink that combined carbohydrate and protein; it has a patent on a 4:1 ratio and delivers simple sugars (e.g., sucrose, fructose) in combination with whey protein (e.g., whey protein isolate and whey protein concentrates). Accelerade has funded several research studies that support its claims of improved aspects of performance and recovery (Harmon et al. 2007; Ivy et al. 2003; Saunders et al. 2005, 2006, 2007; Valentine et al. 2006). In one study, 17 cyclists completed a series of four by two kilometer time trials on a cycle ergometer at a load corresponding to their lactate threshold (Harmon et al. 2007). During the challenge, they drank 354 milliliters of either Accelerade or a flavored placebo 15 minutes prior to their first sprint, 472 milliliters after the first sprint, and 295 milliliters after the second and third sprint. After the first sprint, a 60-minute rest interval was provided, and 30 minutes separated the remaining sprints. The average finishing time was 177 ± 12.1 seconds when Accelerade was provided and 181 ± 10.5 seconds when the flavored placebo was provided. It was also reported that the last sprint was statistically faster for the Accelerade trial and the degree of decline in sprint performance was significantly less as well. Blood glucose was greater ($p < .05$) for Accelerade than placebo before and after the third and fourth sprints.

TABLE 11.2

Comparison of Carbohydrate and Protein Content of Common Commercially Available Sport Drinks

Ingredients per 8 fl oz	Carbohydrate Content (%)	Carbohydrates (g)	Protein (g)	Calories	Sodium (mg)	Potassium (mg)	Other Nutrients	Caffeine (mg)
Accelerade® (RTD)	6	15	4	80	120	15	Vitamin E, calcium	0
Amino Vital Endurance® (RTD)	5.5	13	2.4	40	110	35	Vitamin C, magnesium, calcium	0
Cytomax® Performance Plus (RTD)	5	13	0	50	55	30	MCT, vitamin C, chromium	0
Gatorade G®02 Perform	6	14	0	50	110	30		0
Gatorade G®02 Endurance Formula	6	14	0	50	200	90		0
Gatorade G®03 Recover	3	7	8	60	120	45	Calcium	0
Heed Performance (RTM)	5	13	<1	50	20	13	Vitamin B$_6$, calcium, chromium, magnesium, manganese, tyrosine, carnosine, glycine	0
Powerade ION4®	6	14	0 g	50	100	25	Vitamins B$_3$, B$_6$, and B$_{12}$, calcium, magnesium	0
Vitargo S2® (RTM)	10	23	0 g	93	0	0		0

RTD = Ready to drink; RTM = Ready to mix

Accelerade is a registered trademark of Mott's LLP.

Amino Vital is a registered trademark of Ajinomoto.

Cytomax is a registered trademark of Cytosport Inc.

Gatorade and Propel are trademarks of Stokely-Van Camp Inc.

Heed is a registered trademark of Hammer Nutrition Inc.

Powerade is a registered trademark of the Coca-Cola Company.

Propel is a registered trademark of PepsiCo.

Vitargo is a registered trademark of SweCarb.

11.4.4 Summary Guidelines to Consumers

Athletes are in constant pursuit of finding effective, safe, and legal compounds to ingest to improve their performance. With recent advances and the newfound rapidity with which new evidence becomes available, it is imperative that companies and consumers be wary of pitfalls. Namely, when making claims or applying data to products, it is critical that study details are noted correctly and delivered in the appropriate context as misunderstanding the dose, administration procedure (i.e., timing, recipe/concentration), and applicable athletes or sports can lead to deleterious performance, as may occur with alkalizing agents (e.g., sodium citrate or sodium bicarbonate). If the directions for use are not clear, an athlete may inappropriately use a product and judge it as ineffective. This process may lead to product issues down the line even if the product has clinical data to indicate an ergogenic response.

Moreover, athletes need to be aware that it may take more than one use to "get acquainted" with a product. There may be an initial negative response that may resolve itself or the product may be better tolerated with subsequent uses. If a product is truly effective, then there typically is a "side effect" that might be new. For example, the ingestion of caffeine at an effective dose by someone who is caffeine naive may elicit an unpleasant response when first exposed. That response may resolve itself after several exposures.

11.5 CONCLUSIONS

Innovation is a key driver in the sport nutrition industry. Creating specific nutrient forms and formulations that can have an impact on the efficacy of nutrient timing is intriguing to sport nutrition companies for several reasons. First, as mentioned, it strengthens the marketability of products, which in turn can lead to a higher retail price. Second, it allows for the invention of new nutrient concepts or the reinvention of certain high-profile nutrients to market a competitive advantage in an aggressive and crowded, yet highly lucrative, sport nutrition marketplace. The sport nutrition industry has demonstrated several instances of innovation with regard to carbohydrates, proteins, and sport drinks that have direct application to delivery timing and performance. Some companies have been investing in research studies to demonstrate the efficacy of their products. This trend will continue and continue to shape the sport nutrition industry in the twenty-first century, and an ongoing research will lead to a better understanding of nutritional timing and its impact on performance, recovery, and physique.

12 The Impact of Protein Source on Timing Considerations for Health and Performance

Tyler Churchward-Venne and Stu Phillips

CONTENTS

12.1 INTRODUCTION

The benefits imbued on those individuals possessing a large quantity of skeletal muscle mass are numerous and gaining a greater appreciation within the scientific and clinical community. Beyond the well-known relationship between skeletal muscle size and strength, skeletal muscle is thought to play an important role in reducing the risk for diseases such as obesity, osteoporosis, cardiovascular disease, insulin resistance, and diabetes (Wolfe 2006). For example, skeletal muscle represents the largest body reservoir for the disposal of postprandial blood glucose, thus declines in skeletal muscle mass and quality (i.e., ability to transport, store, and oxidize glucose) may play an important role in the etiology of insulin resistance and diabetes. As such, factors capable of enhancing skeletal muscle mass and metabolic quality are likely to be clinically relevant as they may represent effective strategies to attenuate and even reverse the loss of skeletal muscle that is associated with conditions such as cancer, sarcopenia (age-related muscle loss), and bed rest.

The ingestion of intact dietary proteins (Moore, Tang, et al. 2009; Symons et al. 2007; Tang et al. 2009; Tipton et al. 2004; Wilkinson et al. 2007) or ingestion/infusion of free amino acids (Biolo et al. 1997; Bohe et al. 2001, 2003; Tipton, Ferrando, et al. 1999) stimulates the synthesis of muscle proteins, particularly when consumed in the time period following the performance of acute resistance exercise (Biolo et al. 1997; Tang et al. 2009). Recent evidence suggests that the type (i.e., source) of dietary protein consumed is an important consideration, as sources of dietary protein appear to differentially affect the magnitude of protein synthesis both at rest (Boirie et al. 1997; Dangin et al. 2001, 2003; Tang et al. 2009) and after resistance exercise (Tang et al. 2009; Wilkinson et al. 2007). For example, Tang and colleagues (2009) reported that whey protein hydrolysate stimulated an increase in muscle protein synthesis that was significantly greater than micellar casein protein at rest and both casein and soy protein after acute exercise.

These acute findings may explain why sources of dietary protein have also been reported to differ in their ability to support resistance exercise-induced increases in skeletal muscle mass and strength following chronic resistance training (Cribb et al. 2006; Hartman et al. 2007). Cribb and colleagues (2006) reported that supplementation with whey protein in conjunction with resistance exercise resulted in gains in lean mass that were approximately fivefold greater than those that were observed following supplementation with casein. Hayes and Cribb (2008) have suggested that the type of dietary protein consumed may influence the response to resistance exercise based on fundamental differences in (1) the constituent amino acid profile of the protein, (2) the rate of digestion/absorption and thus peripheral amino acid availability, (3) the hormonal response following protein ingestion (i.e., insulinogenic response following protein ingestion), and (4) antioxidant properties of the protein.

Indeed, the branched-chain amino acid leucine is independently able to stimulate muscle protein synthesis and phosphorylate factors associated with initiating messenger RNA (mRNA) translation (Anthony et al. 2002; Crozier et al. 2005). Thus, small differences in leucine concentration even between sources of "high-quality" (according to protein digestibility-corrected amino acid scores, PDCAASs) dietary proteins may have important implications from the perspective of maximizing the response of muscle protein synthesis following resistance exercise. In addition, sources of dietary protein have been shown to have differential rates of digestion/ absorption (Boirie et al. 1997), and the digestion rate of a protein has been established to be an independent regulator of postprandial whole-body protein synthesis and breakdown (Dangin et al. 2001).

Thus, the aim of this chapter is to highlight the significance of dietary protein source in maximizing muscle protein anabolism and to examine some of the underlying mechanisms that may explain the differential effects on protein turnover that are observed following ingestion of different protein sources. Current evidence suggests that consumption of fluid bovine milk or whey protein in the early time period after exercise is more advantageous than consumption of soy protein, casein protein, or simply increased energy (i.e., carbohydrate) in terms of promoting muscle accretion (Cribb et al. 2006; Tang et al. 2009; Willoughby et al. 2007). Further, the acute responses that are observed with whey and milk appear to be representative, at least qualitatively, of resistance exercise-induced gains in lean mass that occur following the application of chronic training or feeding with whey or milk ingestion postexercise (Cribb et al. 2006; Hartman et al. 2007).

12.2 NET PROTEIN BALANCE: TIPPING THE SCALE IN FAVOR OF PROTEIN ACCRETION

The balance between protein synthesis and breakdown, net protein balance, is ultimately responsible for determining a net gain or loss of skeletal muscle mass. In the fasted state, the rate of muscle protein breakdown is elevated above the rate of muscle protein synthesis, resulting in a net loss of skeletal muscle protein (muscle catabolism). However, provision of a source of amino acids acts to stimulate muscle protein synthesis, resulting in a positive net protein balance and tissue accretion (Biolo et al. 1997). Interestingly, only the essential amino acids are required for protein synthesis (Tipton, Gurkin, et al. 1999; Volpi et al. 2003), and the absence of nonessential amino acids does not appear to reduce muscle protein synthesis (Volpi et al. 2003). Of the net protein balance equation, protein synthesis is subject to changes in magnitude that may be approximately 10- to 20-fold greater than any measured change in protein breakdown when considering typical fasted- to fed-state transitions in healthy persons (Biolo et al. 1997; Volpi et al. 2003). Thus, interventions capable of augmenting the magnitude or duration of muscle protein synthesis, and not manipulating muscle protein breakdown, are likely to be the most relevant and have much greater phenotypic success in terms of promoting increases in skeletal muscle mass.

When performed in the fasted state, resistance exercise can lead to an increase in both muscle protein synthesis and muscle protein breakdown that is quite prolonged (Phillips et al. 1997); however, net protein balance remains negative because the absolute rate of muscle protein breakdown exceeds that of muscle protein synthesis (Biolo et al. 1995). Provision of both amino acids (Biolo et al. 1997; Tipton, Ferrando, et al. 1999) and carbohydrate (Borsheim et al. 2004) is able to completely attenuate the exercise-induced increase in muscle protein breakdown. Provision of a source of amino acids in close temporal proximity to a bout of resistance exercise has a synergistic effect on muscle protein synthesis, such that the increase in muscle protein synthesis is greater than that elicited from either stimulus alone (Biolo et al. 1997). Thus, the robust increase in muscle protein synthesis and attenuation of muscle protein breakdown in response to combined feeding and exercise results in a positive net protein balance and allows for muscle protein accretion (muscle anabolism). However, to ultimately achieve a detectable increase in skeletal muscle cross-sectional area, resistance exercise must be performed chronically (i.e., several times per week) for multiple weeks. Under such circumstances, the acute periods of positive net protein balance brought about by exercise and feeding summate, such that there is a net gain in muscle protein content and eventually muscle hypertrophy (Phillips 2004).

12.3 INGESTION OF PROTEIN: TIMING RELATIVE TO EXERCISE

As mentioned, provision of a source of amino acids is required after resistance exercise to shift net protein balance from negative to positive (Biolo et al. 1997). Strategically planned intake of dietary proteins in the temporal period immediately surrounding resistance exercise has been reported to enhance training-induced gains in lean mass as compared to the provision of these nutrients at other times, even when daily dietary protein intake is adequate (Andersen et al. 2005; Burk et al. 2009; Cribb et al. 2006; Esmarck et al. 2001; Hartman et al. 2007; Josse et al. 2010). An acute bout of resistance exercise, even in the absence of postexercise feeding, stimulates an increase in mixed muscle protein synthesis that persists for at least 48 hours (Phillips et al. 1997). Thus, it has been suggested (Burd, Tang, et al. 2009) that feeding any time within this 48-hour window should theoretically promote an additive response and elevate protein synthesis to a greater extent than feeding in the absence of exercise. In fact, Burd and colleagues (Burd, Staples, et al. 2009) have shown that an acute bout of resistance exercise, regardless of the load, confers an enhanced "sensitivity" of skeletal muscle to the anabolic effects of amino acids that persists for at least 24 hours after exercise. That is, the acute increase in muscle protein synthesis following ingestion of 15 grams of whey protein isolate was significantly greater 24 hours after acute resistance exercise as compared to the feeding response during resting conditions (Burd, Staples, et al. 2009). However, early provision of a source of amino acids after resistance exercise would appear to confer greater benefit than delayed consumption, as exercise-stimulated increases in the rate of muscle protein synthesis are elevated to a greater extent early (three hours) after resistance exercise than at later time points (i.e., 24 and 48 hours) (Phillips et al. 1997). In addition, it has been shown that cell signaling proteins involved in increasing translation initiation of muscle protein synthesis after resistance exercise, such as mTOR and p70S6 kinase, are activated early and appear to undergo peak phosphorylation (i.e., activation) within 30 to 60 minutes after exercise (Camera et al. 2010). Thus, to take advantage of the so-called anabolic cell-signaling pathways involved in translation initiation that are activated early after resistance exercise, feeding should occur in close temporal proximity to the training stimulus, ideally less than one hour following the cessation of exercise, to potentiate the large increase in muscle protein synthesis that occurs early after exercise.

12.4 PROTEIN SOURCE: ACUTE STUDIES

At the whole-body protein level, ingestion of casein promotes a greater net balance of leucine than whey in young subjects, an effect primarily due to greater suppression of whole-body protein breakdown following casein ingestion (Boirie et al. 1997). Casein represents approximately 80% of the protein found in most commercial bovine milk, with whey protein constituting the other 20%. Whey protein is acid soluble; thus, it passes through the stomach relatively quickly and results in large but transient levels of hyperaminoacidemia (Boirie et al. 1997). In contrast, casein forms a clot in the stomach, resulting in delayed digestion/absorption of the protein and subsequently a more moderate but sustained rise in plasma amino acids (Boirie et al. 1997). Thus, whey has been called a "fast" protein because it induces large but transient levels of hyperaminoacidemia, whereas casein is considered a "slow" protein as it is associated with a moderate but sustained rise in plasma amino acids during the postprandial period (Boirie et al. 1997).

Work by Dangin and colleagues (2001) established that the rate of protein digestion is an independent variable affecting whole-body protein kinetics. For example, casein and repeated boluses of whey (slow digestion paradigm) increased whole-body protein retention in young subjects to a greater degree than a large bolus of whey protein or an amount of free amino acids equivalent to that found in the casein bolus (fast digestion paradigm) (Dangin et al. 2001). However, the elderly respond in the opposite fashion; whole-body protein retention (assessed via leucine balance) is increased to a greater extent in response to an isonitrogenous bolus of whey protein than casein (Dangin et al. 2003). The mechanism(s) explaining the age-related differences in whole-body protein metabolism are not entirely clear, but given that the whey protein beverage contained substantially more leucine than that found in the casein drink (Dangin et al. 2003), it is possible that an elevated requirement for amino acids (leucine in particular) to trigger skeletal muscle protein synthesis exists in the elderly.

How the rate of protein digestion regulates skeletal muscle protein synthesis (as opposed to whole-body protein synthesis) remains to be fully elucidated. For example, ingestion of fat-free fluid milk (745 kilojoules, 18.2 grams of protein, 1.5 grams of fat, and 23 grams of carbohydrate) after an acute bout of resistance exercise has been reported to increase muscle protein synthesis, net amino uptake, and net protein balance measured across the leg to a greater degree than an isonitrogenous, isoenergetic, macronutrient-matched soy protein beverage (Wilkinson et al. 2007). As mentioned, typical bovine milk is composed of both casein (approximately 80%) and whey (approximately 20%) protein. Presumably due to its relatively high casein content, milk is digested somewhat slowly, inducing a more moderate rise in plasma amino acids than soy (Wilkinson et al. 2007). Soy, on the other hand, is a plant-based protein composed of a single homogeneous protein source that induces a more rapid rise in plasma amino acids than milk (Wilkinson et al. 2007). The findings of Wilkinson and colleagues (2007) may be explained in part by previous research showing that digestion rate appears to influence the partitioning of amino acids within the body for use.

For example, soy appears to be preferentially directed toward the splanchnic tissues to support protein synthesis, while milk proteins are partitioned toward peripheral tissues (i.e., skeletal muscle) to support protein synthesis (Bos et al. 2003; Fouillet et al. 2002; Morens et al. 2003). Exactly why the amino acids from milk proteins might be preferentially partitioned to peripheral tissues to support protein synthesis is not entirely clear but may relate to the digestion/absorption kinetics of milk proteins. However, the leucine content of milk proteins is much higher than that of soy, and while total aminoacidemia was more rapid for soy proteins, the leucinemia was actually greater with milk (Wilkinson, S.B. and Phillips, S.M., 2007, unpublished observations). This thesis fits with the concept of some kind of leucine "trigger" existing in muscle (Burd, Tang, et al. 2009).

Interestingly, the type of milk consumed also appears to be an important consideration as Elliot and colleagues (2006) reported differences in net amino acid uptake across the leg after resistance exercise following ingestion of whole milk versus fat-free milk. For example, when comparing whole milk (237 grams), fat-free milk (237 grams), and fat-free milk isocaloric with whole milk (393 grams), net threonine uptake after exercise was positive for all drinks but was 2.8-fold greater with whole milk and 2.5-fold greater with isocaloric fat-free milk than with fat-free milk (Elliot et al. 2006). When expressed as the amount of threonine taken up by the muscle relative to the amount ingested, whole milk was superior to both fat-free milk and an isocaloric amount of fat-free milk (Elliot et al. 2006). How the ingestion of whole milk increased the utilization of available amino acids is not entirely clear; however, additional energy in the form of fat may have played a role as there were no differences in plasma insulin levels following the different drinks (Elliot et al. 2006).

Tang and colleagues (2009) compared the effects of soy protein isolate, whey protein hydrolysate, and micellar casein on rates of skeletal mixed muscle protein synthesis both at rest and after an acute bout of resistance exercise (see Figure 12.1). The increase in mixed muscle protein synthesis at rest following whey hydrolysate was significantly greater than that following micellar casein, but not soy protein isolate. However, following acute exercise, the increase in mixed muscle protein synthesis with whey was significantly greater than both casein and soy (Tang et al. 2009). Whey hydrolysate resulted in significantly greater levels of blood essential amino acids and leucine at 60 minutes postexercise as compared to that seen with soy or casein, suggesting that a more rapid hyperaminoacidemia is important in the whey-induced stimulation of muscle protein synthesis (Tang et al. 2009).

However, Tipton et al (2004) compared the effects of 20 grams of whey protein with an equivalent amount of casein after resistance exercise and were unable to demonstrate a difference in net muscle amino acid balance (using arteriovenous amino acid exchange across the limb) between the two protein sources, despite whey resulting in a significantly greater blood leucine concentration than casein. However, the methodology used in this study (Tipton et al. 2004) precluded the ability to differentiate the specific contribution of protein synthesis and breakdown to the resulting positive net balance following ingestion of each protein source after exercise.

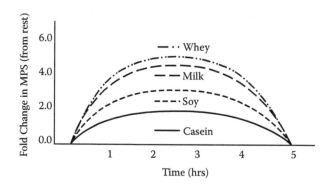

FIGURE 12.1 Feeding-induced change in skeletal muscle protein synthesis (MPS) at rest following ingestion of (1) whey protein, (2) bovine fluid milk, (3) soy protein, and (4) micellar casein protein. (Based on data from Tang, J.E., D.R. Moore, G.W. Kujbida, M.A. Tarnopolsky, and S.M. Phillips. Ingestion of Whey Hydrolysate, Casein, or Soy Protein Isolate: Effects on Mixed Muscle Protein Synthesis at Rest and Following Resistance Exercise in Young Men. *J Appl Physiol* 107(3):987–92, 2009; Wilkinson, S.B., M.A. Tarnopolsky, M.J. Macdonald, J.R. MacDonald, D. Armstrong, and S.M. Phillips. Consumption of Fluid Skim Milk Promotes Greater Muscle Protein Accretion after Resistance Exercise than Does Consumption of an Isonitrogenous and Isoenergetic Soy-Protein Beverage. *Am J Clin Nutr* 85(4):1031–40, 2007.)

Thus, whey may have resulted in a greater stimulation of protein synthesis, whereas casein may have resulted in a greater attenuation of protein breakdown.

Lending additional credence to the notion that an accelerated rate of protein digestion and amino acid availability is an important factor in the postprandial stimulation of muscle protein synthesis is work by Koopman and colleagues (2009) in elderly men. This work shows that ingestion of casein protein hydrolysate is associated with a more rapid protein digestion/absorption rate (and subsequent rate of hyperaminoacidemia) and a trend toward a greater increase in muscle protein synthesis.

Thus, hydrolyzed casein protein tends to exhibit qualities similar to that observed following ingestion of whey; however, whether hydrolyzed whey is any more efficacious at promoting an increase in muscle protein synthesis, at rest or after resistance exercise, as compared to intact whey protein isolate is currently unknown. It is interesting to note, however, that when compared to its constituent essential amino acid content, ingestion of 15 grams of whey protein appears to result in greater protein accretion, at least in elderly subjects (Katsanos et al. 2008). These results suggest that the anabolic properties of whey protein extend beyond its constituent amino acid composition, possibly relating to the insulinotropic properties of whey (Katsanos et al. 2008).

Overall, despite their somewhat divergent digestion/absorption kinetics, fluid milk and whey protein appear to promote a greater postexercise increase in muscle protein synthesis than do soy or micellar casein protein (Tang et al. 2009; Wilkinson et al. 2007). The responses observed with whey and milk in terms of their ability to promote muscle protein anabolism during acute interventions appear to hold up over the long term, as both milk and whey have been reported to promote significantly greater gains in lean mass following chronic resistance training as compared to that achieved with soy protein or carbohydrate consumption (for review, see Phillips et al. 2009).

12.5   PROTEIN SOURCE: CHRONIC STUDIES

A valid question regarding the results generated from acute feeding/exercise studies is whether these findings can be extrapolated to predict, at least qualitatively, the phenotypic response following a period of chronic feeding/exercise. For example, although milk appears to promote greater anabolism than soy in the acute period following resistance exercise (Wilkinson et al. 2007), does chronic milk consumption following a period of resistance exercise training actually result in greater lean mass accrual than chronic soy consumption after exercise? Chronic consumption of fat-free fluid skim milk following 12 weeks of resistance exercise training has been reported to result in greater whole-body lean mass accrual and greater fat mass loss than consumption of soy protein or an energy-matched carbohydrate (Hartman et al. 2007). In addition, studies have documented other examples in which acute findings qualitatively predicted a long-term phenotypic adaptation (West et al. 2009, 2010). Thus, the acute response of muscle protein synthesis to feeding and exercise appears to be qualitatively predictive of the long-term phenotypic adaptations that occur in response to feeding and exercise; however, more studies are required to fully confirm this thesis.

Several studies to date have shown that protein/amino acid supplements, when consumed in close temporal proximity to a bout of resistance exercise, enhance resistance exercise-induced gains in lean mass relative to a placebo or simple carbohydrate following chronic training (Burke, Chilibeck, et al. 2001; Candow, Burke, et al. 2006; Cribb, Williams, Stathis, et al. 2007; Hartman et al. 2007; Josse et al. 2010; Kerksick et al. 2006; Willoughby et al. 2007). However, only a few studies (Brown et al. 2004; Candow, Burke, et al. 2006; Cribb et al. 2006; Hartman et al. 2007) have directly compared the ability of different sources of supplemental dietary protein to augment resistance exercise-based adaptations (see Figure 12.2). For example, Cribb and colleagues (2006) reported that gains in muscle mass were approximately five-fold greater (5.0 kilograms vs. 0.8 kilograms) with supplemental whey protein versus

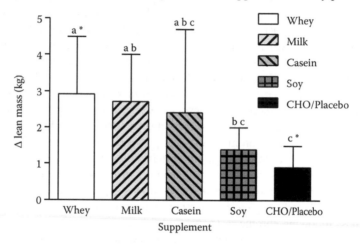

FIGURE 12.2 Resistance exercise training-induced changes in lean body mass in studies of subjects receiving supplemental protein from different sources. A total of 11 studies (Brown et al. 2004; Burke, Chilibeck, et al. 2001; Candow, Burke, et al. 2006; Chromiak et al. 2004; Cribb et al. 2006; Cribb, Williams, Stathis, et al. 2007; Demling and DeSanti 2000; Hartman et al. 2007; Kerksick et al. 2006; Maesta et al. 2007; Rankin et al. 2004) are incorporated ($N = 306$ subjects for all studies; $N = 247$ men and 43 women) into Figure 12.2 with protein supplements of fluid milk (3 studies, $N = 42$ total subjects); whey protein (8 studies, $N = 91$ total subjects); casein protein (2 studies, $N = 20$ total subjects); isolated soy protein (4 studies, $N = 65$ total subjects); or carbohydrate (8 studies, $N = 78$ total subjects). Studies in which other components were included in the supplement (i.e., creatine or crystalline amino acids) were omitted from this analysis unless these compounds were present in all supplements in addition to the protein source itself. All studies were at least 6 weeks in duration and up to as long as 16 weeks (mean = 11.2 weeks). Mean gains in muscle mass as a result of resistance training and protein supplementation were as follows (means ± SD): whey = 2.9 ± 1.6 kilograms (range −0.2 to 5 kilograms); milk = 2.7 ± 1.3 kilograms (range −1.9 to 3.9 kilograms); casein = 2.4 ± 2.3 kilograms (range −0.8 to 4.1 kilograms); soy = 1.4 ± 0.6 kilograms (range −1.1 to 2.0 kilograms); and carbohydrate (CHO)/placebo = 0.9 ± 0.6 kilograms (range −0.3 to 1.8 kilograms). Means were compared with a one-way analysis of covariance adjusting for length of study and age of participants, which showed a main effect for supplement on gains in lean mass. Means were subsequently compared using a Tukey post hoc test. Means with different letters are significantly ($p < .05$) different. Means were also compared to the mean overall gain in lean mass by unpaired t-test assuming unequal variances. An asterisk (*) indicates a significant difference from the overall mean ($p < .05$).

supplemental casein protein following 10 weeks of resistance training in recreational bodybuilders (Cribb et al. 2006).

In addition, Hartman and colleagues (2007) conducted a large ($n = 56$) 12-week resistance exercise training study comparing the effects of postexercise milk consumption relative to an isonitrogenous, isoenergetic, and macronutrient-matched soy protein beverage or a simple carbohydrate drink calorically equivalent to both the milk and soy beverages. Type II muscle fiber area increased with training in all groups; however, the increase was greatest in the group consuming milk after exercise. Similarly, the increase in type I fiber area was greater with milk consumption than soy protein consumption after exercise (Hartman et al. 2007). As might be expected based on the changes in fiber area, whole-body gains in lean mass were also greater in the milk group (6.2% increase) compared to both the soy (4.4% increase) and carbohydrate (3.7% increase) groups (Hartman et al. 2007).

However, Candow and colleagues (2006) examined the effects of whey protein versus soy protein supplementation in conjunction with six weeks of resistance exercise training and reported that, while supplemental protein resulted in greater gains in lean mass than that observed with supplemental carbohydrate, there was no difference in lean mass accrual between the two protein sources (whey = 2.5 kilograms vs. soy = 1.7 kilograms) (Candow, Burke, et al. 2006). These findings are in agreement with earlier work (Brown et al. 2004) that found no difference in lean mass gains between those consuming whey protein bars or those consuming soy protein bars following nine weeks of resistance exercise training. However, the aforementioned studies (Brown et al. 2004; Candow, Burke, et al. 2006) utilized short training periods (six to nine weeks) and experimental groups consisting of a relatively small sample size ($n = 9$). Thus, it is possible that combining training and supplementation for a longer duration (i.e., 12 to 16 weeks and beyond) or increasing the number of subjects to increase statistical power may have resulted in the ability to detect differences in lean mass gains between whey and soy. A review of resistance training-induced gains in lean mass in studies of subjects receiving supplemental protein from different sources concluded that supplemental whey or milk protein ingestion results in greater gains in lean muscle mass than supplemental soy protein or a carbohydrate/placebo (Phillips et al. 2009).

12.6 LEUCINE: A NUTRIENT REGULATOR OF MUSCLE PROTEIN SYNTHESIS

Leucine is a branched-chain amino acid that has been shown to be a key regulator of protein synthesis (Anthony et al. 2002; Crozier et al. 2005). In rats, the independent provision of leucine is able to stimulate muscle protein synthesis and phosphorylate factors associated with initiating mRNA translation through the mTOR signaling pathway, such as p70S6k and 4E-BP1 (Anthony et al. 2002; Crozier et al. 2005). In humans, leucine infusion alone, provided as a large flooding dose, was able to stimulate muscle protein synthesis (Smith et al. 1992). Work in C2C12 myotubes by Atherton and colleagues (2010) has clearly shown that leucine is unique among all of the essential amino acids in its ability to activate anabolic signaling pathways.

For example, of the essential amino acids, only leucine was shown to increase the phosphorylation of mTOR and 4E-BP1, while resulting in the greatest stimulation of p70S6k (Atherton et al. 2010). Thus, given the anabolic potency of leucine as a key regulator of muscle protein synthesis, research has focused on utilizing this amino acid as part of a nutritional strategy to promote muscle protein synthesis (with the ultimate goal of increasing muscle mass) in conditions such as the sarcopenia of aging as well as disuse atrophy.

For example, although elderly muscle has been reported to be resistant to the amino acid-induced increase in muscle protein synthesis following feeding (termed *anabolic resistance*) (Cuthbertson et al. 2005), studies in humans (Katsanos et al. 2006; Rieu et al. 2006) have shown that an increased concentration of leucine is able to restore rates of protein synthesis in the elderly. As an example, Katsanos and colleagues (2006) showed that a 6.7-gram mixture of essential amino acids (26% leucine or 1.74 grams) did not promote an increase in muscle protein synthesis above resting rates in elderly subjects but did increase muscle protein synthesis in young subjects. However, when the leucine content was increased (41% leucine or 2.75 grams), muscle protein synthesis was stimulated above resting rates in the elderly to the same extent as was observed in young subjects (Katsanos et al. 2006) (Figure 12.3).

These data suggest that the leucine content of a protein may be an important factor determining the anabolic response following protein ingestion, particularly in aged muscle. As shown in Table 12.1, milk solids and whey protein are higher in leucine (77 and 108 milligrams of leucine per gram of protein, respectively) than soy protein (62 milligrams of leucine per gram of protein). The higher leucine content of milk protein and whey may explain, at least in part, the greater anabolic response

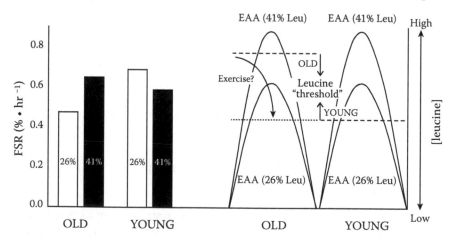

FIGURE 12.3 Increased leucine concentration restores the fractional synthetic rate (FSR) of mixed muscle during resting conditions in elderly humans. The dashed line depicts the elevated extracellular "leucine threshold" in elderly muscle relative to young. EAA = essential amino acids. (Adapted from Katsanos, C.S., H. Kobayashi, M. Sheffield-Moore, A. Aarsland, and R.R. Wolfe. A High Proportion of Leucine Is Required for Optimal Stimulation of the Rate of Muscle Protein Synthesis by Essential Amino Acids in the Elderly. *Am J Physiol Endocrinol Metab* 291(2):E381–87, 2006.)

TABLE 12.1

Amino Acid Composition, Calculated PDCAAS Score, and NPU for Whey, Milk Solids, Casein, and Soy Protein

Amino Acid Content (mg amino acid/g protein)	Whey[a]	Milk Solids (Nonfat)[b]	Casein[c]	Soy[d]
Histidine	20	20	27	28
Isoleucine	76	63	54	44
Leucine	108	77	82	62
Lysine	101	54	73	62
Methionine (+ Cys)	48	33	28	20
Phenylalanine (+ Tyr)	67	48	100	88
Threonine	44	37	54	32
Tryptophan	26	15	12	10
Valine	72	55	64	54
PDCAAS	115[e]	121[f]	123[e]	104[g]
NPU	92[e]	86[e]	78[e]	72[h]

Note: All values are in milligrams of amino acids per grams of protein. NPU = net protein utilization (proportion of protein intake that is retained); PDCAAS = protein digestibility corrected amino acid score. The indispensable amino acid pattern used in the PDCAAS scores was taken from the Dietary Recommended Intakes for protein with protein digestibilities of 95 for milk proteins, 99 for whey and casein, and 97 for soy (Institute of Medicine 2005) Data from acid hydrolysis carried out as described by Wilkinson et al. (2007) of commercially available isolated whey proteins, skim milk powder, micellar casein, and isolated soy protein.

[a] Isolated whey proteins.
[b] Skim milk powder.
[c] Micellar casein.
[d] Isolated soy protein.
[e] From Schaafsma (2000).
[f] From Miller et al. (2006).
[g] Calculated according to Castellanos et al. (2006).
[h] Estimated based on net postprandial protein utilization and reported nutritional values of NPU for soy protein from Bos et al. (2000, 2003).

that is observed following ingestion of these protein sources relative to that observed with soy protein and suggests that these proteins may be particularly suitable for the elderly, who appear to require a greater amount of leucine to stimulate muscle protein synthesis (Katsanos et al. 2006).

Verhoeven and colleagues (2009) examined the efficacy of long-term leucine supplementation as a nutritional intervention capable of promoting increases in skeletal muscle mass in elderly subjects. Supplemental free-form leucine (7.5 grams per day with meals) for a three-month period had no effect on skeletal muscle mass or muscle strength compared to an energy-matched placebo (Verhoeven et al. 2009). However, other studies have reported that supplemental essential amino acids used over longer periods (3 to 16 months) are able to promote an increase in lean muscle mass in the elderly population (Borsheim et al. 2008; Dillon et al. 2009; Solerte et al. 2008). Regardless, any benefit of protein or amino acid supplements on skeletal muscle mass is likely to be enhanced when used in conjunction with a program of resistance exercise training.

For example, Moore and colleagues (Moore, Tang, et al. 2009) reported that the combination of protein and resistance exercise promoted the synthesis of predominantly the myofibrillar (i.e., the contractile proteins actin and myosin) fraction of muscle proteins, while feeding in the absence of resistance exercise increased the synthesis of both myofibrillar and sarcoplasmic proteins. Thus, future studies should examine if leucine supplementation is able to augment gains in lean muscle mass and strength in the elderly when consumed in close temporal proximity to resistance exercise.

In summary, as sources of dietary protein, whey and milk proteins are among the richest in the branched-chain amino acid leucine. As such, these protein sources may be of particular relevance to the elderly, who appear to require meal feedings containing a greater absolute leucine concentration to stimulate muscle protein synthesis (Katsanos et al. 2006). Although more research is needed to fully clarify the role of leucine supplementation as a nutritional intervention to promote muscle protein accretion in the elderly, it is likely that any benefit of leucine supplementation to skeletal muscle will be increased by the concurrent performance of resistance exercise. Thus, the elderly may benefit by consuming high-quality leucine-rich proteins such as milk or whey in the time period immediately following resistance exercise and ensure that adequate protein (approximately 30 grams) is consumed with each meal in an attempt to maximize muscle protein synthesis and preserve skeletal muscle.

12.7 MEASURES OF PROTEIN QUALITY: TIME TO REAPPRAISE?

Sources of dietary protein are evaluated regarding their quality based on their potential nutritive value and their ability to contribute to meeting nitrogen and amino acid requirements during periods of growth or maintenance in people of different ages or physiological conditions (Moughan 2005). Different assays for determining protein quality include the protein efficiency ratio, biological value (BV), net protein utilization (NPU), and the PDCAAS (see Table 12.1). Of these, the PDCAAS is the preferred measure of protein quality currently used to assess the value of a protein in human nutrition (Schaafsma 2000). In the PDCAAS system, protein sources with PDCAAS values over 100% are not considered to contribute any additional benefits in humans (Schaafsma 2000); thus, these proteins are listed and are artificially truncated at 100%. However, the concept of artificially truncating the PDCAAS score at 100% has been challenged, and protein sources that are by arbitrary standards considered of equal value may not be.

For example, as highlighted by Phillips and colleagues (2009), the matched consumption of high-quality proteins with PDCAAS scores of 100% (actually higher but artificially truncated at 100%) is associated with significant differences in skeletal muscle hypertrophy following a period of chronic resistance training (Phillips et al. 2009). For example, despite whey and casein having PDCAAS scores of 100%, Cribb and colleagues (2006) reported that individuals supplementing with whey protein in the time period surrounding resistance exercise achieved gains in lean muscle mass that were approximately fivefold greater than those supplementing with casein (Cribb et al. 2006).

In addition, Figure 12.2 illustrates the average change in lean mass compiled from different resistance exercise training studies ($n = 11$) (Brown et al. 2004; Burke, Chilibeck, et al. 2001; Candow, Burke, et al. 2006; Chromiak et al. 2004; Cribb et al. 2006; Cribb, Williams, Stathis, et al. 2007; Demling and DeSanti 2000; Hartman et al. 2007; Kerksick et al. 2006; Maesta et al. 2007; Rankin et al. 2004) in which supplemental protein sources were provided. As can be seen, the results suggest that supplemental whey protein is associated with gains in lean body mass that are significantly greater than soy protein. Also, lean body mass gains that occurred after ingestion of whey were also greater than the average gain in lean mass when all protein sources were combined. Lastly, one can conclude from this review that milk ingestion promotes greater lean mass gains than simple carbohydrate. Thus, from the perspective of promoting muscle protein anabolism with resistance exercise, dairy-based protein sources such as whey appear to be more effective than plant-based protein sources such as soy, despite being considered equivalent based on their PDCAAS.

12.8 SIGNIFICANCE AND FUTURE DIRECTIONS

The provision of intact dietary food source proteins such as soy (Tang et al. 2009; Wilkinson et al. 2007), whey (Tang et al. 2009), casein (Tang et al. 2009), beef (Symons et al. 2007), and egg (Moore, Robinson, et al. 2009) have all been shown to be capable of stimulating muscle protein synthesis. However, the response of protein synthesis, both in magnitude and duration, is affected by the source of protein consumed (Boirie et al. 1997; Dangin et al. 2001, 2003; Tang et al. 2009; Wilkinson et al. 2007). Supplemental whey protein and bovine milk appear to be particularly beneficial at promoting resistance exercise-induced gains in lean mass; however, the physiological mechanisms responsible for their efficacy are not entirely understood. Milk and whey are particularly rich in the branched-chain amino acid leucine, and given its role as a key regulator of translation initiation of muscle protein synthesis, small differences in the leucine concentration of different protein sources may explain some of the observed differences in the muscle protein synthesis response. However, human work needs to be undertaken to fully elucidate the role of leucine relative to the other essential amino acids in regulating muscle protein synthesis and anabolic signaling. Further, although an elevated leucine concentration appears to help ameliorate the reduced anabolic sensitivity of aged skeletal muscle to acute amino acid feeding (Katsanos et al. 2006), long-term (12 weeks) free-form leucine supplementation in the absence of resistance exercise does not appear to promote increases in lean body mass or increase strength (Verhoeven et al. 2009). Thus, more work is needed to fully clarify the situations under which supplemental leucine is most efficacious in the elderly population; we propose it is in the time period immediately following acute resistance exercise and in combination with appropriate amounts of the other essential amino acids.

The rate of protein digestion also appears to be an important variable affecting the magnitude and duration of protein synthesis (Boirie et al. 1997; Dangin et al. 2001, 2003). Generally, fast proteins such as whey result in a greater fold change increase in protein synthesis than slow proteins such as micellar casein

(Boirie et al. 1997; Dangin et al. 2001, 2003; Tang et al. 2009). However, fluid bovine milk (approximately 80% casein) results in a greater stimulation of muscle protein synthesis after resistance exercise than soy protein, despite being digested at a relatively slower rate (Wilkinson et al. 2007). The high leucine content of the whey component of fluid milk (approximately 20%) may in part explain its efficacy relative to soy in promoting a robust anabolic response after resistance exercise; however, the slower rate at which the amino acids from milk proteins enter peripheral circulation may also serve to prolong the duration of the feeding-induced rise in muscle protein synthesis relative to soy. By extension, it would be interesting to examine how different sources of dietary protein affect the feeding-induced suppression of skeletal muscle protein breakdown; whole-body data suggest that casein is better able than whey to inhibit protein breakdown likely of rapidly turning over gut proteins (Boirie et al. 1997).

Finally, although the acute response of muscle protein synthesis following ingestion of different sources of dietary protein appears to be qualitatively predictive of the long-term changes in muscle mass that occur following a period of chronic resistance exercise (Hartman et al. 2007; Wilkinson et al. 2007), additional definitive studies are needed to determine if the acute responses in muscle protein synthesis that are observed following resistance exercise and feeding correlate with the magnitude of muscle hypertrophy following several weeks of training. It is plausible that individuals who demonstrate the greatest acute rise in muscle protein synthesis following resistance exercise and feeding are likely those who will achieve the greatest levels of hypertrophy following a period of chronic training, but this remains to be tested.

13 Nutrient Timing Programs in Sport

A Case Study Approach

Bob Seebohar

CONTENTS

13.1   INTRODUCTION

Nutrient timing strategies are an important consideration in the field of sports nutrition and athletics. Due to the great diversity in sporting types, body types, food availability, travel schedules, and so on, the ability to translate the findings into a tangible, workable nutrition plan may be a cumbersome task for some athletes and coaches. In addition and due to logistical requirements of individual sports, nutrient timing protocols must be customized based on the gender, age, body weight, and body composition goals of the athlete; sport; sport position (if applicable); and the different cycles of the training year.

The goal of this chapter is to "bring to life" the research and recommendations using the recently published dietary reference intakes (*Dietary Reference Intakes for Energy, Carbohydrate, Fiber, Fat, Fatty Acids, Cholesterol, Protein, and Amino Acids*) and other professional references by the authors Austin and Seebohar (2011). Eight different "athletes" are outlined, and a much more detailed look is provided into how an athlete or coach can take the many different recommendations and apply them to an eating schedule that not only meets nutrient timing guidelines but also has enough practicality that it can reasonably be implemented. There is a blend of both quantitative and qualitative nutrition implementation strategies among the case studies. One approach is not particularly favored over the other. However, the use of each method will depend largely on the athlete. For example, an athlete's nutrition goals may not support a more advanced, quantitative approach if the athlete is less experienced with using performance nutrition principles. Age will sometimes contribute, but usually it is the knowledge level of the athlete that helps to determine if a quantitative or qualitative approach should be used. Athletes who have a better understanding of the impact nutrition has on their bodies may find quantitative nutrient timing strategies more applicable for their specific performance goals. In addition, an athlete's readiness to change should be evaluated prior to placing quantitative nutrition goals on them. If an athlete is not ready to make a nutritional change that has a positive impact on his or her performance, using quantitative nutrition strategies will not help because the athlete simply may not be ready for numbers. Athletes who fall into this category can begin their performance nutrition journey by using the qualitative nutrition guidelines with progressive movement toward quantitative nutrition recommendations when the time is right and their goals support their use.

The following case studies provide different opportunities to understand and apply nutrient timing strategies and provide a hands-on approach of taking the information presented in research and applying it to real-life athlete scenarios. Regrettably, it is not possible for scenarios to be built that can match all combinations. The examples provided have been developed as a means to illustrate how much eating as well as timing strategies can change what is consumed by the athlete and when. It is hoped that enough similarities exist between the athletes so that considerations from one athlete can be adapted and matched in an athletic scenario that is not detailed in this chapter. For example, it is our contention that enough similarities exist between the metabolic challenges of a male football player who plays receiver and defensive back and a male soccer player that subtle changes can be made in the soccer player's plan that will result in the development of an effective nutrient timing program for the football player.

13.2 FEMALE BASKETBALL PLAYER

13.2.1 DEMOGRAPHIC INFORMATION

- Age: 20 years old, sophomore in college
- Height: 6 feet 0 inches

- Weight: 205 pounds, 93.2 kilograms
- Position: Forward
- Other notes: Division I collegiate team; lives on campus with roommates

13.2.2 Training

- Goal: To reduce body weight and body fat and optimize performance through ideal management of her body composition.
- Cycle: Early preseason
- Strength cycle: Traditional, nonexplosive, little to no Olympic movements or plyometrics

13.2.3 Nutrition Implementation Strategies: Major Concepts

Most important, this athlete's chronological and developmental age regarding nutrition and the messages provided on the topic must be considered. This key consideration is one that should be made for all athletes college age and younger. Normally, young athletes do not have much experience cooking, shopping, or putting together certain foods to elicit the most beneficial performance benefit. In this respect, the focus of nutrition education should be on major concepts and building education on the foundational aspects of nutrition knowledge. This includes the following:

- Classifications of carbohydrate, protein, and fat and outlining which foods contain these nutrients. Emphasis should be placed on antioxidant-rich carbohydrates that include fruits, vegetables, and whole grains; the difference between refined starches and whole grains; source of lean versus higher-fat protein and the types of fat, including saturated and unsaturated fats, and their performance effects on the body.
- The different blood sugar responses that each nutrient alone and paired together have on the body and how this relates to body composition and energy control. Specific education should be centered on combining protein- and fiber-rich foods to exhibit favorable weight and body composition changes and appropriateness for the frequency of eating.
- Proper daily hydration techniques as well as hydration strategies before, during, and after practice.
- The differences between biological, habitual, and emotional hunger and when the body needs food versus when there are other factors that trigger food consumption. Specific emphasis will be placed on teaching the athlete what biological hunger is, how to identify it, and how to structure her eating based on her biological hunger while minimizing her emotional and habitual hunger eating times.

13.2.4 Nutrition Implementation Strategies: The Numbers

Due to the athlete's age and developmental stage, an overreliance on specific numbers will likely yield little success and should be minimized as much as possible

TABLE 13.1

Daily Nutrition Guideline for Female Basketball Player in Preseason with a Goal to Lose Body Fat and Improve Body Composition Prior to Her Competitive Season

Training Cycle	Carbohydrate	Protein	Fat
Grams per kilogram of body mass (g/kg)	3–4	2.0–2.5	0.8–1.0
Grams per pound of body mass (g/lb)	1.36–1.8	0.91–1.14	0.36–0.45
Total grams consumed (g)	280–370	85–106	75–93
Number of calories consumed (kcal)	1,120–1,480	340–424	675–837

Total projected daily caloric intake: 2,539 calories

throughout the nutrition prescription. This information will only be confusing to the athlete, and the qualitative information, emphasizing major concepts of healthy eating and effective food choices, should form the foundation of the nutrition plan.

The numbers presented in Table 13.1 are provided for the benefit of any knowledgeable, appropriately trained individual (e.g., coach, athletic trainer, manager, nutritionist) to understand the basis by which the athlete should be provided certain amounts of macronutrients based on her training cycle and her physical training goals. They should only be used as background information to assist these types of individuals in reinforcing the qualitative aspects of the nutrition program to the athlete.

The athlete should set a goal to eat three meals and two snacks each day. Based on the fact that she has two practices each day (morning is strength training, and afternoon is sport-specific practice), energy levels will need to remain consistent; thus, the message of frequency of eating is extremely important for this type of athlete to understand so she will not miss meals.

13.2.5 DAILY MENU

The athlete has access to an on-campus cafeteria for all of her meals and snacks. Morning practice is from 6:30 to 7:30 a.m.; her first class is at 8:30 a.m., and afternoon practice begins at 4:00 p.m. and lasts until 6:00 p.m. Because of this athlete's training program, training cycle, and weight loss and body composition goals, specific nutrient timing strategies for before and after practices are minimized (Table 13.2). Her goal should be to meet her nutrient requirements with her meals, with the only exception her morning strength training. Prior to this workout, sipping or light ingestion of a sports drink or water should be recommended. An overreliance on getting calories from these sources should be minimized. Water will be the preferred beverage, with the goal of eating breakfast immediately after the training session.

13.2.6 NUTRIENT TIMING CONSIDERATIONS

As mentioned, specific nutrient timing strategies for this athlete and her phase of training should allow for meals and feedings that promote recovery and still allow

TABLE 13.2
Sample Meal Plan for a Female Basketball Player in Preseason with a Goal to Lose Body Fat and Improve Body Composition Prior to Her Competitive Season

Meal	Food
Morning workout (6:30 a.m.)	• Fluid replacement with water
Breakfast (7:45 a.m.)	• Egg omelet (at least 4 eggs)
	• Small handful of mushrooms, tomatoes, and bell peppers
	• Three pinches of cheddar cheese
	• Medium glass of low-fat milk
	• One piece of whole-wheat toast with peanut butter
Snack (10:00 a.m.)	• Small cup of yogurt
	• Handful of blueberries, strawberries, etc.
Lunch (12:00–1:00 p.m.)	• Turkey sandwich with mustard, lettuce, and tomato
	• Apple with peanut butter
	• Medium glass of low-fat chocolate milk
Prepractice (4:00 p.m.)	• Sip on sports drink or water
Postpractice (6:00 p.m.)	• Replace lost fluids with sports drink or recovery drink
Dinner (6:30–7:30 p.m.)	• Large piece of chicken
	• Medium serving of broccoli, lightly salted
	• Small-to-medium serving of brown rice
Evening snack	• Handful of peanuts and raisins
	• Replace lost fluids with water

her to reach her goals of losing fat, improving body composition, and improving her conditioning. Depending on environmental practice conditions, fluid maintenance will be an important factor for this athlete and her coaches to consider. An adequate amount of fluids should be available, and athletes should be given dedicated breaks for fluid ingestion and encouraged to drink during these times. Fluid replacement of three to eight ounces every 20 minutes should be encouraged for this athlete during practice sessions. Refraining from fluid replacement in an attempt to lose weight is not an effective strategy and should not be considered. Also, when an athletic individual is trying to minimize caloric intake to allow for weight and body fat loss, focused efforts should be made to promote recovery of liver and muscle glycogen. Postpractice fluids and meals should be emphasized along with an awareness of how many calories are consumed late in the evening that might tip her daily balance of energy (see Chapter 16) in the wrong direction and consequently minimize the amount of fat and weight loss that occurs.

13.3 MALE LONG-DISTANCE TRIATHLETE

13.3.1 DEMOGRAPHIC INFORMATION

- Age: 41 years old
- Height: 5 feet 10 inches
- Weight: 160 pounds, 72.7 kilograms
- Ironman athlete; has completed three Ironmans in the past

13.3.2   TRAINING

- Goal: Implement nutrient timing system to optimize performance
- Cycle: Precompetition, building volume and intensity
- Workouts: Two aerobic sessions per day plus a strength session every other day

13.3.3   NUTRITION IMPLEMENTATION STRATEGIES: MAJOR CONCEPTS

The major concepts to be emphasized with this athlete are minimized since their main goal is to implement a nutrient timing system before, during, and after training sessions to improve performance. However, daily nutrition is still an important aspect to his performance; thus, the following nutrition messages are emphasized:

- Emphasizing antioxidant-rich foods can reduce the damage of free-radical production due to high-volume and high-intensity training. Example foods to be consumed in plentiful amounts throughout all parts of every day are fruits, vegetables, and whole grains.
- Controlling blood sugar to have steady energy levels throughout the day to support multiple training sessions. Emphasis will be placed on consuming a source of lean protein, healthy fat, fruit, vegetables, and whole grains at most meals and snacks.
- Beginning the day with good hydration practices to remain in fluid balance.
- Identifying foods rich in omega-3 fats for their anti-inflammatory effects on the body. An increased training load will shift the body to a more proinflammatory state, and including omega-3 rich foods such as salmon, tofu, walnuts, and flax products becomes important.

13.3.4   NUTRITION IMPLEMENTATION STRATEGIES: THE NUMBERS

Specific numbers and guidelines will be useful to this athlete since his goal is to implement specific nutrient timing strategies before, during, and after training sessions (Table 13.3).

TABLE 13.3
Daily Nutrition Guidelines for a Male Triathlete with a Goal to Implement Nutrient Timing Program to Improve Performance

Training Cycle	Carbohydrate	Protein	Fat
Grams per kilogram of body mass (g/kg)	5–12	1.4–2.0	1.0–1.5
Grams per pound of body mass (g/lb)	2.25–5.4	0.63–0.9	0.45–0.68
Total grams consumed (g)	364–872	102–145	73–109
Number of calories consumed (kcal)	1,456–3,488	408–580	657–981
Total projected daily caloric intake: 3,393 calories			

13.3.5 Proposed Daily Menu

The athlete will eat three meals and four snacks throughout the day to fuel his two or three daily training sessions (Table 13.4). As discussed, the timing of meals is important for this type of athlete to ensure adequate digestion time has been provided. As volume of training goes up and down, the amount of food/size of serving should be adjusted upward or downward.

13.3.6 Nutrient Timing Considerations

13.3.6.1 Before Training

Because this athlete is in his precompetition training cycle that includes a higher training load, nutrient timing implementation strategies are very important. The athlete's nutrition plan before training will vary because of the logistics of the three disciplines in the sport of triathlon. He can tolerate only liquids and semisolids before swimming, solid foods before cycling, and nothing for one hour before running.

13.3.6.2 During Training

His nutrition during training will depend largely on the type of training session that he performs. For any session under 60 minutes, he will not need to consume anything since his pretraining nutrition will supply enough nutrients. Depending on environmental conditions, fluid replacement strategies with water ingestion should

TABLE 13.4

Sample Meal Plan for a Male Triathlete with a Goal to Implement Nutrient Timing Program to Improve Performance

Meal	Food
Snack before training (5:30 a.m.)	• Milk-based fruit smoothie, large serving (12–16 fl oz)
Breakfast (7:45 a.m.)	• One large bowl of oatmeal with 2% milk • Small handful of blueberries • Three small scoops of walnuts • Whey protein isolate powder • One small banana
Snack (10:00 a.m.)	• Large bowl of plain yogurt • Handful of strawberries
Lunch (12:00–1:00 p.m.)	• Large spinach salad with one chicken breast on top with cucumbers, carrots, tomatoes, avocado, and oil/vinegar dressing
Snack (4:00 p.m.)	• Natural energy bar • Whey protein ready-to-drink smoothie
Dinner (6:30–7:30 p.m.)	• Large serving of salmon • Medium serving of brown rice or other whole-grain-based starch (couscous, quinoa, etc.) • Medium serving of asparagus
Snack (10:00 p.m.)	• Small bowl of ice cream

be strongly considered to prevent dehydration. For glycogen-depleting workouts that are longer than two hours or high-intensity workouts that are longer than one hour, the recommendations in Table 13.5 are made to provide adequate fuel throughout the exercise bout.

13.3.6.3 After Training

For training sessions with a duration of two hours or longer of moderate to relatively high intensity, the posttraining feeding guidelines in Table 13.5 are suggested. Because of time constrictions and taste preferences, ready-to-mix postworkout powder that contains a mixture of carbohydrates and high-quality protein are advised. Food sources containing a similar balance of these nutrients are suitable (i.e., low-fat chocolate milk, a lean-meat sandwich with whole-grain breads, or a milk-based fruit smoothie);

TABLE 13.5

Before, During, and After Training Fuel Considerations for a Male Triathlete with a Goal to Implement Nutrient Timing Program to Improve Performance

Timing	Food (Timing, Amount, Type)
	Before Training
Before swimming	• 30–60 minutes prior • 200–300 calories • Liquid, milk-based fruit smoothie
Before cycling	• 60–120 minutes prior • Meat-based sandwich, piece of fruit, water
Before running	• Liquid smoothie, banana with peanut butter, or small cup of yogurt 60–90 minutes before
	During Training
Swimming	• Having a sports drink on the pool deck during swims will meet energy and fluid needs. Drink ad libitum between sets.
Cycling	• Consume up to 24 ounces of fluid per hour, preferably a sports drink, each hour depending on sweat rate. • Additional carbohydrates can be added to reach the recommended 30–90 grams of carbohydrate intake per hour. • This can be accomplished by consuming energy gels, chews, or bars.
Running	• Consume up to 12 ounces of fluid per hour. • If a sports drink is tolerable to the gut during the run, then it is recommended to drink this for the carbohydrate and electrolytes. • Goal is to consume 50 grams of carbohydrate per hour depending on individual gut response.
	After Training
Fluid	• 24 ounces for every pound of body weight that is lost
Carbohydrate	• 1–1.2 grams of carbohydrate per kilogram of body weight (73–87 grams or 292–348 calories based on his body weight)
Protein	• 10–20 grams total (40–80 calories)
Sodium	• Up to 500 milligrams

however, it is likely the athlete's appetite may be blunted, making supplemental ingestion in the form of a drink or shake more amicable to adequate nutrient ingestion.

13.4 FEMALE SAILOR

13.4.1 DEMOGRAPHIC INFORMATION

- Age: 28 years
- Height: 5 feet 5 inches
- Weight: 140 pounds, 63.6 kilograms
- Internationally competitive athlete

13.4.2 TRAINING

- Goal: Improve lean muscle mass and increase body weight to optimize sailing performance on the water.
- Cycle: Competition. Her training varies depending on travel, but she is on the
  water four to five times per week for between three to six hours per session.
- Workouts: Resistance training three times per week (hypertrophy focus) and
  cardiovascular exercise two times per week for 60 to 90 minutes per session.

13.4.3 NUTRITION IMPLEMENTATION STRATEGIES: MAJOR CONCEPTS

Both a focus on increasing foundational knowledge through major concepts and
quantitative strategies will be implemented to support her body weight and composition goals. Her daily nutrition messages will be qualitative and emphasize the
following points:

- Using antioxidant-rich foods to reduce the damage of free-radical production due to high-volume and high-intensity training. Foods to be included
  are fruits, vegetables, and whole grains.
- Controlling blood sugar throughout the day to account for the long period of
  time spent on the water and eating a combination of carbohydrate, protein,
  and healthy-fat foods while on the water.
- Identify and increase intake of foods rich in omega-3 fats for their anti-
  inflammatory effects on the body. An increased training load will shift the
  body to a more proinflammatory state, and including omega-3-rich foods
  such as salmon, tofu, walnuts, and flax products becomes important.
- Having a good source and quantity of protein before strength and higher-
  intensity workouts to improve the body's net protein synthesis rate and
  remain in protein balance to support lean muscle mass goals.

13.4.4 NUTRITION IMPLEMENTATION STRATEGIES: THE NUMBERS

Quantitative numbers will be useful to this athlete at times due to her goal of improving lean muscle mass. However, her desire to increase muscle mass will require a

balanced focus between a conceptual framework and getting specific quantities of certain foods and food types (Table 13.6).

13.4.5 PROPOSED DAILY MENU

The athlete will attempt to eat three meals and two snacks throughout the day, but the frequency will depend largely on how often and long she is on the water sailing (Table 13.7). This is one reason to explain the wide range of potential caloric intake seen in Table 13.6.

TABLE 13.6
Daily Nutrition Guideline for Female Internationally Competitive Sailor Whose Goal Is to Improve Lean Muscle Mass and Increase Body Weight to Optimize Sailing Performance on the Water

Competition Training Cycle	Carbohydrate	Protein	Fat
Grams per kilogram of body mass (g/kg)	5–12	1.4–2.0	1.0–1.5
Grams per pound of body mass (g/lb)	2.27–5.45	0.67–0.91	0.45–0.68
Total grams consumed (g)	318–763	89–127	64–95
Number of calories consumed (kcal)	1,272–3,052	356–508	576–855

Total projected daily caloric intake: 2,204–4,415 calories

TABLE 13.7
Sample Meal Plan for Female Internationally Competitive Sailor Whose Goal Is to Improve Lean Muscle Mass and Increase Body Weight to Optimize Sailing Performance on the Water

Meal	Food
Breakfast	• One medium bowl of a whole-grain cereal with skim milk and a banana • One medium glass of a protein-rich fruit smoothie
Snack	• Handful of almonds and walnuts • One handful of grapes
Lunch	• Two medium-size chicken fajitas with guacamole, tomatoes, lettuce, onions, and cheese • One medium bowl of green beans • One small glass of low-fat milk
Snack (on the water)	• Peanut butter and jelly sandwich • Trail mix • Banana
Dinner	• Medium-size buffalo or lean-beef burger on a whole-wheat bun with ketchup, lettuce, tomato, and avocado • One medium-size sweet potato • Large glass of skim milk

13.4.6 Nutrient Timing Considerations

13.4.6.1 Before Training

Specific nutrient timing strategies will need to be implemented because this athlete is in her competition training cycle and has specific body weight and composition goals. These strategies will be particularly important surrounding her strength training sessions to facilitate lean muscle mass gains and promote a net positive protein synthesis rate. The athlete's nutrition plan before training will vary between her training on the water, strength training, and cardiovascular work. Table 13.8 outlines nutrient timing strategies, discussed next, to be employed before training.

13.4.6.2 During Training

Her nutrition during training will depend largely on the type of training session that she performs. When she is on the water, her nutrition will differ markedly from when she is completing strength and cardiovascular training. Table 13.8 outlines the nutrient timing strategies to be employed during training.

13.4.6.3 After Training

Posttraining nutrition recommendations will have different goals depending on the mode of exercise. Because of her overall goal of increasing body weight and lean mass, restoring muscle glycogen and preventing loss of muscle protein will be the main nutrition goals. These goals can be accomplished through the strategies outlined in Table 13.8.

13.5 MALE SOCCER PLAYER

13.5.1 Demographic Information

- Age: 29 years
- Height: 5 feet 10 inches
- Weight: 170 pounds, 77.3 kilograms
- Goal: Support performance on the field, improve body composition and lean muscle mass in preseason
- Position: midfielder

13.5.2 Training

- Goal: Improve body composition (decrease body fat and increase lean muscle mass)
- Cycle: Precompetition, building volume and intensity
- Workouts: One 90-minute practice and one 90-minute conditioning session (weights and cardiovascular) per day, six days per week

TABLE 13.8
Before, During, and After Training Fuel Considerations for Female Internationally Competitive Sailor Whose Goal Is to Improve Lean Muscle Mass and Increase Body Weight to Optimize Sailing Performance on the Water

Timing	Food (Timing, Amount, Type)
Preworkout Considerations	
Before sailing	• 45–60 minutes prior to getting on the water • 200–300 calories • Peanut butter and jelly sandwich • Higher-protein (20 grams) energy bar • Water
Before strength training	• 30–60 minutes prior to lifting • 250–300 calories • Ready-to-drink or homemade smoothie that contains at least 25 grams of protein and 40 grams of carbohydrate
Before cardiovascular training	• 45–60 minutes prior to workout • Small bowl of yogurt and berries • Water
During-Workout Considerations	
Sailing	• A focus should be made toward maintaining blood sugar levels for optimal physical and mental performance. • Sports drinks are a consideration and should be consumed regularly throughout activity when she has a break. • Foods that are either difficult to open or perishable are not useful. • Sandwiches can be premade and used along with a regular supply of trail mix and fruit such as apples or bananas. • Ideally, fuel every 60–90 minutes.
Strength training	• If adequate prefeeding was accomplished, during strength training strategies should largely consist of water or sports drink consumption.
Cardiovascular	• If adequate prefeeding was accomplished and workout will be less than 90 minutes, she will only need water and possibly a sports drink (which contains valuable electrolytes) if workout is performed in a warm climate to promote optimal fluid balance.
After-Workout Considerations	
Sailing	• Consume 24 ounces of fluid immediately on finishing training as she is sailing back to the dock. • Once at the dock, consume a protein- and carbohydrate-rich (15–20 grams and 50–75 grams, respectively) energy bar before tearing down the boat. • After the boat is put away and any debriefing is done with her coach, sit down to a well-balanced meal consisting of carbohydrate, lean protein, and healthy fat, preferably within one to two hours after getting off the water.
Strength training	• Consume 15–20 grams of protein with at least 50–75 grams of carbohydrate with fluid immediately after strength training to improve protein synthesis rates. • This can be composed of a milk-based fruit smoothie, lean meat sandwich with a glass of milk, or a preformulated postworkout nutrition powder.
Cardiovascular training	• Ideally, she would schedule a meal or snack immediately after her aerobic training session to consume the necessary fluid, carbohydrate, protein, and sodium as stated previously. • Because these sessions will likely not be glycogen depleting, the main goal is to consume a balance of these four key nutrients as soon as possible following training.

13.5.3 Nutrition Implementation Strategies: Major Concepts

An emphasis on major concepts will be effective and will be implemented along with quantitative strategies to support his body composition goals. His daily nutrition messages that will be emphasized from a qualitative standpoint include the following:

- Using antioxidant-rich foods to reduce the damage from free-radical production due to high-volume and high-intensity training. Foods to be included are fruits, vegetables, and whole grains.
- Controlling blood sugar throughout the day to improve the oxidation of fat stores for energy by eating a combination of carbohydrate, protein, and healthy-fat foods at every feeding. This will also assist him in controlling his daily calorie intake.
- Identifying foods rich in omega-3 fats for their anti-inflammatory effects on the body. Including omega-3-rich foods such as salmon, tofu, walnuts, and flax products will be important.
- Listening to the body's hunger and satiety responses will be extremely important for this athlete during his preseason. Controlling hunger and avoiding mindless eating and overeating will be the main goals.

13.5.4 Nutrition Implementation Strategies: The Numbers

Quantitative numbers will be useful to this athlete at times due to his goal of improving body composition (Table 13.9). However, an enhanced understanding of the major concepts should be the primary focus. A focus on specific numbers becomes important after the athlete has developed a full understanding of his biological hunger cues and responses.

13.5.5 Proposed Daily Menu

The athlete will eat three meals and one snack throughout the day (Table 13.10). His typical workout day will consist of one practice lasting for two to three hours. For this type of athlete, the timing of meals is not as important as for others, except

TABLE 13.9

Daily Nutrition Guidelines for a Male Soccer Player Looking for Ways to Support Performance on the Field and Improve Body Composition and Lean Muscle Mass in Preseason

Training Cycle	Carbohydrate	Protein	Fat
Grams per kilogram of body mass (g/kg)	3–4	2.0–2.5	0.8–1.0
Grams per pound of body mass (g/lb)	1.36–1.8	0.91–1.14	0.36–0.45
Total grams consumed (g)	232–309	155–193	62–77
Number of calories consumed (kcal)	928–1,236	620–772	558–693
Total projected daily caloric intake: 2,106–2,701 calories			

TABLE 13.10

Sample Meal Plan for a Male Soccer Player Looking for Ways to Support Performance on the Field and Improve Body Composition and Lean Muscle Mass in Preseason

Meal	Food
Breakfast	• Four-egg omelet (4 egg whites, 1 egg yolk) with tomatoes, mushrooms, bell peppers, onions, and cheddar cheese • Bowl of fresh fruit
Lunch	• Turkey wrap with ample turkey (5–6 ounces) on a thin tortilla with tomato, cucumber, lettuce, and a splash of olive oil • Blueberries and strawberries
Snack	• Handful of almonds and walnuts • Whole-wheat bagel • 12–16 ounces of sports drink
Dinner	• Steak (at least 4–5 ounces) • Asparagus • Mashed potatoes or brown rice

in situations when strategies surrounding strength training workouts should be employed to promote a positive balance of net muscle protein.

13.5.6 Nutrient Timing Considerations

13.5.6.1 Before Training

Because this athlete is in his preseason and wants to improve his body composition as a primary goal, eating out of biological hunger and keeping satiated will be the main goals before training. While he is training twice a day, meals and snacks will be used to prepare and recover his body before and after training sessions. Thus, specific nutrient timing recommendations can become important during times when a busy schedule may keep him from getting adequate food intake to facilitate recovery. Depending on environmental situations, an emphasis by the athlete will need to be made prior to exercise to make sure an adequate level of hydration is achieved prior to practice or competition. This can be accomplished by having a fluid source in the prepractice snack or meal. The athlete's conditioning practice will take place midmorning, and his traditional practice will happen after his afternoon snack and before dinner. By timing his sessions in this manner, he will be well fueled for his morning practice, having just eaten breakfast, and his afternoon session will be fueled by his lunch and small afternoon snack. His afternoon practice nutrition recovery will be his dinner.

13.5.6.2 During Training

Because he will be well fueled before practices, he will focus only on drinking water (three to eight fluid ounces every 20 minutes) during workouts that last less than 60 minutes or do not take place in particularly hot and humid environments. As the duration of practice increases and environmental conditions become hotter and more humid, the need for regular consumption of a sports drink at the same rate of water consumption mentioned is needed to maintain optimal fluid balance.

13.5.6.2   After Training

Eating out of biological hunger will be his main goal while improving satiety. Thus, he will depend on his lunch and dinner as his postworking nutrition recovery meals. He will make sure to eat these within 60 minutes of finishing his practices. Practically speaking, if the athlete cannot consume an adequate meal due to the schedule or a lack of desire to eat after a workout, postworkout ingestion of a milk-based fruit smoothie or a recovery drink providing a combination of carbohydrates and protein in a ratio of four grams of carbohydrate for every gram of protein is recommended.

13.6   MALE FOOTBALL PLAYER

13.6.1   Demographic Information

- Age: 19 years old
- Height: 6 feet 5 inches
- Weight: 300 pounds, 136.4 kilograms
- Position: Offensive lineman

13.6.2   Training

- Goal: Gain body mass, improve body composition, gain lean muscle mass, reduce body fat
- Cycle: Preseason
- Workouts: One 60-minute strength-and-conditioning session per day, six days per week, along with one 2-hour practice session five times per week

13.6.3   Nutrition Implementation Strategies: Major Concepts

Because this athlete will also have a readily available supply of healthy foods, emphasis should be made toward foods that provide valuable energy and an effective array of nutrients. As a result, major concepts to be reinforced to this athlete are outlined as follows:

- Eating frequently to support the high-energy expenditure from training and practice sessions and his desire to gain lean muscle mass. Each meal should consist of some form of carbohydrate as well as some form of protein source, with slightly more carbohydrates (e.g., pastas, potatoes, grains, etc.) than protein sources (e.g., meats, dairy, eggs, etc.).
- Using antioxidant-rich foods to reduce the damage from free-radical production due to high-volume and high-intensity training. Foods to be included

are fruits, vegetables, and whole grains. The athlete should be encouraged to consume a wide variety of foods that consist of a wide variety of colors.

- Staying well hydrated throughout the day to remain in fluid balance.

13.6.4 Nutrition Implementation Strategies: The Numbers

As a result of this type of athlete likely having an available strength-and-conditioning staff to offer support, an outline of required quantities could be valuable to this athlete (Table 13.11). It is important to provide continual focus on the qualitative or educational aspect of the nutritional program to help further educate the athlete on healthy food choices. However, to help guide the athlete through the massive amount of food that must be consumed to achieve goals, a numbers-based approach may also be effective to help the athlete "add" up how well they are meeting their required needs.

13.6.5 Proposed Daily Menu

As part of the heavy training and the goal to increase body mass and lean muscle mass and to improve body composition, a relatively frequent schedule of eating should be adopted (Table 13.12). It is planned for this athlete to eat three meals and three snacks throughout the day. His relatively large body mass and his goal to get even bigger demands a high intake of energy, requiring a relatively frequent pattern of eating.

13.6.6 Nutrient Timing Considerations

13.6.6.1 Before Training

This athlete's preseason goal is to add lean mass, add body mass, and improve body composition. As a result, the frequency and volume of eating along with the quality of food consumed are primary factors for this athlete to consider. A nutrient timing strategy including appropriately timed meals and snacks will be used to prepare and recover his body before and after training sessions to optimize his body weight, lean mass, and performance goals. The athlete's strength-and-conditioning practice will

---

TABLE 13.11
Daily Nutrition Guidelines for a Male Football Player (Offensive Lineman) with a Goal of Increasing Body Mass, Improving Body Composition, Reducing Body Fat, and Improving Performance

Training Cycle	Carbohydrate	Protein	Fat
Grams per kilogram of body mass (g/kg)	8–10	1.6–1.8	1.0–1.3
Grams per pound of body mass (g/lb)	3.64–4.55	0.73–0.82	0.45–0.59
Total grams consumed (g)	1,091–1,364	218–246	136–177
Number of calories consumed (kcal)	4,364–5,456	872–984	1,224–1,593
Total projected daily caloric intake: 6,460–8,033 calories			

TABLE 13.12

Sample Meal Plan for a Male Football Player (Offensive Lineman) with a Goal of Increasing Body Mass, Improving Body Composition, Reducing Body Fat, and Improving Performance

Meal	Food
Breakfast	• Four scrambled eggs with cheddar cheese and salsa • One large bowl whole-grain cereal with 2% milk • One medium-size bowl oatmeal with a banana
Snack	• Protein- and carbohydrate-rich fruit smoothie or protein shake (the added fiber and nutrients of a smoothie are preferred)
Lunch	• Two roast beef sandwiches with cheese, lettuce, tomato, and mustard • Banana • Strawberries • One medium glass of 1–2% milk
Snack	• Protein- and carbohydrate-rich energy bar • One medium-size glass of juice
Dinner	• Two rotisserie chickens • One medium bowl of green beans • One corn on the cob • One medium serving of mashed potatoes
Snack	• One large glass of low-fat chocolate milk

take place midmorning, and his traditional football practice will happen in the afternoon before dinner. By timing his sessions in this manner, he will be well fueled for his morning practice, having just eaten breakfast, and his afternoon session will be fueled by his lunch. Recovery from his afternoon practice will include immediately having a postpractice recovery shake (containing three to four more carbohydrates than protein), then his dinner with a postdinner snack included to account for his late-day, more strenuous training session and high-energy needs.

13.6.6.2 During Training

The athlete should not need anything except for a few gulps of water every 15 to 20 minutes during his strength-and-conditioning indoor practice but should consume a sports drink at regular intervals (three to eight ounces every 20 minutes) throughout his afternoon outdoor practice. As environmental conditions become hotter and more humid, the regular ingestion of fluids becomes more important to help ensure adequate hydration and prevent dehydration.

13.6.6.3 After Training

Hydration and the quality of food will be the two main goals for this athlete following training. Implementing nutrient timing strategies within the first 30 to 60 minutes that include fluid, carbohydrate, protein, and sodium will be of utmost importance, and in most cases his meals or snacks can be used to satisfy these requirements. However, if the athlete will not be able to consume these nutrients in 30 to 60 minutes posttraining, a sports drink (20 to 24 ounces) and energy bar with at least 10 grams of protein and 30 grams of carbohydrate or a recovery shake containing similar levels of nutrients can be used to start the nutrition recovery process. Postpractice meetings, hygiene, injury management, and media obligations may prevent athletes from getting a meal in a desired time frame. In these situations, a postworkout complex carbohydrate and whey protein isolate shake is recommended along with a couple of pieces of fruit and a whole-wheat bagel to meet immediate timing needs and "buy time" until a meal is consumed.

13.7 FEMALE MARATHON RUNNER

13.7.1 DEMOGRAPHIC INFORMATION

- Age: 32 years old
- Height: 5 feet 2 inches
- Weight: 120 pounds, 54.5 kilograms

13.7.2 TRAINING

- Goal: Reduce body weight and fat while optimizing performance
- Cycle: Off-season
- Workouts: One running session per day, six days per week, and one functional/core strength session three times per week

13.7.3 NUTRITION IMPLEMENTATION STRATEGIES: MAJOR CONCEPTS

Because this athlete is in her off-season, qualitative strategies will be implemented and favored over quantitative strategies to support her weight loss goals. Her daily qualitative nutrition messages that will be emphasized include the following:

- Focus on biological hunger and satiety cues and eat according to these. Minimize habitual and emotional eating and identify triggers and solutions to emotional eating.
- Emphasize foods rich in antioxidants for their ability to help minimize cellular damage and oxidative stress. Fresh fruits and vegetables are critical considerations in this regard and can also be a good source of water.
- Focus on foods that contain omega-3 fatty acids for their ability to help control inflammation.
- Identify foods that provide a good balance of carbohydrates to continually be feeding carbohydrates throughout the day to promote recovery and support training.

13.7.4 NUTRITION IMPLEMENTATION: QUANTITATIVE APPROACH

Quantitative numbers take a backseat for this athlete since it is her off-season, and she is not training to compete (Table 13.13). The qualitative approach will be favorable as she will need to learn her hunger cues once again rather than eating to support her exercise energy expenditure as she did in her competition cycle. Qualitative emphasis will also allow her to focus on healthy, nutritious natural foods versus sports nutrition products ingested as part of workouts.

13.7.5 DAILY MENU

The athlete will eat three meals and two snacks throughout the day (Table 13.14). Although her exercise frequency is high at six days per week, her less-structured program has reduced volume and intensity, thus minimizing needs for specialized nutrient timing. Postexercise recovery of lost muscle glycogen will be important but will not be as critically important during this phase of training due to her lower training load.

13.7.6 NUTRIENT TIMING CONSIDERATIONS

The athlete's running sessions will take place first thing in the morning before breakfast. Her runs will range from five to ten miles and will never exceed 90 minutes in

TABLE 13.13
Daily Nutrition Guidelines for a Female Marathon Runner with a Goal of Reducing Body Weight and Fat while Striving to Increase Performance

Training Cycle	Carbohydrate	Protein	Fat
Grams per kilogram of body mass (g/kg)	3–4	1.5–2.3	1.0–1.2
Grams per pound of body mass (g/lb)	1.36–1.82	0.68–1.05	0.45–0.54
Total grams consumed (g)	164–218	98–125	54.5–65
Number of calories consumed (kcal)	656–872	392–500	491–585
Total projected daily caloric intake: 1,633–1,957 calories			

TABLE 13.14
Sample Meal Plan for a Female Marathon Runner with a Goal of Reducing Body Weight and Fat while Striving to Increase Performance

Meal	Food
Breakfast	• One large bowl of Greek yogurt with a large handful of blueberries and a half handful of walnuts, with 10 grams (half of one scoop) of whey protein isolate added
Snack	• One large bowl of part-skim cottage cheese • Two handfuls of strawberries
Lunch	• Large spinach salad with cucumbers, carrots, bell peppers, mushrooms • Chicken strips (at least 5 ounces) • Light drizzle of olive oil on top
Dinner	• One large serving of salmon • Two servings of asparagus, broccoli, or other steamed vegetable • One small serving of brown rice
Snack	• One large glass of low-fat chocolate milk

length. The intensity is aerobic. Her functional strength training sessions will take place in the afternoon between lunch and dinner.

13.7.6.1 Before Training

Because this athlete is in her off-season and her energy expenditure from training is significantly reduced, specific nutrient timing strategies will not be implemented. Rather, focusing on preexercise blood sugar stabilization prior to exercise and timing of preexercise feedings will be important.

13.7.6.2 During Training

Runners are known for not consuming much nutrition during training. Because this athlete is in her off-season and will have significantly less energy expenditure due to less training, fluid balance will be the main goal. The athlete is encouraged to take a few sips of water throughout training sessions and, more importantly, enter training sessions well hydrated. However, care and concern should be taken when training will greatly exceed 60 minutes and even more so when this type of training session will occur in hot and humid environmental conditions. In these cases, fluid consumption should follow the guidelines of 8 to 12 ounces every 20 minutes.

13.7.6.3 After Training

Because this athlete's goals center on weight and body fat loss, her posttraining nutrition plan will include having a meal or snack immediately after a training session. She will not implement strict nutrient timing strategies that would provide unnecessary calories. A fine line must be walked in these scenarios because adequate carbohydrate stores are required to ensure optimal recovery of muscle and liver glycogen, but an excessive amount will keep her from meeting her body composition goals. Thus, she is encouraged to consume a balance of lean protein, healthy fat, and carbohydrates in the posttraining meal or snack.

13.8 MALE WRESTLER

13.8.1 Demographic Information

- Age: 22 years
- Height: 5 feet 10 inches
- Weight: 164 pounds, 77.5 kilograms
- Position: Competes in the 157- to 165-pound weight class; already at competition weight and does not need to go through weight cutting

13.8.2 Training

- Goal: Support and improve performance in competitive wrestling tournament that spans two to three days
- Cycle: Competition
- Workouts: Wrestling practice five times per week, dedicated strength-and-conditioning workouts three times per week

13.8.3 NUTRITION IMPLEMENTATION: QUALITATIVE APPROACH

The main goal for this athlete is to provide him adequate energy during a weekend tournament, and considering he is at his competition weight already, daily nutrition outside his tournament is not discussed. It is important to note that each wrestler has specific weight-cutting strategies that are individual, and this case study does not provide in-depth information about weight cutting. In addition, due to weight control, wrestlers normally restrict calories or skip meals. Regardless, food choices and recommendations are similar to those for other athletes, with the goal of providing nutrient-rich foods. Foods rich in vitamins, minerals, and antioxidants are critically important, especially considering the athlete is expending a significant amount of energy and is likely restricting energy intake to maintain weight throughout the tournament. To provide needed fuel, foods rich in complex carbohydrates are advised during meals, but throughout the tournament days these foods might be hard to come by, with the exception of a whole-wheat bagel, premade sandwich, or the like.

13.8.4 PROPOSED DAILY MENU AND NUTRIENT TIMING CONSIDERATIONS

Due to the specific approach for this athlete, the remainder of this case study takes on a different format than the other case studies. This section attempts to replicate a typical day for a wrestler when taking part in a multiday tournament. In effect, this section combines two sections (proposed daily menu and nutrient timing considerations). The proposed timeline for this athlete follows, and proposed nutrient timing programs for days 1 and 2 of competition can be found in Tables 13.15 and 13.16, respectively.

Saturday (day 1)
- 9:00 a.m.: Weigh-in
- 11:30 a.m.: Match 1
- 4:00 p.m.: Match 2

Sunday (day 2)
- 8:30 a.m.: Weigh-in
- 10:00 a.m.: Match 1
- 6:00 p.m.: Match 2

13.9 FEMALE SWIMMER

13.9.1 DEMOGRAPHIC INFORMATION

- Age: 20 years
- Height: 5 feet 8 inches
- Weight: 130 pounds, 59.1 kilograms

TABLE 13.15
Day 1 of a Nutrient Timing Program for a Male Wrestler with a Goal to Support and Improve Performance in Competitive Wrestling Match that Spans Two to Three Days

Timing	Food (Timing, Amount, Type)
Day 1 preevent meal	• 1 cup water • 2 slices white bread with honey *Note:* The precompetition meal is necessary, but due to weigh-in, it should be low in calories. Salt intake should be minimized; eat 3–4 hours before weigh-in with familiar foods and one to two cups of water. Meal should be comprised of moderate carbohydrates and be low in fat and protein.
	9:00 a.m.: Weigh-in
Snack	• To be consumed five to ten minutes after weigh-in (9:05–9:15 a.m.) • 1 white bagel with jelly • 1 bottle of sports drink • 1 banana • 1 cup water between 9:15 and 11:00 a.m.
	11:30 a.m.: Match 1
11:50 a.m. Postmatch 1	• 1 bottle sports drink immediately following match 1
12:00 p.m. Postmatch 1 meal	• Baked potato with salsa • 1 cup water • 1 cup low-fat yogurt
2:00–3:00 p.m.	• 1 bottle sports drink
	4:00 p.m.: Match 2
4:30 p.m. Postmatch 2 meal	• Postworkout recovery powder mixed with 16–20 ounces of water containing relatively high amounts of carbohydrate (at least 50–75 grams), moderate protein (15–25 grams), and low fat (less than 8 grams)
7:00 p.m. Postmarch 2 dinner	• Large bowl of white rice • Baked chicken breast • Small glass of skim milk • 1 dinner roll with honey

13.9.2 TRAINING

- Goal: Achieve optimal performance during peak competition season and implement nutrient timing principles.
- Cycle: Competition.
- Workouts: She swims five to six days per week, twice per day, with meets every weekend. She swims both individual and relay events in meets.

13.9.3 NUTRITION IMPLEMENTATION: QUALITATIVE APPROACH

Qualitative strategies for this athlete are important and due to her age should be a major focus to ensure this athlete increases her knowledge and understanding of

TABLE 13.16

Day 2 of a Nutrient Timing Program for a Male Wrestler with a Goal to Support and Improve Performance in Competitive Wrestling Match that Spans Two to Three Days

Timing	Food (Timing, Amount, Type)
7:00 a.m. Day 1 preevent meal	• 1 cup water • 2 slices white bread with jelly *Note:* The precompetition meal is necessary, but due to weigh-in, it should be low in calories. Salt intake should be minimized; eat 3–4 hours before weigh-in with familiar foods and one to two cups of water. Meal should be comprised of moderate carbohydrates and be low in fat and protein.
	8:30 a.m.: Weigh-in
Snack	• To be consumed five to ten minutes after weigh-in (8:35–8:45 a.m.) • 1 white bagel with jelly • 1 bottle of sports drink • 1 banana • 1 cup water between 9:00 and 9:30 a.m.
	10:00 a.m.: Match 1
11:00 a.m. Postmatch 1	• Postworkout recovery powder mixed with 16–20 ounces of water containing relatively high amounts of carbohydrate (at least 50–75 grams), moderate protein (15–25 grams), and low fat (less than 8 grams)
11:30 a.m. Postmatch 1 meal	• 2 slices white bread with honey • 1 cup water • 1 cup low-fat yogurt • 1 bottle sports drink
	6:00 p.m.: Match 2
7:00 p.m. Postmatch 2 meal	• Eat freely for his dinner meal, comprised of carbohydrates, protein, and fat with adequate fluids

many aspects of her nutrition. Due to her being in the competition phase of her training cycle, an enhanced focus on numbers, or a quantitative approach, is considered. Her main goal is focused solely on performance and using a nutrient timing system before, during, and after weekend competitions. However, daily nutrition is an important aspect to her performance; thus, the following nutrition messages are emphasized from a qualitative standpoint:

- Using antioxidant-rich foods to reduce the damage from free-radical production due to a high training and competition load. Foods to be included in this message are fruits, vegetables, and whole grains.
- Controlling blood sugar to have steady energy levels throughout the day to support multiple training sessions. Emphasis is placed on consuming a source of lean protein, healthy fat, fruits, vegetables, and whole grain at most meals and snacks.

- Focusing on hydration both in and out of the water to ensure her body is hydrated.
- Identifying foods rich in omega-3 fats for their anti-inflammatory effects on the body. Due to a higher training load, her body's inflammatory state will be higher; thus, including omega-3-rich foods such as salmon, tofu, walnuts, and flax products will be important.

13.9.4 NUTRITION IMPLEMENTATION: QUANTITATIVE APPROACH

Quantitative numbers will be useful to this athlete since her goal is to improve performance, and she is swimming multiple events during a meet (Table 13.17).

13.9.5 DAILY MENU

Like other collegiate athletes, this athlete will have access to on-campus dining in addition to fluid and snack opportunities inside the athletic training and strength-and-conditioning area. She trains two times per day in addition to taking classes and competing on weekends. Combining this busy schedule with a sport that burns an exceptional amount of calories, the athlete needs to be given a plan that provides three meals and four snacks throughout the day to fuel her body (Table 13.18).

13.9.6 NUTRIENT TIMING CONSIDERATIONS

This athlete is in her competition cycle and competes weekly. During meets, she swims both individual and relay events throughout the day. This presents a challenge to her due to the high frequency of competitions along with short rest intervals between events. The athlete's nutrition plan before training will be based on what her gut can handle before getting in the water. Familiar food, which should be consumed before training sessions, should be emphasized as detailed previously. Table 13.19 provides a sample nutrition plan for a competition day for this athlete.

TABLE 13.17

Daily Nutrition Guideline for a Collegiate Female Swimmer Who Has a Goal to Achieve Optimal Performance during Peak Competition Season and Implement Nutrient Timing Principles

Training Cycle	Carbohydrate	Protein	Fat
Grams per kilogram of body mass (g/kg)	5–10	1.4–1.7	1.0–1.2
Grams per pound of body mass (g/lb)	2.27–4.54	0.64–0.77	0.45–0.55
Total grams consumed (g)	296–591	83–100	59–71
Number of calories consumed (kcal)	1,184–2,364	332–400	531–639

Total projected daily caloric intake: 2,047–3,403 calories

TABLE 13.18
Sample Meal Plan for a Collegiate Female Swimmer with a Goal to Improve Performance and Implement Nutrient Timing Principles

Meal	Food
5:00 a.m. Preworkout snack	• ½ banana with peanut butter • Small glass of orange juice
5:30 a.m., Training Session 1: Sports Drink or Water Throughout	
7:30 a.m. Postworkout snack	• 1 glass low-fat chocolate milk
8:00 a.m. Breakfast	• Three scrambled eggs with tomatoes, onions, and a small amount of grated cheese • Two slices of toast with peanut butter • One grapefruit • One large glass of skim milk
11:30 a.m. Lunch	• Lean turkey sandwich with lettuce, tomato, and mustard • Large fruit smoothie (made with skim milk)
2:30 p.m., Training Session 2: Sports Drink or Water Throughout	
4:45 p.m. Postworkout snack	• 1 glass low-fat chocolate milk
5:30 p.m. Dinner	• Large serving of lean roast beef • Large serving of mashed potatoes • Large salad with greens, nuts, and vinegar/oil dressing • Glass of skim milk
Evening snack	• Handful of peanuts and raisins • Replace lost fluids with water

TABLE 13.19
Sample Nutrient Timing Program for a Collegiate Female Swimmer with a Goal to Improve Performance and Implement Nutrient Timing Principles

Meal	Food
Normal breakfast	• Foods to which her gut is accustomed • Minimize heavy milk, creamy or fatty foods • Minimal fat, moderate carbohydrate content, low in protein • 3–4 hours before first event
30 minutes before first event	• 150–200 calories • Sports drink with or without protein • A fruit smoothie • Bagel with fruit
Event 1	
Snack after event	• Medium-size chocolate milk • Minimum of 30 minutes before event 2 (if possible)

TABLE 13.19 (continued)

Sample Nutrient Timing Program for a Collegiate Female Swimmer with a Goal to Improve Performance and Implement Nutrient Timing Principles

Meal	Food
	Event 2
Snack after event	• Peanut butter and jelly sandwich
	• Sports drink
	• Banana
	• At least one hour prior to next event; if closer, minimize solid food intake and emphasize fluids, easily digested foods
	Event 3: 1–2 hours later
Snack after event	• 16–20 ounces of sports drink
	Event 4: 15–20 minutes later
Snack after event	• Apple
	• Low-fat chocolate milk
Dinner	• Chicken breast
	• Mixed vegetables seasoned with salt and pepper
	• Sweet potato
	• Iced tea
	Multiday Considerations
Within 1 hour postcompetition	• Fluid: 24 ounces for every pound lost
	• Carbohydrate: 1–1.2 grams of carbohydrate per kilogram of body weight (59–71 grams or 236–284 calories based on body mass)

13.10 SUMMARY AND CONCLUSIONS

This chapter attempts to provide a real-life look at how nutrient timing strategies, found and supported by research, are utilized by different athletes and sports. It is important to remember that the physical periodization cycles of athletes along with their body weight, composition, and performance goals will largely dictate their nutrition plan. The case studies presented offer a method to understand how to deliver the nutrient timing quantitative numbers into food patterns of athletes. By seeing how different areas of focus are applied depending on the factors identified, it is very likely a coach or athlete could easily adapt the principles to their specific athletic scenario. The focus of this chapter was to provide a balance of nutrient timing scenarios but in no way could all situations be highlighted.

14 Incorporating Nutrient Timing as Part of a Complete Recovery Program

Amanda Carlson-Phillips and Craig Friedman

CONTENTS

14.1 REGENERATION: ENHANCING RECOVERY FOR OPTIMAL PERFORMANCE

Achieving success in the world of sport is often associated with scoring the most points, achieving the best record, finishing with the fastest time, and most importantly winning. At first glance, all of these metrics relate to the effort exerted on the particular field of play; however, when looking into the movement and activity exhibited, the athlete's daily training and practice become important elements that have an

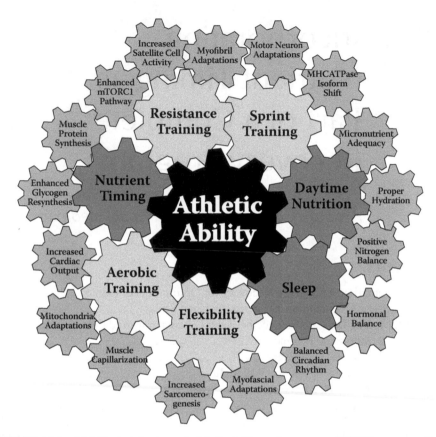

FIGURE 14.1 Multifactorial nature of athletic ability and recovery. mTORC1 = mammalian target of rapamycin complex 1; MHCATPase = myosin heavy chain adenosine triphosphatease enzyme. (Diagram concept adapted from Wenger, H.A., and G.J. Bell. The Interactions of Intensity, Frequency and Duration of Exercise Training in Altering Cardiorespiratory Fitness. *Sports Med* 3:346–56, 1986.)

impact on the resulting performance. When examined even further on a physiologic level and as the level of competition increases or as the athlete's body naturally ages, the recovery and adaptation steps the athlete adopts emerge as a critical element. Therefore, maintaining excellence is much more than just skill or scoring the most points; it also involves an enhanced ability to cope with, adapt to, and recover from the physical and mental stress that results from training and competition.

A true champion is not someone who can achieve success one time, but someone who can perform at an extremely high level mentally, physically, and emotionally time and time again. Therefore, although many factors have an impact on performance (Figure 14.1), an athlete's ability to recover and adapt to training and competition represent a defining predictive factor of success. Recovery strategies are designed to help decrease injury potential, increase career longevity, and create a sustainable level of elite performance over the course of an athlete's career. For these reasons, recovery can be looked at in two ways:

1. Long-term recovery strategies that operate as a function of periodization
2. Short-term/acute recovery strategies that are comprised within a training session or competition

This chapter has two primary goals. The first is to define and describe how the process of recovery as well as a number of different strategies are employed to promote recovery. Second, we introduce, if not speculate, how nutrition, particularly nutrient timing, should be considered as part of a complete recovery program. The chapter brings some perspective and protocol into an area of performance that is underresearched as a whole to improve understanding of various recovery strategies, put together an effective recovery program, and create real-world nutrition solutions to optimize the recovery protocol.

14.2 RECOVERY, OVERTRAINING, OVERREACHING, AND STRESS

Recovery and regeneration are being studied with increasing frequency each year (Bishop et al. 2008), and strategies have evolved in an attempt to decrease soreness, improve hormonal balance, speed return to play, rehydrate, and refuel. Recovery is often considered the physiologic process, while regeneration consists of the many steps or activities completed in an attempt to facilitate recovery. While more scientific information is available regarding the impact of recovery strategies, athletes often need to be educated on how and when they should be implemented. Athletes tend to turn toward regeneration modalities when they are sore, tired, or injured. Instead, recovery needs to be integrated on a daily basis and thought of as equally important as the training itself. For most athletes and coaches, regeneration strategies should take place after a workout or competition. In reality, however, recovery is a continual cycle (Figure 14.2) in which an organized approach is required and should be considered a process that takes place throughout the entire day. The many aspects of recovery play a significant role in the physiological adaptations that occur in response to training and sport. As with any training program that is designed to

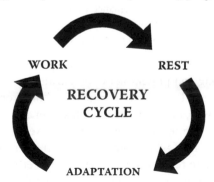

FIGURE 14.2   The recovery cycle. Recovery results from the constant interplay of work and rest that optimizes adaptation. Periodization will dictate a well-thought-out plan for delivery of stress. Recovery will complement the periodized program and optimize performance and prevent inadequate recovery. Adaptation is the product of the correct dose of work and rest.

achieve a specific goal, the process of recovery should be viewed in much the same light. High training loads are often associated with underrecovery and overreaching, which can lead to recurring periods of underperforming. Recovery could therefore be reframed and thought of as a preventive measure in that, if performed consistently, it could prevent some of the detrimental effects of overreaching, overtraining, and underrecovering (Robson-Ansley et al. 2009).

14.2.1 The Delicate Balance between Overreaching and Overtraining

The external loads and various stresses applied as a result of training break the body down, and it is the planned regeneration, rest, and recovery between training sessions that allow the athlete to achieve maximal performance and supercompensation. Within this equation, the proper planning and periodization of work are just as important as the planned regeneration sessions used to enhance recovery (Figure 14.3). Recovery through regeneration sessions and proper planning is critical to the success of every athlete. *Periodization* is classically defined as programmed variation in the training stimuli with the use of planned rest periods to augment recovery and restoration of an athlete's potential (Haff 2004).

The risk for overtraining increases when proper regeneration methods are missing from a training program. Overreaching and overtraining are loosely defined in the literature, but Kuipers and Keizer (1988) defined *overtraining* as "an imbalance between training and recovery"; Lehmann and colleagues (1999) described it as "an imbalance between stress and recovery." More recently, Halson and Jeukendrup (2004) suggested the following definitions:

> **Overtraining:** An accumulation of training and/or nontraining stress resulting in a long-term decrement in performance capacity with or without related physiological and psychological signs and symptoms of overtraining in which restoration of performance capacity may take several weeks or months.
>
> **Overreaching:** An accumulation of training and/or nontraining stress resulting in a short-term decrement in performance capacity with or without related physiological and psychological signs and symptoms of overtraining in which restoration of performance capacity may take several days to weeks.

According to Kraemer and Ratamess (2005) repeated periods of overreaching will lead to overtraining and present not only detriments to physical performance but also neuroendocrine balance. Overtraining, resulting from chronic increases in volume and underrecovery, has been shown to result in elevated cortisol and reductions in both total and free testosterone. Moreover, exercise-induced elevations in total testosterone are blunted when high-volume training is occurring, while acute catecholamine response to resistance exercise was exacerbated in overtrained men. In this respect, the overtraining syndrome was broken down by Smith (2004) into three major categories (Figure 14.4):

> **Tissue trauma:** Recurring, mild episodes of tissue trauma in the absence of appropriate regeneration occur that eventually increase in severity.

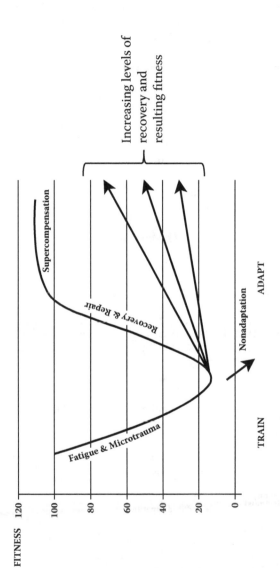

FIGURE 14.3   Role of optimal recovery in classical model of periodization and supercompensation. Increases in training intensity and volume result in fatigue and microtrauma. Effective recovery results in recovery and repair, resulting in improved physiological ability (also termed supercompensation). Notice the downward-pointing arrow intended to depict the resultant level of performance due to no recovery or inappropriate recovery.

Acute and chronic inflammation: The body's response to tissue damage is the upregulation of acute inflammation. Insufficient recovery can be a driver in causing acute inflammation to move into chronic inflammation (Buckley et al. 2001; Smith 2004).

Cytokines: Cytokines are molecules that assist in the communication of information between cells. They are not detected in the blood in normal/healthy conditions, but when there is an injury or our bodies are exposed to trauma

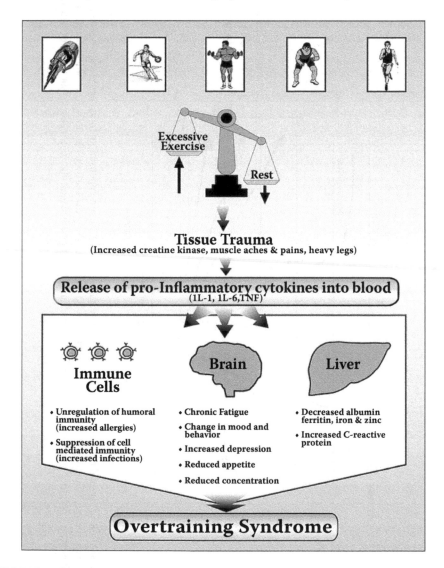

FIGURE 14.4 Proposed mechanism of the sequence of events that may result in the overtraining syndrome. IL = interleukin; TNF = tumor necrosis factor. (From Smith, L.L. Tissue Trauma: The Underlying Cause of Overtraining Syndrome? *J Strength Cond Res* 18(1): 185–93, 2004. Used with permission.)

or an abundance of stress, circulating levels of cytokines increase. As concentrations increase, they tend to communicate with the whole body to ensure that different organs are contributing what is necessary for the healing process (Maier and Watkins 1998). Smith's (2000) hypothesis is that insufficient recovery may result in chronic injury and subsequently a period of chronic inflammation as a result of the body's attempt to heal itself.

In conclusion, how the athlete feels during a training session or competition is a key factor to consider. Initially, an exercise session may feel harder than it should, or it takes longer for the athlete to recover. Eventually, heart rate levels could be elevated, appetite could be negatively impacted, and the athlete may likely adopt a rather apathetic attitude toward the sport. These types of changes in addition to a loss of body mass and changes in circulating concentrations of various blood markers (e.g., cortisol, creatine kinase, testosterone, cytokines) can also be signs of overtraining syndrome. Overall, the main purpose of recovery strategies is to prevent the downward cycle of overtraining syndrome. Proper periodization, regeneration solutions, and nutrient timing can all serve important roles in the recovery process (Halson and Jeukendrup 2004).

14.2.2 STRESS AND FATIGUE

Currently, two theories exist that attempt to explain the impact of stress on the body and how it adapts to that stress. The classic theory, general adaptation syndrome, was developed by Hans Selye in 1946 and was further characterized through a book published in 1956. Briefly, Selye suggested that all forms of biological stress were nonspecific in nature but resulted in specific and quantifiable adaptations to the body. This response by the body consists of three distinct phases (1) the alarm phase, which consists mainly of general biological responses in the body and a mobilization of available resources; (2) the resistance or adaptation phase, during which the body unveils a variety of specific adaptations to cope with the stressors; and (3) the exhaustion phase, in which the available resources in the body are overwhelmed, resulting first in an overtrained or stressed state, which leads to continual stress, further sickness, and eventual death.

More recently, the fitness-fatigue model attempts to explain physiologically how programmed variation through proper periodization can enhance resulting performance (Haff 2004). Briefly, the fitness-fatigue model characterizes the short-term fatigue that results from common exercise and training sessions. This anticipated response provides the necessary "overload" to invoke the desired physiological adaptation seen as a result of regular exercise training. Finally, the model outlines the long-term fitness or performance effect that is specific to the type of work being completed (i.e., maximal strength vs. hypertrophy). Importantly, if work is reapplied during the short-term fatigue state too soon or too often, then performance will continue to fall, resulting in an enhanced potential for overtraining (Chiu and Barnes 2003).

Fatigue is a multifactorial state impacted at the central, peripheral, and parasympathetic/vagal levels. *Central fatigue* is a commonly discussed theory of fatigue. In this respect, proponents of central fatigue state that muscles are capable of greater mechanical output than what is produced, but negative feedback from the central nervous system blocks continued muscular effort, which is purported to serve as a potential mechanism for protection from injury or some other self-sacrificing purpose (Bishop et al. 2008; Taylor et al. 2000). For example, sustained contractions inside a muscle decrease motor neuron activity, resulting in submaximal levels of force production, while motor cortex output is reduced during times of fatigue (Gandevia 1998). *Peripherally,* fatigue has been reported to occur when the homeostatic mechanisms inside muscle are disrupted to the point that the muscle is biochemically or mechanically incapable of responding effectively when compared to a typical response at rest (Bishop et al. 2008; Lainer 2003). Finally, parasympathetic or vagal fatigue is thought to result in increased fatigue, feelings of apathy and an altered mood state along with decrements in immune and reproductive function (Halson and Jeukendrup 2004). *Parasympathetic fatigue* is suggested to be the most common form of fatigue and is most often linked to overtraining (Lehman et al. 1998), often resulting from an imbalance between high-volume training, underrecovery, and other stressors. For this reason, a common recovery goal is to improve or restore the balance between parasympathetic and sympathetic activity.

Regardless of the type of fatigue, a number of stressors arise within any given training session, and fatigue should be viewed as a combination of both central and peripheral fatigue in addition to depletion of fuel stores that overall is dependent on the type of session or activity (Bishop et al. 2008; Enoka 1995; Kay et al. 2001). Regarding fatigue and the type of activity or the nature of training, specific sites of fatigue have been identified: (1) *nutritional* (fluid balance and availability of fuel stores); (2) *physiological* (nerve, muscle, bone, connective tissue cells); (3) *neurological* (peripheral nervous system); and (4) *psychological* (central nervous system) (Cochrane 2004). As such, the highest-to-lowest determinants of fatigue for endurance athletes were nutritional, physiological, neurological, and psychological, while for strength/power or speed athletes these were neurological, physiological, nutritional, and psychological (Calder 1995). While theoretical, this suggestion holds important implications for those who are working with different types of athletes and designing recovery solutions for a diverse array of athletes. While all components need consideration, it stands to reason that the solution should be driven by what is needed based on the stress of the training or activity.

14.2.3 THE STRESS OF EXERCISE

When thinking in terms of recovery from a nutritional and physical standpoint, various forms of negative stress caused by a training session, practice, or game exist. Recovery considerations include an assessment of the amount of tissue trauma, degree of dehydration, and most importantly the amount of fuel and nutrient depletion as all of these factors interact with biochemical adaptations and dictate what the nutritional requirements are within the body. In essence, the amount of repletion should always be driven by the amount of trauma or depletion that the body endures. Certainly, the intensity of exercise then becomes a critical factor that must be monitored and carefully considered. Strenuous exercise (>70% VO_2Max [maximum oxygen consumption]) is known to increase neural humoral factors that increase the hormonal output of epinephrine, norepinephrine, and glucagon while decreasing the release of insulin. These actions stimulate glycogen breakdown in the liver and active muscle, in effect resulting in the primary means by which fuel is provided to the working muscle. In addition, intense exercise oxidizes tremendous amounts of carbohydrate as fuel and increases the breakdown of protein. As the duration of high-intensity exercise continues, hepatic release of glucose supplies up to 30% of the total energy required by the exercising muscle, with the remaining fuel needs coming from intramuscular glycogen. For example, it has been shown that just one hour of high-intensity exercises ($>75\%$ VO_2Peak) decreases liver glycogen by about 45%, while a duration of two hours exhausts both hepatic and skeletal muscle stores of glycogen (McArdle et al. 2001). Similarly, moderate and prolonged exercise (50–60% VO_2Max) is fueled predominantly by glycogen stored in active muscles. Within the first 20 minutes of moderate-intensity exercise, liver and muscle glycogen supplies between 40% and 50% of the energy requirement. The remainder is provided by fat breakdown. As exercise continues and the immediate muscle glycogen stores diminish, blood glucose from the liver becomes a major supplier of carbohydrate energy (McArdle et al. 2001).

14.3 BASIC OVERVIEW OF RECOVERY MODALITIES

As mentioned, promoting a positive balance of parasympathetic and sympathetic involvement should be a primary goal of recovery. It is well established that exercise decreases parasympathetic activity and increases sympathetic activity. Sympathetic activation induces myriad responses, including release of noradrenalin and adrenaline, which increases myocardial contractility and acceleration of heart rate. Vasoconstriction in other tissues (skin, gut, liver, kidneys, etc.) increases blood pressure, vasodilation of heart and skeletal muscle vasculature facilitates venous return, while dilation of airways promotes gas exchange (McArdle et al. 2001). Regular, chronic overstimulation of sympathetic activity, without adequate recovery, is hypothesized to result in overreaching and overtraining. Several modalities exist that when used independently and synergistically can potentially assist in reestablishing parasympathetic/sympathetic balance and speeding physiological recovery.

14.3.1 ACTIVE RECOVERY

Active recovery is a common recovery modality that can increase metabolic rate and promote systemic blood flow (Barnet 2006; Martin et al. 1998), thereby allowing for increased removal of accumulated metabolic waste. Other factors, such as local blood flow, chemical buffering, and lactate conversion to pyruvate in the liver, muscle, and heart, all are thought to have an impact on the extent that accumulation occurs in the blood (Cochrane 2004; McArdle et al. 2001). These considerations, along with other findings that illustrate increased removal of lactate after active recovery versus passive recovery (Cochrane 2004; Martin et al. 1998), lead to the recommendation of utilizing a period of active recovery after the stress-inducing training session or competition (Menzies et al. 2010).

A number of active recovery techniques exist. Dodd et al. in 1984 found that a 40-minute recovery period of continuous moderate-intensity (35% VO_2Max) exercise produced faster removal of lactate in comparison to passive recovery, and that the combination of high intensity (65% VO_2Max) and low intensity (35% VO_2Max) was equally effective. Studies have shown beneficial active recovery intensities ranging from 25% to 63% of VO_2Max (Menzies et al. 2010).

Interestingly, current literature suggests that an active recovery intensity relative to lactate threshold may be more beneficial as it may more effectively link lactate accumulation to the workload at which lactate production exceeds lactate removal (Greenwood et al. 2008). For example, lactate clearance was determined after similar-duration exercise periods at 100%, 80%, 60%, 40%, and 0% of lactate threshold (Menzies et al. 2010). Lactate removal was found to be most effective between 60% and 100% of lactate threshold, and that recovery within this range was statistically more effective at clearing lactate than recovery at 40% of lactate threshold. Also, recovery at 40% of lactate threshold was no better than passive recovery (Menzies et al. 2010). Therefore, utilizing an athlete's lactate threshold and corresponding heart rate appears to be an effective consideration to facilitate recovery.

Certainly, the importance of lactate clearance is a matter of debate, but it has been recognized that elevated blood concentrations of skeletal muscle and blood lactate are associated with impaired muscle function (Menzies et al. 2010), and although a direct correlation between lactate and fatigue is lacking, when looked at indirectly, lactate accumulation is associated with increased release of H^+, a key factor leading to metabolic acidosis. In addition, increases in metabolic acidosis lead to the subsequent inhibition of glycolytic rate-limiting enzymes, lipolysis, and contractility of skeletal muscles (Brooks 2002; Menzies et al. 2010). Consequently, whether or not an increased removal of lactate will directly enhance performance remains in question, strategies to improve blood flow and remove lactate are associated with improved recovery and enhanced adaptation (Menzies et al. 2010).

14.3.2 HYDROTHERAPY

Water can be used as a medium during both active and passive recovery. Ice baths, whirlpools, warm baths, cold plunges, and even hotel bathtubs filed with ice water have become popular as recovery modalities (Cochrane 2004). The physiology of cooling involves temperature decreases in the skin and connective and muscle tissues (Enwemeka et al. 2002). Decreases in tissue temperature result in vasoconstriction of sympathetic fibers, ultimately resulting in decreases in swelling and inflammation (Cochrane 2004; Enwemeka et al. 2002).

Thermotherapy, also called heat therapy, has been shown to increase tissue temperature, local blood flow, and muscle elasticity while causing local vasodilation. Heat therapy decreases sympathetic nerve activity, which results in vasodilation of local blood vessels and increased circulation. Increases in blood flow result in an increased supply of oxygen and antibodies and the ability to clear metabolites (Zuluaga et al. 1995). Finally, thermotherapy can also serve as a psychological unloading or relaxation tool. Thermotherapy, however, is not recommended for the initial three to four days after an acute injury, such as a sprained joint or severely strained muscle, due to its ability to increase circulation, which in this scenario would result in an increase in swelling, a contraindicated response. However, chronic or regular aches, pains, tenderness, tightness, and so on can effectively be managed with thermotherapy.

Cryotherapy, also called cold therapy, is likely the most commonly employed therapeutic modality for its ability to decrease pain, swelling, and inflammation and promote general recovery as well as recovery from acute injuries. While a number of investigations have attempted to identify the impact of various types of ice, size of application, combination with other modalities, and so on, it remains that cryotherapy is an important consideration to promote recovery from acute injuries as well as chronic overuse injuries (Bleakley et al. 2004; Meeusen and Lievens 1986; Swenson et al. 1996). Vaile and colleagues (2008) reported that cold water immersion lowered body temperature to a greater degree than contrast therapy while similarly restoring performance.

Contrast therapy, or intermittent exposure to thermotherapy (heat) and cryotherapy (cold), is a commonly used modality as well. This modality is thought to play a role in inducing a superficial flush of vascular/lymphatic tissues through repetitive vasodilation and vasoconstriction, resulting in increased blood flow, removal of metabolites, muscle repair, and slowing of the metabolic process (Cochrane 2004). Like the other forms of hydrotherapy, a number of studies have reported on the impact of contrast therapy. For example, Gill and colleagues indicated that acute contrast hydrotherapy decreased creatine kinase, a predominant marker of muscle damage, in rugby players (Gill et al. 2006), while a soreness-inducing protocol utilizing a leg press failed to have an impact on creatine kinase changes but did effectively improve the recovery of other markers, as seen by an overall smaller reduction as well as faster restoration of strength and power lost after completing the soreness protocol. Finally, Ingram and colleagues (2009) used a simulated 80-minute team sport activity followed by a 20-meter shuttle run to exhaustion and compared cold water immersion and contrast therapy. While both modalities effectively reduced muscle soreness and recovery of performance, contrast therapy was found to be superior.

14.3.3 Soft Tissue

Massage and soft tissue work or myofascial release are used as another common modality to help manage pain, improve tissue quality, and facilitate recovery. Massage is theorized to facilitate displacement of accumulated fluid that results after injury and leads to an increase in pressure levels that act on pain sensors inside tissues, resulting in an increased sensation of pain. As such, longitudinal massage is thought to result in increased drainage of venous, lymphatic, and tissue fluids as well as metabolites and pain agents. On removal of these components, oxygenated blood can be put back in its place (Sandler 1999). However, the research on massage falls to serious methodological flaws (Ernst 1998) in which reported studies in which recommendations are derived have failed to contain necessary controls and adequate number of subjects and conclusions drawn from speculative versus objective interpretations of the data (Chiu et al. 2001; Moyer et al. 2009). Regardless, the practice of massage in sport is widespread.

Immediate kneading massage performed after maximal running was not found to enhance lactate clearance in comparison to passive recovery (Gupta et al. 1996), a modality that has been discussed in this chapter as inferior to active forms of recovery. Similar outcomes were found in cyclists after multiple wingate tests (Martin et al. 1998), while a massage immediately after boxing performance was found to have psychological (perceived recovery), but no physiological, benefits (lactate removal) when compared to passive recovery (Hemmings et al. 2000). Interestingly, massage performed immediately after maximal exercise had no impact on changes in creatine kinase, neutrophil changes, and cortisol levels, but when delayed for two hours, greater outcomes were reported (Smith et al. 1994). For this reason, delayed use of massage by a few hours or integrating massage into a recovery day a few times a week may be a more efficient use of massage on recovery.

14.3.4 WHOLE-BODY VIBRATION

Whole-body vibration is another increasingly popular recovery modality used in enhancing the body's adaptation to exercise. A number of studies have outlined various neuromuscular, physiological, and biochemical changes that occur on exposure to whole-body vibration. In 2006, Kvorning et al. compared the combination of whole-body vibration with resistance training, resistance training only, and vibration training only. No changes were reported in any neuromuscular variables, but the groups undergoing conventional strength training and vibration plus strength training increased their maximal force production capabilities on the squat exercise. Testosterone increased in a similar fashion in all groups after exercise (as expected), but the combination of strength training and vibration the only modality that failed to elicit changes in growth hormone, but it did see changes in cortisol. The authors concluded that the combination of vibration and strength training did not exert any additional effect over traditional resistance training, and that the combination of strength training and vibration training may result in unfavorable hormonal changes.

Other studies have reported that whole-body vibration may result in an improved anabolic profile. For example, whole-body vibration increased circulating IGF-1 (insulin-like growth factor 1) when strength exercises were combined with vibration (Cardinale et al. 2010), but these effects were seen in a nonathletic, aged population, so how well these outcomes translated to young, healthy athletes are unknown.

Finally, studies have suggested that vibration training may reduce postexercise soreness. Whole-body vibration massage has been shown to significantly increase blood flow and to decrease perceived soreness; therefore, it is suggested to be used as a tool for reducing pain, muscle soreness, and tightness after strenuous training. In this respect, Rhea and colleagues (2009) completed a study that concluded that whole-body vibration can reduce perceived pain within 24 hours of ending a training session in comparison to a control group.

In summary, Marin and Rhea completed two impressive reviews on vibration training and its impact on strength (Marin and Rhea 2010b) and power (Marin and Rhea 2010a). Their conclusions are as follows:

- Chronic improvements in strength compare favorably with conventional resistance training for vertical vibration platforms. A moderate treatment effect of whole-body vibration exists over an average of 13.5 weeks of training.

- Vertical vibration platforms were found to be more effective in comparison to oscillating platforms for chronic strength improvements.
- A linear increase in effect was demonstrated with an increase in vibration frequency. Frequencies between 40 and 50 Hz with amplitudes between 8 to 10 millimeters resulted in the greatest improvements in strength. Maximum strength gains were seen when total whole-body vibration totaled 12 to 15 total minutes per session.
- No positive effect on acute power output was noted on either vertical or oscillating platforms.

14.3.5 Breathing/Visual Relaxation

An additional commonly used modality is meditative breathing and visualization. It is widely recognized that relaxation/visualization can influence parasympathetic tone and autonomic balance, which effectively creates the foundation for its inclusion as a potential regenerative technique. In this respect, heart rate variability has become a popular tool used to evaluate and study the neural control of the heart and the interaction between sympathetic and vagal influence on the heart (Aubert et al. 2002). Within the measurements of heart rate variability, changes in vagal modulation and sympathetic tone can be detected because they are associated with different frequency regions (Aubert et al. 2002). When using heart rate variability as a marker of adaptation, it has been shown that breathing at a frequency of six breaths per minute assisted by biofeedback can improve the variability of cardiovascular function. For this reason, deep breathing is considered to be an important regenerative strategy to improve autonomic balance (Vaschillo et al. 2002, 2004).

14.4 NUTRITION AND ITS INCLUSION IN RECOVERY

A number of factors play a role in the acute and chronic adaptation to exercise, including appropriate training, and nutrition, as well as regeneration and recovery techniques. Unfortunately, research investigating the synergistic effects of nutrition integrated into a recovery program is lacking; however, by taking a look at the science behind each method, we can see the potentially synergistic effect of employing the science of nutrient timing in conjunction with recovery solutions. It has been known for some time that the quality, quantity, and timing of dietary intake around the workout allow for the body to adapt most efficiently (Figure 14.5) (Volek 2004). However, there is a clear need for additional research on the combined effects of recovery modalities and practices with the timing on nutrients; however, it is concluded that if athletes can combine the right nutrients at the right time while there is an increase in nutritive blood flow (Clark et al. 2000), they should be able to maximize the ability of their body to refuel, recover, and rebuild.

Nutrient timing in relation to recovery nutrition and the prevention of overtraining is often viewed only in the window of recovery, which is pre-, during, and after workout/activity. This window is extremely important in promoting adaptation and stimulating recovery (Hawley et al. 2006), but it is consistent nutrition and other recovery strategies that help athletes to maximize adaptations to training and keep

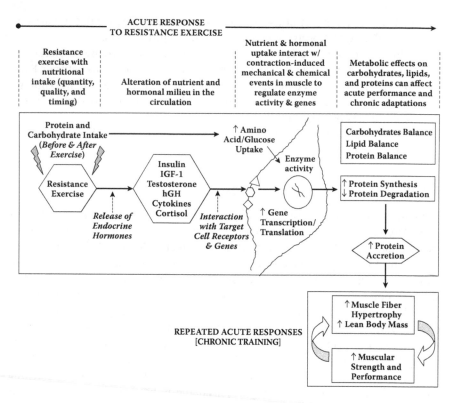

FIGURE 14.5 Acute response to resistance training. (From Volek, J. Influence of Nutrition on Responses to Resistance Training. *Med Sci Sports Exerc* 36(1):69–96, 2004. Used with permission.)

the athlete healthy through the duration of a season. In this respect, studies have reported that athletes who are undernourished and inadequately fueled on a day-to-day basis are at a higher risk for overtraining (Gleeson and Nicolette 2000; Lowery and Forsythe 2006). While this text is devoted to providing nutritional timing recommendations as a part of various aspects of sport, the following sections provide broad and general recommendations for all athletes.

14.4.1 Daily Nutrition

- Carbohydrate: Five to seven grams of carbohydrate per kilogram of body mass per day for general training needs and seven to ten grams of carbohydrate per kilogram of body mass per day for increased needs due to endurance training or strength and power athletes enduring multiple training sessions per day (Burke, Cox, et al. 2001; Manore et al. 2000).
- Protein: 1.2 to 1.7 grams of protein per kilogram of body mass per day depending on sport and intensity of training (Manore et al. 2000; Phillips 2006).

- Fat: Remainder of needed calories. The amount of fat should be at least one gram of fat per kilogram of body mass per day and no less than 15% of total calories (Manore et al. 2000).
- Hydration: The Institute of Medicine's recommendations for fluid intake are 2.7 liters per day for women and 3.7 liters per day for men. Determine an exact amount of fluid for your athlete to consume. A range of 0.5 to 1 fluid ounce per pound per day depending on activity throughout the day will help to give greater direction for fluid intake.
- Multivitamin, fish oil ergogenic aids: Must be determined on an as-needed basis from the analysis of dietary intake. These recommendations should be made under the supervision of a dietitian, sports nutritionist, or a physician knowledgeable in nutrition and need to be in accordance with the rules on banned substances for the athlete.

In this respect, fish oil has been found to improve many recovery markers for athletes. Prolonged intensive exercise results in suppression of immune function, and supplementation with long-chain polyunsaturated fatty acids—eicosopentaenoic acid (EPA) and decosahexaenoic acid (DHA)—contained in fish oil can mediate production and accumulation of leukotrienes and prostaglandins and subsequently decrease inflammation. Elite swimmers taking 1.8 gram of EPA/DHA per day for six weeks had lower levels of arachidonic acid, a precursor to inflammation, and lower values of cytokines specific to immune stress (Andrade et al. 2007). EPA/DHA supplementation has also been found to improve the perception of pain in athletes with chronic tendinitis and rheumatoid arthritis (Lewis and Sandford 2009; Mavrogenis et al. 2004). Finally, in comparison to an antioxidant mixture, 2.4 grams of EPA/DHA supplementation was found to superiorly improve markers of oxidative stress after six weeks of intense cycling training (McAnulty et al. 2010). Therefore, a minimum of 1.8 grams of EPA/DHA is recommended on a daily basis to assist athletes in controlling inflammatory and immune markers.

14.4.2 Recovery Nutrition

14.4.2.1 Pretraining or Practice

As outlined in Chapters 6 and 9 of this text, the optimal carbohydrate and protein content of a preexercise meal is dependent on a number of factors, including exercise duration and fitness level:

- General guidelines recommend ingestion of one to two grams of carbohydrate per kilogram of body mass and 0.15 to 0.25 grams of protein per kilogram of body mass three to four hours before exertion (Kerksick et al. 2008).
- Preexercise ingestion of essential amino acids or protein alone increases muscle protein synthesis. In addition, ingesting protein and carbohydrate preexercise has been shown to maximally stimulate muscle protein synthesis while promoting rapid resynthesis of muscle and liver glycogen (Kerksick et al. 2008).

- Ingest 17 to 20 fluid ounces of water or a sports drink in the two hours prior to training and then an additional 10 fluid ounces 10 to 20 minutes prior to training (Casa et al. 2000).

14.4.2.2 During Training or Practice

Fluid intake is critical during training and practice, particularly in hot and humid conditions, and should comprise a major focus of an athlete's nutrition and recovery efforts. Other factors to consider include

- Copious and regular fluid ingestion at a rate of 12 to 16 fluid ounces of water if the exercise session will take less than 45 to 60 minutes. This recommendation is employed to help the athlete make sure he or she drinks enough fluid to prevent no more than a 2% decrease in body weight during the workout or competition (Casa et al. 2000).
- If exercise duration increases beyond 60 minutes, a sports drink containing carbohydrate and electrolytes is beneficial. This carbohydrate source should supply 30 to 60 grams of carbohydrate per hour and can typically be delivered by drinking one to two cups of a 6–8% carbohydrate solution (8 to 16 fluid ounces) every 10 to 15 minutes (Kerksick et al. 2008).
- Mixing different forms of carbohydrate has been shown to increase muscle carbohydrate oxidation from 1.0 gram of carbohydrate per minute to levels ranging from 1.2 grams to 1.75 grams of carbohydrate per minute, an effect associated with an improvement in time trial performance; therefore, glucose, fructose, sucrose, and maltodextrin can be used in combination, but large amounts of fructose are not recommended due to the greater likelihood of gastrointestinal problems (Kerksick et al. 2008).
- The research suggests that carbohydrate alone or in combination with protein during resistance exercise increases muscle glycogen stores, offsets muscle damage, and facilitates greater training adaptations after acute and prolonged periods of resistance training (Kerksick et al. 2008).
- Food and fluids should be palatable and easy to digest.

14.4.2.3 After Training or Practice

Postexercise recovery has been shown to be a critical period for the athlete as a number of athletes do not eat anything in the postworkout period. A general guideline then is to add a meal, chocolate milk, or a whole-food snack as soon as possible after a training session or competition to facilitate the recovery process. The postworkout nutrition beverage or food should consist of both carbohydrate and protein (Kerksick et al. 2008). Liquid is often better tolerated than solid food because some athletes experience appetite suppression with intense exercise and for this reason they are recommended; however, when tolerance and appetite are not an issue, solid foods are a viable consideration. Engineered supplements, like protein shakes and bars, are commonly utilized during this time period because of their convenience. However, other less-expensive alternatives like chocolate milk have been shown to be effective in helping with recovery (Karp et al. 2006). Regardless, any combination of carbohydrate and protein as soon as possible but within the first 30 minutes after the completion of training is advised. A final recommendation is to keep things simple. To an athlete or coach, particularly a young athlete, nutrition can seem overwhelming when looked at over the course of a whole day's meals, a week's plan, or a yearly schedule, but providing a good source of fuel in a convenient, easy-to-administer format may be the easiest and most consistent way to jumpstart the body's recovery process.

14.5 CONCLUSION

The proper recovery solution will take into account all levels of distress on the body: environmental, physiological, psychological, social, biochemical, anatomical, and structural. An approach of education and empowerment should be taken with active individuals to ensure understanding and control of sustainable strategies. From a foundational aspect of nutrition recommendations, considerations such as meal spacing and timing and portion control based on goals, grocery shopping, preworkout nutrition, during-workout nutrition, hydration, travel strategies, and most importantly, postworkout nutrition are key factors to consider.

The practice of sports nutrition and coaching is somewhere between science and art. It is important not to get bogged down in the specific clinical findings and create a system that works for the athletes with whom you work. If you do not have a cold plunge and a whirlpool, use an ice bath and a warm shower. If you cannot meet exact protein needs postworkout, find the closest thing possible. Getting athletes to change the way they act and eat can have a positive impact on performance, although impacting behavior change is not always easy. By using a systematic approach to assessment, evaluation of needs, and intervention/education and then building deep relationships with an athlete, you will be able to change his or her systems and improve recovery. Integrating nutrition with other regeneration techniques will help to meet the body's need to combat the distress on the body from environmental, psychological, social, physiological, biochemical, anatomical, and structural sources. There are many other strategies for creating recovery solutions, but contained within this chapter are sustainable suggestions that can put an athlete in the best possible position to perform every time they step into a competitive or training scenario. In the end, the best methods are those that the athlete believes in, feels empowered to complete independently, and improves the athlete's performance.

15 Nutrient Timing Considerations for the Military, Aged, Metabolically-Challenged Populations, and Children

Vincent J. Dalbo, Jeffrey R. Stout, and Chad M. Kerksick

CONTENTS

15.1 INTRODUCTION

The majority of research investigating the impact of nutrient timing has focused on metabolic changes and adaptations associated with various types of exercise. On considering the potential impact for nutrient timing in sporting scenarios, interest has developed to explore how nutrient timing may have an impact on other specialized groups or populations. In this respect, available research suggests that nutrient timing strategies may exert a positive effect in aged (>50 y) populations and their current or future battle with sarcopenia. In addition, nutrient availability and timing have become an area of special interest for military personnel, metabolically challenged, and athletic children.

15.2 NUTRITION AND NUTRIENT TIMING IN AN AGED POPULATION

Sarcopenia is known as a progressive loss of skeletal muscle mass with age, resulting in reductions in strength (Giresi et al. 2005), mobility (Giresi et al. 2005), quality of life (Evans 1997), and increases in injury risk (Evans 1997; Giresi et al. 2005). The prevalence of sarcopenia in the Unites States is impressive as approximately 45% of adults 60 years of age and older have been estimated to be sarcopenic, with approximately 20% classified as functionally disabled (Janssen et al. 2004). The most recent estimate of the economic impact of sarcopenia was published in 2000, with estimated direct health care costs at $18.5 billion. As such, a 10% reduction in the prevalence of sarcopenia could save the United States $1.1 billion per year in health care costs (Janssen et al. 2004).

Numerous factors contribute to the age-related loss of skeletal muscle mass, including: (1) hormonal adaptations that occur at rest (Copeland et al. 1990; Gray et al. 1991; Kern et al. 1996; Kraemer et al. 1999; Lamberts et al. 1997; Roberts et al. 2009) and following resistance exercise (Craig et al. 1989; Hakkinen and Pakarinen 1995; Nicklas et al. 1995; Roberts et al. 2009); (2) decrements in myofibrillar protein synthesis (Welle et al. 1995); (3) reduced number of total (Roth et al. 2001; Verdijk et al. 2007) and active satellite cells (Roth et al. 2001; Verdijk, Gleeson, et al. 2009); (4) denervation and reinnervation of skeletal muscle fibers (Lexell and Downham 1991); and (5) decreased physical activity (Sallis 2000).

15.2.1 NUTRITIONAL CONSIDERATIONS FOR AGED POPULATIONS

A sedentary lifestyle and nutritional deficiencies are two primary factors that contribute to the development of sarcopenia. Multiple investigations have indicated that the regular dietary intake of older individuals is deficient in a number of important nutrients. For example, Foote and colleagues (2000) reported that 1,740 healthy older adults (51 to 85 years) did not get adequate amounts of vitamin D, vitamin E, folate, and calcium, and only 10% consumed recommended amounts of dairy, grains, fruits, and vegetables.

15.2.1.1 Protein Considerations for the Aged

The need for adequate protein is well established (Paddon-Jones 2006; Paddon-Jones et al. 2004; Walrand and Boirie 2005). Although the current Recommended Dietary

Allowance (RDA) for protein is 0.8 grams of protein per kilogram of body mass per day, reports have suggested that 15% to 38% of adult men and 27% to 41% of adult women consume less than this recommended amount (Campbell et al. 2001). This is particularly problematic when a number of studies have suggested that older adults are less efficient at utilizing protein and for this reason may require a greater daily amount of protein (Cuthbertson et al. 2005; Rousset et al. 2003; Walrand and Boirie 2005). Continued debate exists as a number of studies have suggested that 0.8 grams of protein per kilogram of body mass per day of protein is an adequate amount of protein (Millward 1999; Millward et al. 1997; Zanni et al. 1979), while other investigations have suggested that a protein intake between 1.0 and 1.3 grams of protein per kilogram of body mass per day may be necessary to maintain nitrogen balance and counteract lower energy intake, decreased protein synthetic efficiency, and impaired insulin sensitivity characteristics of older adults (Campbell et al. 2001; Cuthbertson et al. 2005; Morais et al. 2006; Paddon-Jones et al. 2008).

Although no widespread consensus exists, many studies suggest that a minimum of one gram of protein per kilogram of body mass per day is necessary (Houston et al. 2008; Paddon-Jones and Rasmussen 2009; Wolfe and Miller 2008). In this regard, Rousset et al. concluded that older individuals who consume 0.8 grams of protein per kilogram of body mass per day are at greater risk for disease than older adults who consume over 1.2 grams of protein per kilogram of body mass per day (Rousset et al. 2003).

An interesting concept regarding protein intake with aged individuals is the total amount of protein consumed per meal or, more specifically, the total amount of essential amino acids per meal (Table 15.1). For starters, ingesting a 25- to 30-gram

TABLE 15.1
Protein/Amino Acid Profile of Commonly Consumed Meats

	95% Lean Ground Beef (85 g)	Pork Loin (85 g)	Light Meat Chicken with Skin (79 g)	Turkey Breast with Skin (112 g)	Whey Protein Isolate (100 g)	Soy Protein Isolate (100 g)
Protein (g)	22.3	21.6	22.9	32.2	100	100
Isoleucine (mg)	979	1,009	1,152	1,621	6,800	4,900
Leucine (mg)	1,741	1,729	1,674	2,509	10,900	8,200
Lysine (mg)	1,861	1,938	1,875	2,941	9,500	6,300
Methionine (mg)	589	570	613	908	3,100	1,300
Phenylalanine (mg)	858	860	893	1,261	2,500	5,200
Threonine (mg)	882	984	949	1,408	8,300	3,800
Tryptophan (mg)	132	274	258	356	2,000	1,300
Valine (mg)	1,094	1,169	1,116	1,680	6,400	5,000
Histidine (mg)	745	861	678	972	1,800	2,600
Tyrosine (mg)	702	750	743	1,228	3,100	3,800

dose of protein has been shown in both young and older adults to maximally stimulate muscle protein synthesis (Paddon-Jones and Rasmussen 2009). Studies primarily in younger individuals, however, have suggested that it is the essential amino acid content, in a dosage of five to eight grams, that favorably dictates stimulation of muscle protein synthesis (Volpi et al. 2003, 148). In older adults, however, a dosage of 7.5 grams is too low to stimulate an anabolic response (Paddon-Jones and Rasmussen 2009). Interestingly, when a large dose is provided (10 to 15 grams of essential amino acids), older adults respond in a similar fashion as younger adults (Katsanos et al. 2005; Paddon-Jones et al. 2004). Finally, smaller doses of protein (20 to 30 grams) are recommended for older adults after Symons and colleagues (2007) reported that increases in muscle protein synthesis were similar after ingesting a 90-gram dose and a 30-gram dose, a conclusion also supported by the findings of Moore and coworkers, who reported that no further increase in muscle protein synthesis was seen after ingestion of 40 grams of egg protein when compared to 20 grams of egg protein in young individuals (Moore, Robinson, et al. 2009).

15.2.1.2   Creatine Monohydrate and the Aged

Creatine supplementation has been suggested to enhance skeletal muscle hypertrophy through a variety of mechanisms, all of which act to reduce whole-body proteolysis and amino acid oxidation (Berneis et al. 1999), favorably altering the expression of myogenic transcription factors (Hespel et al. 2001; Ingwall 1976; Willoughby and Rosene 2001; Young and Denome 1984); increase satellite cell activity (Dangott et al. 2000; Olsen et al. 2006); and allow for increased exercise volume to be completed secondary to favorable alterations to various components of the phosphocreatine energy system (Casey et al. 1996; Rawson and Volek 2003). Interestingly, limited evidence does suggest that creatine may exert hypertrophic effects independent of an exercise stimulus, albeit the increases in type II muscle fibers were the ocular muscles (Sipila et al. 1981). More commonly, daily creatine administration (six grams per day) over a 12-week period along with resistance training increased myosin heavy-chain isoform messenger RNA (mRNA) and protein expression to a greater extent than training alone in college-aged men (Willoughby and Rosene 2001). This study along with other seminal reviews and position statements on creatine monohydrate support its efficacy as an ergogenic aid to improve strength and endurance and promote muscle hypertrophy (Buford et al. 2007; Kreider 2003).

In this respect, studies suggest that when creatine supplementation is combined with a regular resistance training program in older adults, significant increases in skeletal muscle mass (Candow et al. 2008; Chrusch et al. 2001; Gotshalk et al. 2008; Rawson and Clarkson 2000); strength (Brose et al. 2003; Candow et al. 2008; Chrusch et al. 2001; Gotshalk et al. 2008; Rawson and Clarkson 2000); and skeletal muscle endurance (Stout et al. 2007) are the result. Of particular interest are the studies of Gotshalk et al. (2002, 2008), who reported creatine supplementation at a dose of 0.3 grams of creatine per kilogram of body mass per day for a period of seven days significantly increases the ability of older adults to perform functional tasks.

The typical dosing regimen for creatine supplementation is traditionally a two-stage approach. During the loading phase, a daily creatine dosage of 20 grams per day (approximately 0.3 grams of creatine per kilogram of body mass per day) is achieved by ingesting four doses of five grams each throughout the day. After five to seven days of loading, a maintenance dose of two to four grams each day (0.03 g/kilogram of body mass) is ingested indefinitely. The loading phase is not necessary (Brose et al. 2003; Chrusch et al. 2001; Gotshalk et al. 2002, 2008) unless rapid increases of intramuscular creatine stores are desired.

Using an older population, Stout and colleagues (2007), over a 14-day period, had older men and women supplement with either a placebo or creatine monohydrate and complete a series of performance assessments. Creatine supplementation increased upper body grip strength and physical working capacity on a cycle ergometer, an outcome also found by Brose et al. (2003). Over a longer period of time, Candow et al. (2008) had 35 older (59 to 77 years) men who resistance trained three days per week for 10 weeks. Participants were randomly assigned in a double-blind fashion to one of three groups: creatine-protein (0.1 grams of creatine per kilogram of body mass + 0.3 grams of protein per kilogram of body mass); creatine (0.1 grams of creatine per kilogram of body mass); or a placebo group. Supplements were only consumed on training days. Creatine and creatine-protein supplementation resulted in significantly greater gains in body mass and total muscle thickness and less bone resorption as assessed by cross-linked N-telopeptides of type I collagen (NTx) when compared to the placebo group. The combination of creatine and protein, however, resulted in significantly greater increases in bench press strength than the creatine-only and placebo groups, suggesting that some level of synergistic action was occurring. Incidentally, similar outcomes were reported by Kerksick and colleagues (2007) in a population of young resistance-trained males, leading one to speculate that this combination may be of equal benefit to both young and older populations.

15.2.1.3 Whey Protein and the Aged

As mentioned, maintaining an appropriate level of protein intake in the diet is physiologically important and many times a challenge for older populations. For this reason, whey protein is considered a key source of protein because of its relatively high quality, ease of digestion, and bioactive capabilities (Phillips et al. 2009). These factors, in addition to a relative lack of desire to eat and chewing difficulties with other common protein (meat) sources (Paddon-Jones et al. 2008), make whey protein a popular consideration.

Relative to the timing of these nutrients, the work of Cribb and Hayes (2006) in young, resistance-training males suggest the combination of protein, creatine, and carbohydrates immediately prior to and following each resistance training session over 10 weeks is a powerful stimulus to increase lean body mass, strength, and type II muscle fiber cross-sectional area compared to consuming the same supplement in the morning and late evening in young men. Interestingly, Verdijk et al. (Verdijk, Jonkers, et al. 2009) completed a similar study comparing the effect of ingesting protein immediately before and immediately after bouts of resistance training and compared them to a control group over a 12-week period. Each week, 26 healthy, older participants (72 ± 2 years) resistance trained three days per week and consumed a protein drink containing 10 grams of protein. No differences between groups for strength, muscle mass, or skeletal muscle hypertrophy of type I or type II skeletal fiber size were found following training, suggesting that timing of a protein supplement surrounding resistance exercise may not have the same benefits as seen in younger participants. On the other hand, the relatively small dose of protein might not have adequately stimulated protein synthetic mechanisms in the older population (Paddon-Jones and Rasmussen 2009). This study and another study with younger, college-aged participants suggest that as long as an adequate amount of protein is being consumed daily (1.1 grams of protein per kilogram of body mass per day), protein supplementation surrounding resistance training may offer limited additional benefit.

This last point is important because a number of studies revealed that many positive changes result when protein intake in older populations is adequate, although studies do suggest that many older people have difficulty consuming higher amounts of protein. In a recommendation somewhat related to timing, it does appear that a key factor to maximize muscle protein synthesis is the consumption of 25 to 30 grams of protein with each meal (Paddon-Jones and Rasmussen 2009) and for these meals to be spread out across the entire day.

15.2.1.4 Leucine and the Aged

Leucine is an essential amino acid that has been found to promote muscle protein synthesis by modulating intracellular kinases that activate the translation of mTOR (Dardevet et al. 2000; Kimball et al. 1999), a key molecule implicated in building more protein. In light of other dietary recommendations, several investigations have suggested the acute consumption of leucine with normal mixed-nutrient meals may improve or normalize muscle protein synthesis in aging muscle of animals (Combaret et al. 2005; Dardevet et al. 2000; Rieu et al. 2003) and humans (Layman 2002; Rieu et al. 2006).

Using an animal model, leucine addition to a high-fat diet resulted in a 32% reduction of weight gain, 25% reduction in adiposity, 27% reduction in total cholesterol, 53% reduction in low-density lipoprotein (LDL) cholesterol, and an improvement in insulin sensitivity when compared to mice fed a high-fat diet with no additional leucine (Zhang et al. 2007). These findings were not replicated in healthy older men (71 ± 4 years; 26.1 ± 0.5 kg/m^2) who consumed 2.5 grams of leucine with breakfast, lunch, and dinner for a period of three months; the authors reported no improvements in skeletal muscle mass, strength, indices of whole-body insulin sensitivity, or plasma lipid profiles (Verhoeven et al. 2009). Nevertheless, leucine supplementation has been found to acutely improve muscle protein synthesis in older adults (Rieu et al. 2006) and animals supplemented with leucine for a period of 10 days (Rieu et al. 2003), suggesting the long-term use of leucine may provide a nutritional mechanism to slow the rate of skeletal muscle aging. Finally, the consumption of leucine and protein may work synergistically, as Koopman et al. (2005) reported the consumption of carbohydrate, protein, and leucine significantly increased whole-body net protein balance to a significantly greater degree than protein and carbohydrate or carbohydrate alone.

Based on the findings of Zhang et al. (2007) and Koopman et al. (2005), it appears that regular ingestion of a whey protein and a leucine-containing drink may optimize amino acid delivery. In addition, a relatively high dose of leucine (16 grams) was shown to have an effect in the Koopman study, while a smaller dose (2.5 grams) three times per day had no effect over strength and hypertrophy in healthy older adults (Verhoeven et al. 2009).

In conclusion, research suggests that older adults may need to consume more than 7.5 grams of essential amino acids per dose to optimize muscle protein synthesis (Paddon-Jones and Rasmussen 2009), and that a single 16-gram dose of leucine in a 33-gram dose of whey protein may be needed to optimally stimulate whole-body protein synthesis (Koopman et al. 2005).

15.2.2 Putting It All Together

As an individual ages, a number of physiological maladaptations occur, many of which specifically target skeletal muscle mass and function. While more research needs to be conducted, a number of studies have suggested that nutritional interventions can help to mitigate some of these negative outcomes. Particularly, optimal protein intake appears to be a primary consideration as studies suggest that many older individuals have trouble even consuming the RDA (Campbell et al. 2001), a statistic that is particularly troubling when one considers other reports suggest that *more* protein may be needed in an aged population due to a loss of efficiency with metabolic processes that results in muscle protein synthesis (Cuthbertson et al. 2005). In this respect, it is recommended that 25 to 30 grams of high-quality protein sources are consumed during each feeding period, and that a minimum of 10 grams of leucine are provided per meal (Layman 2002; Rieu et al. 2006). In addition to optimal protein and leucine intake, a diet high in antioxidants (fruits and vegetables) and fiber (vegetables, whole grains, etc.) and low in saturated fat and cholesterol can help minimize the development of cardiovascular disease, cancer, and oxidative stress-related problems (Slavin 2005).

Outside of general nutritional recommendations, a few studies have been conducted to suggest that purposeful timing of nutrients may be an effective strategy. Candow et al. suggest the consumption of protein in approximately 25-gram doses immediately before resistance training exercise over 12 weeks significantly increases knee extensor hypertrophy to a greater extent than when ingested after exercise (Preexercise ingestion = 21% increase vs. Postexercise ingestion = 12% increase) (Candow, Chilibeck, et al. 2006). However, other measures of hypertrophy did not yield similar results in the same subjects, a point that requires careful interpretation of the data. Similarly, Esmarck and colleagues (2001), in what is likely the most well-known study investigating a nutrient timing question in older adults, concluded that ingesting a small amount of protein (approximately 10 grams) with a small amount of carbohydrate (7.7 grams) and fat (3.3 grams) immediately after resistance training sessions versus waiting two hours significantly increased hypertrophy and strength. Careful interpretation of these data is required, a point that was highlighted nicely in Chapter 10 of this text.

Finally, Koopman and colleagues (2005) fed older adults a drink containing whey protein (33 grams) with a large dose of leucine (16 grams) before and after an exercise bout and reported significantly greater levels of muscle protein synthesis, a response that was not found when smaller doses of leucine (7.5 grams) and protein were consumed without any exercise stimulus over a three-month period (Verhoeven et al. 2009). Table 15.2 outlines a hypothetical diet that would allow an older individual to achieve these stated dietary goals; however, particular challenges result when

TABLE 15.2

Theoretical Diet for Older Adults to Optimize Muscle Protein Synthesis

Meal	kcal	PRO (g)	CHO (g)	Fat (g)	Saturated Fat (g)	Fiber (g)
Breakfast (7:00 a.m.)						
240 g oatmeal (1 serving)	170	7	34	2	0	7
⅓ cup whey protein powder	105	25	1	0.3	0	0
1 cup skim milk	101	10	14	1	0	0
Subtotals	*376*	*42*	*49*	*3.3*	*0*	*7*
Preexercise supplement (9:00 a.m.)						
1 cup skim milk	101	10	14	1	0	0
½ scoop whey protein (2 tbsp)	52.5	12.5	0.5	0.15	0	0
1½ cups of raspberries	51	0	12	0	0	6
½ cup strawberries	49	1	12	0	0	3
5 g leucine						
2.5 g creatine						
Subtotals	*253.5*	*23.5*	*38.5*	*1.15*	*0*	*9*
Postexercise supplement (11:00 a.m.)						
1 cup skim milk	101	10	14	1	0	0
½ scoop whey protein	52.5	12.5	0.5	0.15	0	0
1 cup blackberries	124	4	30	2	0	16
5 g leucine						
2.5 g creatine						
Subtotals	*277.5*	*26.5*	*44.5*	*3.15*	*0*	*16*
Lunch (1:00 p.m.)						
1 large (5 oz) chicken breast	152	32	0	0	0	0
1 cup spinach	21	3	3	0	0	3
1 cup carrots	10	0	2	0	0	0
Fat-free Italian salad dressing	40	0	8	0	0	0
Subtotals	*223*	*35*	*13*	*0*	*0*	*3*
Snack (3:00 p.m.)						
Fiber bar, 1 bar	150	3	29	4.5	1.5	9
Subtotals	*150*	*3*	*29*	*4.5*	*1.5*	*9*
Dinner (5:00 p.m.)						
Large, lean sirloin steak	150	27	0	3	3	0
1 cup broccoli	12	2	2	0	0	0
Subtotals	*162*	*29*	*2*	*3*	*3*	*0*
Snack (7:00 p.m.)						
1 cup skim milk	101	10	14	1	0	0
7.5 g leucine						
Subtotals	*101*	*10*	*14*	*1*	*0*	*0*
Totals	**1,543**	**169**	**190**	**16.1**	**4.5**	**44**

considering reduced hunger and increased lactose intolerance commonly reported in this population.

15.2.3 TAKE-HOME MESSAGES

- Consuming over the recommended daily allowance for protein, 0.8 grams of protein per kilogram of body mass per day in older adults, may help slow the rate of skeletal muscle loss with age.
- Older adults should focus on consuming between 25 and 30 grams of protein per meal to optimize muscle protein synthesis, which should minimize skeletal muscle loss with age.
- Creatine supplementation at a dose of two to four grams per day can increase functional capacity and skeletal muscle strength in older adults.
- The combination of creatine and protein may work synergistically to enhance skeletal muscle strength in older adults.
- Each feeding should contain protein and ideally should be consumed every two hours. Adding leucine to small protein meals (<25 grams) may also help to promote skeletal muscle protein synthesis.

15.3 NUTRIENT TIMING CONSIDERATIONS FOR THE MILITARY

Military, in particular special forces (Navy SEALS, Army Rangers), face unique nutritional challenges during the time in the field when they may be required to perform tasks that need significant energy expenditure, with little sleep and limited supplies of food and water. This section focuses on nutritional aids and interventions that may enhance the field performance of soldiers exposed to conditions in which dehydration and lack of food and sleep could result in decrements in performance.

15.3.1 CALORIC DEPRIVATION

In combat situations, soldiers may be exposed to prolonged bouts of time in the field when access to energy sources is limited, creating situations during which protein breakdown may be increased and glycogen stores are diminished, resulting in decreased physical and cognitive performance. Previous investigations (Brozek et al. 1957; Johnson et al. 1971) have found the majority of weight loss of soldiers during field studies results from reductions in fat (approximately 64%) and water (approximately 21%) rather than skeletal muscle (approximately 15%), a seemingly "positive" response (Johnson et al. 1971). Using a simulated combat course over a four-day period that required soldiers to walk 25 to 35 kilometers each night with limited sleep (three to four hours each night) while carrying approximately 11.0 ± 1.2 kilograms of gear and randomly encountering combat activities, a diet that provided 1,800 calories per day for five days resulted in a 14% decrease in mean aerobic power and an 8% decrease in VO_2Max with no change in anaerobic power. Alternatively, a doubling of energy intake (3,200 to 4,200 kilocalories per day) over a four-day period has been shown to allow soldiers to maintain performance effectively (Guezennec et al. 1994). This finding when compared against a report that indicated average daily caloric intake in the field is approximately 2,775 calories (Marriott 1995), a shortage of required energy is a primary concern for military populations.

Marriott and colleagues reported that the typical dietary intake of soldiers in the field contains 2,775 calories, 110 grams (approximately 15% of calories) of protein, 334 grams (approximately 48% of calories) of carbohydrate, and 281 grams (approximately 40% of calories) of fat (Marriott 1995). While protein intake (1.47 grams of protein per kilogram of body mass per day) in this active population appears adequate, the intake of carbohydrate is inadequate (4.45 grams of carbohydrate per kilogram of body mass per day) (Marriott 1995). When considering that military activities in the field often consist of repeated, short-duration, high-intensity bouts of activity or long-duration marches at moderate intensity, depletion of glycogen stores is a concern (Fink et al. 1975; Marriott 1995) as a failure to replenish muscle and liver glycogen reserves can result in fatigue and disorientation (Costill et al. 1971) and injury risk (Marriott 1995). Thus, increasing the field consumption of carbohydrate could result in notable performance improvements of soldiers, particularly when in the field for extended periods of time. Due to the findings that strength is relatively well maintained with caloric restriction for up to 10 days while absolute VO_2Max starts to significantly decrease during the same period of time (Guezennec et al. 1994), nutritional interventions should focus on providing soldiers with highly palatable, nutrient-dense options that are high in carbohydrate, low in fiber, lightweight, and indestructible and take up limited backpack space. As a result, each of these factors must be taken into account when making suggestions to supplement the field diet of a soldier.

15.3.2 Effects of Dehydration on Performance

There is a general consensus that when dehydration exceeds 2% of body weight, aerobic performance (Cheuvront et al. 2003), muscle strength (Judelson et al. 2007), and muscle endurance (Judelson et al. 2007) decrements occur as a result of impaired cardiovascular, thermoregulatory, central nervous system, and metabolic functioning (Cheuvront et al. 2003; Judelson et al. 2007). An early investigation dehydrated men by approximately 5.5% of initial body weight by overnight exposure to high heat (115°F). On waking, participants were asked to walk and then run in moderate temperature conditions (78°F). Results from the investigation revealed that when dehydrated, pulse rates during and following walking and running were greater, rectal temperature was greater during walking, and dehydration negatively affected VO_2Max when compared to a state of euhydration (Buskirk et al. 1958).

The deleterious effects of dehydration on performance of physical tasks have been well documented (Marriott 1995), and as a result much of the recent research has examined mechanisms to minimize the risk of dehydration and maintain performance during long-duration tasks. For instance, Mudambo et al. (1997) examined the effects of ingesting no water, water, dextrose (7.5 grams dextrose mixed in 100 milliliters water) with electrolytes or fructose/corn solids (7.5 grams mixed in 100 milliliters water) at a rate of 400 milliliters every 20 minutes during a 16-kilometer walk/run in heat (39.4 ± 4°C, 28 ± 2% humidity). Of interest were the findings that drinking fluid significantly reduced ratings of perceived exertion of the task and maintained body weight to a significantly greater degree than when no fluids were ingested.

15.3.3 EFFECTS OF SLEEP DEPRIVATION ON PERFORMANCE

Sleep comes at a premium for soldiers who are out in the field, and for this reason it is critical for soldiers to be able to maintain cognitive and psychomotor performance on little sleep. This poses an interesting challenge as research has found getting less than six hours of sleep per night can have an impact on coordination, reaction time, and judgment. In fact, people who drive a motorized vehicle after being awake for 17 to 19 hours performed worse on a driving test than people with a blood alcohol level of 0.05% (Chattington 2007). The effects of sleep deprivation are well documented in military settings as prior research has found sleep deprivation to have deleterious effects on marksmanship accuracy (Tharion et al. 2003), sighting time (Tharion et al. 2003), time to exhaustion (Martin 1981), vertical jump height (Takeuchi et al. 1985), isokinetic extension force (Takeuchi et al. 1985), ratings of perceived exertion (Martin 1981; Plyley et al. 1987), ventilation during exercise (Martin 1981), and a personal assessment of one's mood (Angus et al. 1985; Lieberman et al. 2002). Interestingly, preliminary research does suggest that nutritional interventions can minimize to some extent the deleterious effects of sleep deprivation (Lieberman et al. 2002; McLellan, Kamimori, Bell, et al. 2005; Tharion et al. 2003), but more research is currently needed in this area.

15.3.4 NUTRITIONAL CONSIDERATIONS FOR THE MILITARY

Research has demonstrated that field consumption of nutrients is notably lower than calories provided (Askew et al. 1987; Marriott 1995), with soldiers reporting inadequate rations of food availability in the field, while other reports suggest that low levels of palatability exist with the rations provided (Marriott 1995). Because of the relatively constant and high-energy demands for a soldier in the field, employing nutritional strategies to provide nutrients is important. For these reasons, a key consideration would be the inclusion of easy-to-pack and easy-to-mix meal replacement powders that provide a balanced breakdown of carbohydrates, protein, fat, and vitamins and minerals. In addition, powdered carbohydrate-electrolyte drinks should be considered as a means to effectively replace lost carbohydrates, fluids, and electrolytes. Relatively recent development of bladder-based personal hydration systems have made fluid ingestion more convenient, a key development when considering previous reports have shown that soldiers hypohydrate themselves throughout the day (Marriott 1995). Reports suggest that supplementation with creatine monohydrate may help to prevent heat-related problems and injuries (Dalbo et al. 2008). In addition, other studies suggest that creatine supplementation may reduce thermal load in the way of reduced heart rate, body temperature, and ratings of perceived exertion following exercise and when compared to a placebo (Easton et al. 2007). Last, regular administration of creatine may help to reduce skeletal muscle catabolism during periods of caloric restriction. In this respect, daily administration of 20 grams of creatine per day in conjunction with a restricted calorie diet (18 calories per kilogram of body mass) helps to preserve greater amounts of lean mass when compared to a placebo (Rockwell et al. 2001).

Caffeine may be the most widely studied supplement to enhance alertness and reduce feelings of fatigue; as a result, numerous investigations have examined the effects of caffeine on performance of tasks that may be required of soldiers while in the field (Lieberman et al. 2002; McLellan, Kamimori, Bell, et al. 2005; McLellan, Kamimori, Voss, et al. 2005; Tharion et al. 2003). Specifically, the consumption of 200 milligrams and 300 milligrams of caffeine one hour prior to a marksman-ship test significantly increased sighting time of soldiers following 73 hours of sleep deprivation during high-stress conditions without compromising shooting accuracy. Of further interest was the finding that 100 milligrams of caffeine were unable to positively influence marksmanship performance (Tharion et al. 2003).

Another investigation reported a dose-dependent effect of caffeine consumption to positively influence visual vigilance, choice reaction time, repeated acquisition, self-reported fatigue, sleepiness, reaction time, and alertness without affecting marksman-ship following 72 hours of sleep deprivation under high-stress conditions (Lieberman et al. 2002). The positive effects of caffeine were most pronounced one hour following administration but were still significant eight hours following consumption, suggest-ing that caffeine may provide an advantage to soldiers facing high-stress situations with limited to no sleep. In addition, repeated administration of caffeine enhanced 6.3 kilometer run times (McLellan, Kamimori, Voss, et al. 2005), observation and reconnaissance vigilance task test score performance (McLellan, Kamimori, Voss, et al. 2005), marksmanship vigilance (McLellan, Kamimori, Bell, et al. 2005), reaction time (McLellan, Kamimori, Bell, et al. 2005), and psychomotor vigilance test scores (McLellan, Kamimori, Bell, et al. 2005) during conditions of sleep deprivation.

Creatine supplementation at a dose of 20 grams per day for five (McMorris et al. 2006) or seven days (McMorris et al. 2007) has been reported to improve perfor-mance in the absence of sleep (McMorris et al. 2006, 2007). Specifically, creatine supplementation resulted in smaller decrements in performance on a random move-ment generation task, choice reaction time, balance, and mood state changes after creatine was added to the diet (McMorris et al. 2006).

From a timing perspective, no studies have examined the impact of caffeine or creatine timing. Fortunately, both nutrients can come in either capsule or chewable tablet form, making them convenient nutrients to consume throughout the day. In addition, caffeine acts rather quickly in the blood on ingestion, typically reach-ing peak levels within 30 to 45 minutes; therefore, a dose can be taken as needed throughout the day. If adequate notice of a planned mission allows for completion of a loading protocol with creatine, this would be suggested as creatine levels remain elevated inside the skeletal tissue for up to four weeks, a period of time likely much longer than any planned mission.

15.3.5 TAKE-HOME MESSAGES

- Military action requires a high level of physical and cognitive function on little sleep under high levels of stress, many times in situations with inad-equate levels of energy and fluid.

- For short-term excursions (≤10 days), loss of skeletal muscle strength resulting from caloric restriction does not appear to be an issue; however, aerobic capacity can significantly decline in this period of time.
- Typical military operations require moderate-intensity, long-duration walks and intermittent, high-intensity bouts of work in which the body runs optimally on carbohydrates as a fuel source. As a result, carbohydrate should provide the bulk (approximately 70%) of the energy consumed for soldiers in the field.
- Meal replacement powders may serve as a lightweight, inexpensive addition to increase the caloric consumption of soldiers in the field.
- A high-carbohydrate powder that can be added to water can be used to increase caloric and carbohydrate intake while providing valuable fluids and needed electrolytes and will function to maintain blood glucose concentrations and spare the loss of muscle and liver glycogen.
- Creatine can maintain skeletal muscle mass during periods of caloric restriction and reduce the risk of dehydration, cramping, and overheating in hot environments.
- Creatine may improve mental acuity during severe-to-moderate states of sleep deprivation.
- Caffeine consumption (200 to 300 milligrams) can enhance performance for up to eight hours and improve tasks such as aerobic performance, reaction time, marksmanship sighting time, ratings of perceived exertion, mood, and alertness during periods of sleep deprivation.

15.4 NUTRIENT TIMING CONSIDERATIONS FOR TYPE 1 DIABETES

Type 1 diabetes occurs as the result of pancreatic β-cell destruction and typically results in absolute insulin deficiency (Devendra et al. 2004). Although type 2 diabetes is more common, type 1 diabetes accounts for 5–10% of the cases of individuals with diabetes (Daneman 2006), with 1 of every 400 to 500 children and adolescents under the age of 20 years diagnosed with type 1 diabetes (Devadoss et al. 2011). Two forms of type 1 diabetes exist: type 1A, which occurs from a cell-mediated autoimmune attack on β-cells (Devendra et al. 2004), and type 1B, which has no known cause (Abiru et al. 2002).

A majority of research surrounding diabetes has focused on type 2 diabetes. The onset and negative effects of type 2 diabetes can certainly be blunted with dietary and nutritional interventions; however, there is a lack of literature concerning suggestions to maintain or promote the health of people with type 1 diabetes.

The American Diabetes Association position statement on physical activity and exercise indicates that all forms of physical activity can be performed by individuals with type 1 diabetes (Zinman et al. 2004), a consensus also supported by a review of type 1 diabetes and athletic activities (Gallen et al. 2011). In fact, studies suggest that type 1 diabetes does not impair physical performance, and resulting work output is comparable between participants with type 1 diabetes and healthy individuals (Fisher et al. 1989; Nugent et al. 1997; Veves et al. 1997; Wanke et al. 1992). The primary concern of people with type 1 diabetes exercising is the increased likelihood of hypoglycemic episodes, which occur secondary to the widespread cascade of hormonal changes that happen during exercise. Risk for hypoglycemia can extend for up to 31 hours as a result of increased insulin sensitivity and glucose extraction for replenishment of muscle and liver glycogen (Guelfi et al. 2007). Interestingly and somewhat confusingly, for a young athlete learning more about his or her condition, intense forms of exercise result in hyperglycemia due to the massive changes in circulating concentrations of catecholamines and hepatic glycogenolysis that occur with intense exercise (Sigal et al. 2000). For this reason, care and attention need to be made within this population to effectively match blood glucose concentrations with insulin dose and duration and intensity of ensuing exercise.

This section provides suggestions in terms of the timing/consumption of nutrients to increase delivery of energy and it is hoped to promote an improved quality of life, training quality, and performance in individuals with type 1 diabetes. The primary consideration in regard to the following recommendations is the maintenance/promotion of health, but suggestions are made with the goal of performance enhancement as there are a number of professional athletes who have been diagnosed with type 1 diabetes.

15.4.1 Professional Athlete Spotlight

Jay Cutler had a successful collegiate football career at Vanderbilt University (Nashville, TN, USA) as a four-year starter and three-time team captain. Among his accomplishments, Cutler set school career records for total offense (9,953 yards), touchdown passes (59), passing yards (8,697), pass completions (710), pass attempts (1,242), and combined touchdowns (76) [Jay Cutler (American Football) 2010]. Cutler was selected with the 11th pick in the NFL draft by the Denver Broncos; he set single season records in the NFL for pass attempts (616), pass completions (384), pass yards (4,526), and 300-yard passing games (8) [Jay Cutler (American Football) 2010]. During the 2007 NFL season, Cutler lost 33 pounds and during the off-season reported being chronically tired. Despite the finding that Cutler possessed the warning signs for diabetes (weight loss, frequent urination, constant thirst, and lack of energy), he never considered he may be diabetic because of a lack of family history. However, in 2008 after being tested, Cutler announced he was diagnosed with type 1 diabetes. Cutler is among numerous current and former professional athletes (i.e., Adam Morrison, NCAA and NBA basketball; Gary Hall, USA Olympic gold medalist in swimming; Billie Jean King, women's tennis) who have competed with diabetes and made the necessary modifications to maintain healthy blood glucose concentrations by monitoring diet and administering insulin to control blood glucose concentrations.

15.4.2 General Nutritional Recommendations for Type 1 Diabetes

The maintenance of healthy concentrations of blood glucose should be a primary goal as uncontrolled blood glucose concentrations can result in organ damage and other complications resulting from diabetes (Koro et al. 2004); as mentioned, the danger of hypoglycemic episodes with type 1 diabetes are of particular concern. No daily specific macronutrient recommendations exist for active people with type

1 diabetes (Gallen et al. 2011). In fact, McKewen and colleagues (1999) provided evidence that simply providing more carbohydrates in the diet (50% vs. 60% of daily calories as carbohydrates) was not an effective strategy in trained male athletes with type 1 diabetes. As a result, nutritional planning should be individualized and made according to each individual's dietary preferences, age, weight, insulin type, insulin dose, fitness status, and so on (Gallen et al. 2011). For these reasons, it is advisable for all athletes with type 1 diabetes to consult with a registered dietician who is knowledgeable in exercise physiology and sports nutrition.

15.4.3 NUTRITIONAL RECOMMENDATIONS SURROUNDING EXERCISE

An initial consideration for any health care practitioner, coach, athlete, or parent for exercising or competitive individuals who have type 1 diabetes is their form of insulin treatment. While a detailed discussion of this topic is beyond the scope of this chapter and is not intended to replace advice from a personal physician, reports have indicated that mode of administration (continuous subcutaneous insulin infusion vs. multiple daily injections), type of insulin (long acting vs. fast acting), and administration site (abdomen, buttocks, arms, etc.) can also exert subtle changes in how the administered insulin performs. As an example, studies suggest that dose modifications of 50–90% may be required depending on the intensity and duration of exercise and previous carbohydrate status in the body (Mauvais-Jarvis et al. 2003; Rabasa-Lhoret et al. 2001). Other key factors more related to exercise involve the timing of exercise commencement relative to their last bolus of insulin. In this respect, it is suggested that if exercise occurs within 90 to 120 minutes of a previous insulin dose, the amount of insulin can be subsequently reduced, and resulting carbohydrate needs during the exercise bout will be reduced. If this is not considered, carbohydrate needs during exercise within two hours of an insulin bolus will be increased from the typically recommended 30 to 60 grams of carbohydrate per hour (Chapter 7 of this text).

Another factor is the blood glucose levels at the beginning of exercise. Because glucose uptake will be rapidly increased at the start of exercise in an individual with type 1 diabetes, blood glucose levels below 7 millimoles per liter (mmol/L) will likely require a small carbohydrate snack (15 to 30 grams), and if greater than 10 millimoles per liter, a carbohydrate feeding can actually be delayed (Gallen et al. 2011).

Yet another factor involves the glycemic status of individuals on days prior to prolonged periods of moderate exercise. In this respect, reports suggest that glucose needs are markedly increased to maintain euglycemia during prolonged exercise a day after prolonged hypoglycemia when compared to a day without hypoglycemia (Davis et al. 2000). This is a key factor for athletes, coaches, and parents to consider as much focus typically falls on the initial hours before and during an activity, while a much a greater period of time might be needed for consideration.

The intensity of exercise is a crucial factor that will dictate glycemic status. Somewhat paradoxically, high-intensity (sprints) and intermittent bouts of high-intensity (football, weightlifting, etc.) activity may stimulate hyperglycemia, and for this reason carbohydrate feedings may actually exacerbate this problem.

Finally, the athletes and their support system must understand that profound metabolic changes occur and often result in postexercise hypoglycemia due to increased insulin sensitivity and the increased uptake of glucose from the blood into the liver for replenishment of internal glycogen stores (Gallen et al. 2011).

As one can imagine, research involving type 1 diabetics and specific nutrient timing questions are scant. Anecdotal reports suggest that an exercise taper, which often is part of a carbohydrate-loading protocol, will require insulin to manage blood glucose levels and consequently may make it a challenge to maintain glycemic levels. This along with the lack of research makes it difficult to recommend any specific nutrient timing strategies for this population. Because of the number of other factors that can dictate glycemic status (as discussed in this section), it is recommended that diabetic athletes regularly ingest recommended amounts of carbohydrate (seven to ten grams of carbohydrate per kilogram of body mass per day). In addition to the previously mentioned concerns regarding maintenance of glycemia during and after exercise, general guidelines are summarized in Table 15.3.

Currently, recommendations and specific strategies to improve anaerobic performance and accretion of lean tissue are not available for athletes with type 1 diabetes. In this respect, the athlete must appreciate and understand the importance

TABLE 15.3
Strategies to Prevent Hypoglycemia Associated with Exercise

Strategy	Advantages	Disadvantages
Reducing preexercise insulin bolus (preferably when exercise is within 90–120 minutes of an insulin bolus)	• Reduced hypoglycemia during exercise • Reduces carbohydrate requirement • Beneficial for weight management	• Requires planning • Not helpful for spontaneous or late postprandial exercise • May result in starting exercise with increased blood glucose
Adjusting preexercise and during exercise basal rate of insulin infusion	• As above	• Requires planning as basal rate adjustments may need to be made at least 60 minutes prior to the start of exercise
Carbohydrate feeding during exercise	• Useful for unplanned or prolonged exercise	• Counterproductive when purpose of exercise is for weight control • Not practical with all sports • Gastrointestinal discomfort
Preexercise or postexercise sprint	• Reduces immediate postexercise hypoglycemia	• Effect limited to shorter and less-intense exercise • No effect on hypoglycemia during exercise
Reducing basal insulin postexercise	• Reduces nocturnal hypoglycemia	• May cause raise fasting blood glucose
Taking caffeine before exercise	• Reduced hypoglycemia during and after exercise • Reduced carbohydrate requirements	• Impairments or alterations of fine motor control and technique • Overarousal (interfering with recovery and sleep patterns)

Source: From S.S. Gidding et al. (2005). Dietary Recommendations for Children and Adolescents: A Guide for Practitioners. *Circulation* 112(13):2061–75. Wolters Kluwer Health Publishing. With permission.

of maintaining optimal glycemic levels and the impact this has on other metabolic considerations. While research involving healthy individuals provides support for the inclusion of nutrients such as creatine (Buford et al. 2007), leucine (Anthony et al. 2000; Kimball et al. 1999), essential amino acids (Rasmussen et al. 2000; Volpi et al. 2003), and whey protein (Campbell et al. 2007) for their ability to promote positive resistance training adaptations, evidence (both scientific and anecdotal) is lacking that provides specific recommendations regarding general nutritional needs and any specific timing strategies for nutrition.

15.4.4 TAKE-HOME MESSAGES

- The first priority for type 1 diabetics is the maintenance of healthy blood glucose concentrations.
- Particular attention should first be made to understanding the differential impact of the type, dose, action, and location of insulin being administered.
- The timing between delivery of an insulin bolus and later ensuing exercise can dictate glycemic responses and resulting perceived exertion and performance.
- Blood glucose levels prior to commencing exercise should be monitored and are suggested to be at a level of seven to ten millimoles per liter. Higher or lower glycemic levels may likely dictate administration or refraining, respectively, from additional carbohydrate feeding.
- Hypoglycemic status several hours and potentially days before prolonged, moderate exercise can and may dictate need for glucose.
- The type, duration, and intensity of exercise can all have an impact on ensuing glycemic status.
- Traditional nutrient timing strategies have yet to be researched in athletes with type 1 diabetes, and for this reason, traditional nutritional recommendations are suggested.
- The inclusion of creatine, leucine, essential amino acids, and other protein sources to facilitate resistance training adaptations are unresearched in type 1 diabetics and should not be primary nutritional considerations.

15.5 NUTRIENT TIMING CONSIDERATIONS FOR CHILDREN

The nutritional needs of children have been outlined by the American Heart Association, and these recommendations are provided in Table 15.4. A discussion surrounding children is particularly challenging. On one hand, an increased prevalence of overweight/obese children continues to be reported (Wang et al. 2002). When considering this, a discussion similar to that in Chapter 16 of this text is required that centers largely on improving the balance between caloric intake and caloric expenditure. Additional topics such as glycemic index or "quality" of carbohydrate sources, feeding frequency, and metabolic cost of various macronutrients would be relevant. However, these discussions are much too complex for a child to understand; for this

TABLE 15.4
Energy and Nutritional Recommendations for Children

Variables	1 Year	2–3 Years	4–8 Years	9–13 Years	14–18 Years
Calories (kcal)					
Females	900	1000	1200	1600	1800
Males	900	1000	1400	1800	2200
Fat (% of kcal)	30–40%	30–35%	25–35%	25–35%	25–35%
Milk (servings)	2 cups[a]	2 cups[b]	2 cups[b]	3 cups[b]	3 cups[b]
Lean meat/beans					
Females	1.5 oz	2.0 oz	3.0 oz	5.0 oz	5.0 oz
Males	1.5 oz	2.0 oz	4.0 oz	5.0 oz	6.0 oz
Fruits (servings)					
Females	4.0	3.0	3.0	3.0	3.0
Males	4.0	3.0	3.0	3.0	4.0
Vegetables (servings)					
Females	3.0	3.0	2.0	4.0	5.0
Males	3.0	3.0	3.0	5.0	6.0
Grains[c] (oz)					
Females	2.0	3.0	4.0	5.0	6.0
Males	3.0	4.0	5.0	6.0	7.0
Fiber (g)					
Females	19.0	19.0	25.0	26.0	29.0
Males	19.0	19.0	25.0	31.0	38.0
Sodium (mg)					
Females	<1,500	<1,500	<1,900	<2,200	<2,300
Males	<1,500	<1,500	<1,900	<2,200	<2,300
Potassium (mg)					
Females	3,000	3,000	3,800	4,500	4,700
Males	3,000	3,000	3,800	4,500	4,700

Source: From S.S. Gidding et al. (2005). Dietary Recommendations for Children and Adolescents: A Guide for Practitioners. *Circulation* 112(13):2061–75. Wolters Kluwer Health Publishing. With permission.

[a] Suggested consumption of 1% milk.
[b] Suggested consumption of fat-free milk.
[c] Half of grains should be whole grains.

reason, an emphasis to increase physical activity and improve the quality of the child's diet should persist as the mainstays of guidance in this scenario.

On the other hand, 36 million children in the United States between the ages of 6 and 17 years of age are reported to participate in at least one team sport every year. For children who routinely train and exercise, calorie and nutrient needs exist in much the same manner as they do for exercising adults. However, coaches and parents must understand that the processes of growth and motor development are energy demanding, thus resulting in a caloric requirement that may be surprisingly high (Bar-Or 2001). Outside of distinct caloric demands, studies suggest that protein needs of active children are increased to satisfy growth requirements (Bar-Or 2001). In this regard, an investigation by Boisseau et al. (2007) examined the protein requirements for adolescent (13.8 ± 0.1 years) male soccer players and found the U.S. RDA for protein (0.8 to 1.0 gram of protein per kilogram body mass per day) was not enough to sustain growth in boys participating in high-intensity exercise. Furthermore, this report suggested that a protein intake of 1.2 to 1.4 grams of protein per kilogram of body mass per day may be required to sustain growth in physically active children.

A final focus of discussion should be centered on the daily needs of calcium and vitamin D. Specifically, 12- to 19-year-old males and females on average consume 1,061 and 789 milligrams of calcium per day ,respectively, values that are below the RDA of 1,200 milligrams per day (Fleming and Heimbach 1994). This is particularly troubling for children during this stage of development, during which approximately 50% of adult bone structure is developed (Hightower 2000), and peak calcium accretion rates in the skeleton occur at approximately 12 to 13 years of age in females and approximately 14 years of age in males (Bailey et al. 2000). In this regard, Lee et al. (1994) found that daily consumption of 300 milligrams of calcium carbonate for 18 months significantly improved bone mineral content and bone width in 162 children consuming low amounts of calcium in their diet (280 milligrams per day).

Also, Volek et al. in 2003 demonstrated the importance of calcium in physically active boys (13 to 17 years of age) who participated in resistance training for 12 weeks and consumed 24 fluid ounces (710 milliliters) of either 1% milk or nonfortified apple juice in addition to their regular diet. Boys who consumed 1% milk experienced a significantly greater increase in bone mineral density than boys consuming apple juice, suggesting the addition of milk to the diet of physically active adolescent boys may improve bone health.

15.5.1 Nutritional Recommendations Surrounding Exercise

Dehydration, particularly among young athletes, is associated with heat-related injuries. Even in professional sports, with well-trained doctors and coaches, athletes routinely fall ill due to heat exhaustion. It is also important to keep in mind that using thirst as a cue to drink is not a reliable way to prevent dehydration. By the time athletes are thirsty, they have already entered the first stage of dehydration. A 2% reduction in body weight from fluid loss can lead to a significant decline in strength, endurance, fine motor skills (i.e., hand-eye coordination), and mental alertness (Judelson et al. 2007). Cramping as a result of dehydration will limit an athlete's ability to participate in an intense exercise session and will likely have a negative impact on subsequent training or competition.

Preventing dehydration is simple. A water bottle should become a part of the young athlete's training gear, just like a towel, shoes, or uniform. Water breaks should become an integrated part of a workout routine. Healthy and competitive athletes should be accustomed to rehydrating periodically, and as a coach or parent, this should be viewed no differently from stressing the importance of dynamic warmups or cool-down stretching. During exercise, young athletes should drink ½ to 1 cup of water, diluted juice, or sports drink every 15 minutes of intense training. A study demonstrated that ingesting a 6% carbohydrate-electrolyte solution before and during exercise improved the intermittent, high-intensity endurance running capacity of adolescent (12 to 14 years) soccer, rugby, and field hockey athletes

(Phillips et al. 2010). Young athletes often do not instinctively drink enough fluids to replace water losses, so their intake should be monitored. Finally, after exercise, athletes should ingest 16 fluid ounces (two cups) for every pound of weight lost over a practice. Therefore, weight should be measured before and after intense practices, with a goal of maintaining body mass. An hour or two before a competition or practice, young athletes should drink until they are no longer thirsty and then drink an additional 8 to 16 ounces (one to two cups) of fluids. Ten to 20 minutes prior to their first competition, they should consume an additional eight ounces (one cup) of fluid (Antonio and Stout 2004).

15.5.2 TAKE-HOME MESSAGES

- Primary and initial concerns for children are to educate them regarding healthy nutrition, provide them with healthy food sources, and help them to build effective nutritional habits.
- For exercising, growing children, the RDA of 0.8 to 1.0 gram of protein per kilogram of body mass per day of protein might not be an adequate amount of protein to promote optimal growth and recovery.
- Adolescent girls and boys underconsume the RDA of calcium of 1,200 mg per day, and as a result calcium and vitamin D consumption should be increased to promote bone and muscle health.
- Hydration is critical to the health and safety of young athletes. Adequate pre-, during-, and postexercise consumption of fluids is recommended.
- Weighing the athlete before and after practice will give the coach or parent a good idea of how the young athlete is doing to maintain weight.
- Consuming a 6% carbohydrate-and-electrolyte beverage during practice or competition may maintain or improve performance.

16 The Impact of Nutrient Timing Considerations on Weight Loss and Body Composition

Colin Wilborn and Chad M. Kerksick

CONTENTS

16.1 INTRODUCTION

Nutrient or meal timing has become an extremely popular topic not only for competitive athletes, but also for weekend warriors and individuals hoping to lose weight. While it has become clearer through years of scientific inquiry that taking advantage of various hormonal and metabolic environments may allow recreationally and competitively active individuals to optimize their training and enhance their recovery, this response for the general population interested in weight loss and body composition is less conclusive. It has been shown in studies utilizing athletic populations that nutrient timing may positively affect body composition and help modulate responses seen while restricting caloric intake. In addition to benefiting athletic performance and other athletic attributes, improving body composition in overweight, obese, and otherwise metabolically challenged populations can improve self-efficacy and reduce risk for various metabolic and cardiovascular diseases.

With an astonishing 68% (Flegal et al. 2010) of Americans overweight, one must ask the question, "Is meal or nutrient timing a worthwhile consideration for someone wanting to lose weight in the general population?" Regular suggestions in the mainstream media champion an increase in meal and breakfast frequency for their positive benefits on appetite, satiety, and glucose and insulin control as well as greater weight loss, improvements in body composition, and a greater ability to maintain weight loss. A number of studies have been conducted since the 1990s examining this question, with a majority of the literature suggesting a general lack of support for these suggestions. This chapter focuses entirely on the impact of meal and breakfast frequency and quality for its ability to facilitate weight loss and other improvements in health.

16.2 ENERGY BALANCE (BASICS OF FAT AND WEIGHT LOSS)

To understand the impact that nutrient timing might have, it is important first to understand how energy balance is derived. Many clinicians, dieticians, and scholars have subscribed to the theory of calories in versus calories out. That is, when one takes in the exact number of calories that one expends, then that individual will maintain their current weight. Calories are taken in via the three macronutrients: carbohydrates, proteins, and fats. Fats have over twice the caloric density of proteins and carbohydrates, and as a result are frequently targeted in association with the weight gain seen since the 1980s, and in some instances for good reason.

A review of 28 clinical trials that studied the effects of reducing energy intake showed that a reduction of 10% in the proportion of energy from fat was associated with a reduction in weight (Bray and Popkin 1998). A 2002 study concluded that energy from fat was associated with obesity, suggesting that high-fat dietary patterns are contributing to the high rates of obesity in U.S. men (Satia-Abouta et al. 2002). However, more recent evidence suggests that differing metabolic costs of macronutrient ingestion (discussed in detail in this chapter) might play a role.

While there are many possibilities with regard to the increasing weight gain, what we do know is that eating excess calories (when compared to how many calories are expended) leads to weight gain (Kopelman 2000). A simple question to ask, then, would be what amount of calories is required, and what amount is considered excessive? Energy expenditure is composed of three categories: basal metabolic rate, thermic effect of food, and caloric expenditure from physical activity. When energy intake is equal to the sum of these three components, body weight should, in theory, stay the same. As is often the case, however, the number of calories consumed is greater than the amount of calories expended, resulting in weight gain and eventual development of obesity.

A 2002 review examined energy intake over a 19-year period (1976 to 1996) and found energy consumption increased by approximately 20% (Nielsen et al. 2002). Interestingly, these data coincide with a 30% increase in obesity, providing further epidemiological support of the concept of calories in versus calories out.

Thermogenesis associated with physical activity accounts for approximately 15% to 50% of total daily expenditure in normal populations, with an inverse relationship existing between physical activity levels and weight gain (DiPietro 1995). For example, a 2005 review by Castaneda et al. reported that minimal amounts of spontaneous physical activity are significant predictors of accumulating fat mass during overfeeding in humans (Castaneda 2005). Furthermore, these authors concluded that increased sedentary behavior represents one reason for the increasing prevalence of obesity. Furthermore, Slentz et al. (2005) reaffirmed that if individuals partake in a modest exercise program similar to what is suggested by the Centers for Disease Control and Prevention, the American College of Sports Medicine, and other national health and medicine-affiliated organizations, significant increases in visceral fat can be avoided, and exercise that is a modest increase beyond the recommendation can facilitate significant decreases in visceral, subcutaneous, and total abdominal fat without changes in daily dietary intake (Slentz 2005).

In a similar light, when energy intake is reduced to levels below caloric expenditure, an individual can expect to lose weight. It is generally recommended that individuals striving to lose weight decrease daily energy intake by a modest amount (e.g., 500 calories), which represents a theoretical rate of weight loss of one pound per week. Alternatively, individuals could choose to increase energy expenditure through increased exercise or physical activity and burn an additional 500 calories a day. With no changes in dietary intake, this increase in exercise should theoretically result in identical rates of weight loss compared to caloric restriction. Finally, this person could also choose to utilize a combined approach, resulting in a net daily deficit of 1,000 calories, which in theory should lead to two pounds of weight loss per week. This combined approach is often the most widely recommended approach by health and fitness professionals.

Thus, the idea of energy balance seems quite simple. However, this equation may not always hold true. While simplistic in nature and good for instructional purposes, this theory continues to receive a wide array of criticisms, such as food type, timing of meals, amino acid intake/protein quality, and metabolic rate as factors that individually and collectively may result in more favorable changes in weight loss and body composition. In addition, the concept is further challenged when individuals (such as athletes) hope to lose only adipose tissue as opposed to losing lean tissue mass. Therefore, it is vital that weight loss occurs at a rate that allows for optimal fat loss but effectively preserves skeletal muscle in the process.

Singularly, this complex paradigm has initiated decades of research studies, debates, and position stands. Positions by many reputable organizations differ greatly in their stance on macronutrient content, meal frequency, and caloric need. For this reason, the implications of the current literature must be critically analyzed to investigate the extent to which nutrient timing can have an impact on fat and or weight loss.

16.3 MEAL FREQUENCY

16.3.1 THE THEORY

Likely the most profound aspect of nutrient timing for weight loss is the frequency of meals. This topic is quite popular in the mainstream media as a number of reports suggest that increased meal frequency favorably impacts metabolism and weight loss outcomes. As discussed, resting energy expenditure and the thermic effect of food are critical factors that help to explain an individual's metabolic response. While some food types have a greater metabolic cost than others (discussed later in this chapter), postprandial increases in energy expenditure are common and exhibit a typical dose-response effect. In recent years, dieticians, nutritionists, and exercise enthusiasts have taken this theory to suggest that if one is to eat more frequently, resulting metabolic activity will be increased and sustained at these higher levels throughout the day. For this concept, in essence, the recommendation is commonly to eat five or six smaller meals a day as opposed to two or three meals each day. It is important to note that this theory would be based on consuming the same amount of calories regardless of the number of meals consumed. Many people believe that if the body is fed at regular intervals, continual feedback is received that energy is available to the body and as a result it does not have to store calories. In contrast, when we skip meals we trigger a nutrient-sparing mode in which metabolism is negatively affected, resulting in a decrease in calorie burning.

16.3.2 FAVORABLE STUDIES

It is commonly regarded that Fabry and coworkers were the first to demonstrate the inverse relationship between meal frequency and body weight in humans (Fabry et al. 1964, 1966; Hejda and Fabry 1964). The first of these three studies reported through an epidemiological, cross-sectional approach that the proportion of 379 overweight subjects aged 60 to 64 years and mean skinfold thickness were inversely related to meal frequency (Fabry et al. 1964). Similar outcomes were reported in a sample of 80 subjects aged 30 to 50 years (Hejda and Fabry 1964). Also, a rather large study by Metzner and colleagues reported an inverse relationship between meal frequency and adiposity in approximately 2,000 men and women aged 35 to 60 years (Metzner et al. 1977). However, metabolism was not assessed, and 24-hour dietary recall tells little of the normal eating patterns of the individuals in this study.

More recent studies report similar findings regarding positive outcomes associated with an increased frequency of eating. A cross-sectional survey indicated men who ate more frequently had lower body fat (Ruidavets et al. 2002). Data from the Seasonal Variation of Blood Cholesterol Study (1994–1998) was used to evaluate the relationship between eating patterns and obesity. On average, 13 dietary recalls over a 24-hour period were used along with body weight measurements to indicate the relationship between meal frequency and body weight while also controlling for energy intake and calories burned from exercise. Results indicated that a greater number of eating episodes each day was associated with a lower risk of obesity (Ma et al. 2003).

In a somewhat related review in 2011, the relationship between energy intake and regular meal consumption was discussed (Ekmekcioglu and Touitou 2011). Researchers concluded that eating on a consistent schedule (sometimes a challenge for shift workers) more frequently facilitated greater energy balance, a relationship that may likely have an impact on outcomes associated with adiposity and weight loss.

An additional consideration discussed further in the chapter is the impact of meal frequency on changes in serum hormones that may have an impact on substrate utilization as well as appetite control. For example, studies have found that when lean, male subjects increased their meal frequency, greater appetite control resulted (Speechly and Buffenstein 1999). Similarly, an artificially manipulated increase of meal frequency acutely reduced the appetite of obese males (Speechly et al. 1999). This might partially explain some of the findings in that individuals who eat more frequently have a reduced appetite.

An important point to consider, however, when evaluating the majority of these studies is that the design of the research was not set up to determine causality. In addition, dietary studies are well known to contain significant error (Black et al. 1993; Lichtman et al. 1992; Prentice et al. 1986). In this respect, many studies often report error magnitudes of 25–30%. Furthermore, studies also suggest that similar or even greater misrepresentation occurs regarding snacking (Heitmann and Lissner 1995; Livingstone et al. 1990), a problem that would particularly influence the accuracy of meal frequency and energy intake. To this end, many of these studies used dietary recall as a primary means to determine energy intake and did little to account or control for exercise, so their ability to truly represent the physiological impact should be viewed with caution. For these reasons, these studies have drawn the ire of skeptics.

Another interesting fact to consider involves a 2002 study that used an experimental approach to investigate the relationship between habitual and manipulated meal frequency on energy intake in partially isolated men (Westerterp-Plantenga et al. 2002). Men who habitually ate more frequently reported higher metabolic rates than those individuals who only manipulated their meal frequency when under laboratory conditions, a response likely to occur when beginning to follow a new dietary program. While seemingly contradictory, this study focused more on the impact of eating regularly or skipping meals. It was concluded that when a meal frequency plan was regularly adopted (whatever the frequency), more favorable adaptations related to metabolic control occurred.

Finally, the topic of meal frequency and endpoint adiposity has been widely discussed. For the most part, experimental approaches do not support this suggestion; however, a review by Leidy and Campbell (2011) did nicely outline studies that suggest that greater meal frequency does afford people greater appetite control and satiating effects. This is a newer idea that is certain to be researched more fully in the years to come.

Two published studies by the same research group explored the impact of providing a drink with a blend of thermogenic ingredients, including taurine, guarana extract, green tea extract, and caffeine, in overweight men (Lockwood et al. 2010) and women (A.E. Smith et al. 2010). Overweight and obese participants were assigned to one of four groups (exercise + active drink, no exercise + active drink, exercise + placebo drink, and no exercise + placebo drink), and those who exercised completed a combined cardiovascular and whole-body resistance training workout five days per week. Drinks were ingested on a daily basis for the entire duration of the study, and on workout days the drinks were ingested 15 minutes before each workout. Changes in body mass, body composition, fitness, and blood markers were determined before and after completion of the study. In the women, exercising individuals increased fitness and some body composition parameters, but when the active drink was provided in combination with the exercise group, improvements in muscle mass, fitness, and lipid profiles resulted (A.E. Smith et al. 2010). Favorable results were also reported in men who completed this study. In this group, when the active drink and exercise program were combined, significantly greater decreases in fat mass and percentage of body fat resulted while greater increases in VO_2Max (maximum oxygen consumption) were also found when compared to the group who exercised and ingested a placebo (Lockwood et al. 2010). While neither of these studies was designed to determine the specific impact of preexercise ingestion of thermogenic ingredients in combination with a daily exercise program, results do suggest this time frame may facilitate favorable outcomes. Certainly, and with the popularity and efficacy of caffeine as a lipolytic agent, future investigations should expand on this preliminary research to identify the independent impact of caffeine in the formulation and to determine if timing of ingestion is important and if its potential favorable effects can be modulated if combined with some form of restricted energy intake.

16.3.3 OPPOSING STUDIES

Not all of the research has been favorable in regard to meal frequency. A 1997 review nicely summarized a number of studies that investigated the concept of meal frequency and its impact on weight loss and adiposity. While a few epidemiological studies are likely the root of the common belief surrounding meal frequency, careful interpretation should be made regarding their findings. In fact, a number of studies highlighted in this review failed to demonstrate any effect to support the inverse relationship between meal frequency and adiposity (Bellisle et al. 1997). To this point, the authors critically highlighted the pitfalls associated with using dietary recall for measures of energy intake as well as a natural response by dieting individuals (people who often have an elevated body mass) to reduce the food they consume (by skipping a meal), thereby creating an instant artifact in the data that overweight people eat fewer meals. In essence, these authors concluded that the epidemiological evidence is at best weak and prone to misinterpretation and further concluded that any effects of meal pattern on the regulation of body weight are likely to be mediated through effects on the food intake side of the energy balance equation (Bellisle et al. 1997).

An effective interpretation of this confounding effect was conducted using data from Kant et al. (1995), which reported a significant inverse relationship between meal frequency and adiposity in 4,567 women. Using previously published energy expenditure prediction equations and a conservative correction for activity levels, Bellisle et al. (1997) illustrated that the self-reported energy intake levels in people consuming meal frequencies ranging from two to seven meals per day were less than their predicted energy needs. More important, the magnitude of underreporting grew to seemingly impossible levels of energy intake as meal frequency decreased. For example, individuals who reported consuming one or two meals had energy intake levels 50% lower than a predicted value, and individuals who consumed three meals per day were ingesting 37% less calories than required by their bodies. Yet, these people were the ones who were gaining weight even though their energy intake was 50% and 37% less, respectively, than what it should have been.

A number of additional studies of varying experimental designs have reported no relationship between meal frequency and adiposity. As such, a 2007 study performed by Yannakoulia and colleagues reported that an increased meal frequency in pre- and postmenopausal women did not influence adiposity in premenopausal women, but an increased meal frequency in postmenopausal women was associated with an increase in adiposity. These findings would suggest that frequency of eating is not a major factor in weight loss and may in fact increase risk of adiposity in postmeno-pausal women.

Similarly, 48 men and 47 women participated in a study to investigate the effects of eating frequency and its impact on body weight as well as identify any influence physical activity or caloric intake may have on this relationship. Using seven-day physical activity diaries and macronutrient intake logs, researchers found men to exhibit a significant negative correlation between eating frequency and both body weight and body mass index (BMI). However, in women, no relationship between eating frequency and body weight status existed. Significant positive correlations between eating frequency and total energy intake (Drummond et al. 1998) were reported. Thus, these differing results seem to cloud the waters.

The basis of support for eating more frequently, as discussed, is to increase energy expenditure or to suppress or control appetite. To examine this question, Dallosso and colleagues (1982) investigated the effects of eating two versus six meals on energy balance as measured by whole-body calorimetry. This study failed to identify any impact of meal frequency on energy expenditure, a conclusion that was observed after 1,987 study participants had thermogenic responses determined after ingesting two versus six meals over a two-day period (Wolfram et al. 1987).

In addition, similar effects have been reported in women as Kinabo and Durnin (1990) investigated the effect of meal frequency on the thermic effect of food in 18 nonobese female subjects using open-circuit indirect calorimetry. Eight subjects consumed a high-carbohydrate and low-fat meal, and ten other subjects consumed a low-carbohydrate and high-fat meal either as one large meal or as two smaller meals. It was determined that meal frequency as well as meal composition did not seem to influence the thermic effect of food.

An investigation of four weeks of dietary variability was completed in 14 female subjects (Verboeket-van de Venne and Westerterp 1993). During four consecutive weeks, 14 female subjects restricted their food intake to 1,000 kilocalories per day, with seven subjects consuming the diet in two meals daily, the others consuming the diet in three to five meals. Body mass and body composition, obtained by deuterium dilution, were measured at the start of the experiment and after two and four weeks of dieting. Sleeping metabolic rate was measured at the same time intervals using a respiration chamber. At the end of the four-week intervention, 24-hour energy expenditure and diet-induced thermogenesis were assessed by a 36-hour stay in a respiration chamber. The authors found that there was no significant effect of the feeding frequency on body composition or metabolic rate. In addition, these results were corroborated by studies that utilized two versus six meals (Taylor and Garrow 2001), six versus four meals (Holmback et al. 2003), and six meals versus a variable number of meals (Farshchi et al. 2005a).

Most recently and in support of these data, 16 obese (34.6 ± 9.5 years and a BMI of 37.1 ± 4.5 kilograms per square meter) men and women were instructed to reduce their energy intake by 700 calories per day and were randomized into two treatment groups. In an energy-matched fashion, one group consumed six meals each day (three traditional meals and three snacks), and the other group consumed three meals each day. Before and after the eight-week intervention, obesity indices, body mass, appetite, and ghrelin were measured, and no significant differences were found (Cameron et al. 2010). This last study is particularly important because it is one of the few studies to utilize a true experimental approach, and it has been shown that under more rigorous conditions, it is consistently reported that an increased meal frequency exhibits no pattern of relationship with overweight, increased adiposity, and so on.

16.3.4 Varied Meal Patterns

A very interesting study was completed in 2005 (Farshchi et al. 2005a) that investigated whether regular meal frequency affects energy intake, energy expenditure, or circulating insulin, glucose, or lipid concentrations versus varied meal frequency. In other words, this study investigated the influence of skipping meals. This randomized crossover trial consisted of three 42-day phases; each phase was broken up into 14 days. For all subjects, the middle 14 days (phase 2) was considered a washout period, and participants followed their typical, everyday dietary pattern. A meal or feeding was considered to be the consumption of any food or drink item that contained energy. The regular meal pattern phase required participants to eat and drink items from their normal diet on six occasions each day with regular intervals between meals. The irregular or "chaotic" meal plan required participants to consume between three and nine meals each day. To standardize the pattern between participants, the exact number of meals each day was predetermined, and all meal frequencies (3 to 9 daily meals) were followed twice during this phase. The results of this study showed that regular meal patterns lowered energy intake and supported greater thermogenesis. The findings from this study support the ascertainments of Bellisle et al. (1997) that greater meal frequency likely leads to a greater energy intake, and if controlled, meal frequency has minimal impact over weight loss and body composition changes. Specifically, it does provide credence to the idea that a more consistent regimen of eating may be favorable when it comes to metabolic and weight-related adaptations.

This last point was also discussed in a 2011 review that outlined studies that explored the relationship between meal timing and time-of-day eating and how it related to appetite. These authors concluded that a regular meal pattern (not necessarily more meals) promoted an overall favorable physiological outcome; interestingly, they also discussed psychobiological areas that were supported by a regular pattern of eating (Ekmekcioglu and Touitou 2011).

16.4   MEAL TYPE/METABOLIC COST

16.4.1 Protein

The most simplified concept of energy balance is energy in versus energy out. If either side changes over a prolonged period of time, body mass will change accordingly. One area that has challenged this long-standing thesis is the impact of varying macronutrient content in the diet. In support, varying thermogenic effects are realized for carbohydrate, fats, and protein (Bray and Popkin 1998; Hermsdorff et al. 2007; Ludwig et al. 1999; Smeets and Westerterp-Plantenga 2008). In other words, all calories may not be equal, and the types of carbohydrate, proteins, and fats one consumes in the diet may influence the propensity to gain or lose weight. Based on their thermogenic properties, proteins may be the most important macronutrient in regard to thermogenesis, weight control, and body composition. In that regard, an increase in thermogenesis could lead to a greater reduction in body fat, improving body composition, or facilitate better maintenance of body mass and body composition.

Certainly, a common theme throughout this text has been the biological importance of how specific timing of key nutrients can be helpful. A 2004 review (Halton and Hu 2004) concluded that there is convincing evidence that a higher protein intake increases thermogenesis and satiety compared to diets of lower protein content. Furthermore, these authors found that high-protein meals lead to reduced subsequent energy intake and increased weight loss and fat loss.

Further support for this was provided by Leidy and colleagues, who had obese men consume isocaloric meals consisting of either 14% or 25% protein, respectively, in three or six eating occasions each day. When higher protein was consumed (25% protein), greater levels of satiety were reported, independent of feeding frequency (Leidy et al. 2010).

Robinson and colleagues (1990) compared the thermogenic effects of consuming isocaloric amounts of high-carbohydrate and high-protein meals and found that the thermic response of consuming a meal higher in protein was significantly greater when compared to a high-carbohydrate meal.

More recently, investigators employed resistance-trained males to determine whether protein supplementation before an acute bout of resistance training would influence postexercise resting energy expenditure and substrate oxidation according to the respiratory exchange ratio (Hackney et al. 2010). The authors found that 24 hours after the exercise bout, resting energy expenditure in response to protein supplementation was significantly greater when compared to a predominantly carbohydrate meal.

Prior to this study, similar findings were realized when protein consumption was investigated before a single strength training session for changes in blood hormones, energy metabolites, respiratory exchange ratio, and excess postexercise oxygen consumption (Hulmi et al. 2005). Briefly, resistance-trained males consumed either 25 grams of whey and caseinate proteins or a noncaloric placebo 30 minutes before a heavy strength training session using a crossover design separated by at least seven days. Changes in postexercise oxygen consumption were significantly greater in the protein condition compared with placebo 90 to 120 minutes after exercise.

Another study (Johnston et al. 2002) evaluated the effects of ingesting a high-protein meal on thermogenesis before being fed a meal either high in protein or high in carbohydrate. Resting energy expenditure was determined following a 10-hour fast and 2.5 hours after ingesting breakfast, lunch, and dinner. After 28 and 56 days of consuming the prescribed diet, subjects repeated the experiment following the alternate diet. When compared to ingesting the high-carbohydrate meals, energy expenditure was 100% greater 2.5 hours after ingesting the high-protein meals. In addition, nitrogen balance was significantly greater when ingesting the high-protein diet. Given this information, one can assume that these increases in energy expenditure, if extrapolated over several weeks, would lead to positive changes in body weight and composition, particularly if caloric restriction is employed.

Indeed, and in addition to the positive effects on acute changes in thermogenesis, other studies have identified regular increased protein intake as being associated with positive effects on weight loss, body composition, health markers, satiety, and energy levels (Layman et al. 2003, 2005; Weigle et al. 2005). For example, a 2005 study (Weigle et al. 2005) found that an increase in dietary protein from 15% to 30% of energy at a constant carbohydrate intake produces a sustained decrease in ad libitum caloric intake. Layman and associates (2003, 2005) provided rather convincing evidence after reporting on a study that examined the efficacy of two weight loss diets with modified carbohydrate and protein ratios in changing body composition in women both with and without regular exercise. Women were assigned to either a carbohydrate group consuming a diet with a carbohydrate-to-protein ratio of 3.5 (68 grams of protein per day) or a group with a protein-to-carbohydrate ratio of 1.4 (125 grams of protein per day). When a higher-protein diet was ingested, significantly greater losses of fat were found when compared to the higher-carbohydrate diet. These authors concluded that increasing the proportion of protein to carbohydrate in the diet of adult women has positive effects on body composition seen by greater losses of fat and greater maintenance of lean tissue.

Finally, a number of researchers then considered the impact of diets comparing different macronutrient ratios (Kerksick et al. 2009, 2010; Noakes et al. 2005). Kerksick and colleagues (2009, 2010) published two separate studies investigating rather large cohorts of participants who were assigned to restricted energy diets with and without following an exercise program. In both of these studies, greater improvements in body composition were found to occur when higher amounts of protein were ingested as part of the 14-week diet-and-exercise program. In addition, when this concept was investigated with and without a regular exercise program, individuals who consumed more protein reported greater improvements in body composition, and a positive synergistic effect was also realized when exercise was added to each diet (Layman et al. 2005). While these studies did not investigate changes directly associated with the timing of nutrients, the macronutrient-specific response in favor of protein are important considerations when evaluating the overall impact of nutrient timing on weight loss and changes in body composition.

16.4.2 CARBOHYDRATES

The most researched macronutrient in regard to sports performance is carbohydrate. In fact, one could argue the entire concept of nutrient timing was created around the ability of postworkout carbohydrate to replenish glycogen stores or carbohydrate "loading" the diet before a prolonged bout of exercise. Biologically, the importance of carbohydrates lies in their role as a primary and immediate source of fuel for working muscles and the brain and a valuable source of water for athletes. Interestingly, and from a weight loss perspective, the rapid increase in blood glucose and insulin levels after carbohydrate ingestion has resulted in scrutiny for this nutrient and any role it may play in weight loss and favorable changes in body composition. As such, low-carbohydrate diets have become popular as a way to lose weight (see previous section).

Three considerations predominate when evaluating carbohydrates in regard to weight loss: the time you eat them, the type you eat, and how much of them are consumed in the diet. Carbohydrates are rated on their glycemic index, which is the degree to which they raise blood sugar (Foster-Powell et al. 2002). Carbohydrates with a high glycemic index increase glucose and insulin levels to a greater degree than those with a low-to-moderate glycemic index. Consuming fewer high-glycemic-index carbohydrate sources or reducing carbohydrate availability in the diet has been shown to improve insulin sensitivity and promote greater weight loss (Abete et al. 2008; Layman et al. 2005). Short-term intervention trials suggest that simply replacing high-glycemic-index foods with low-glycemic-index foods promotes weight loss and improves insulin sensitivity (Brand-Miller et al. 2002; Walberg-Rankin 1997), both favorable metabolic adaptations.

To this point, Scribner et al. (2008) evaluated the effects of glycemic index on fuel metabolism and body fat over a 40-week time period. When a high-glycemic-index diet was consumed, development of body fat was 40% higher, insulin resistance was twofold greater, and physical activity was 45% lower. As a result, the authors concluded that a diet with a high glycemic index negatively impacted body composition, increased development of insulin resistance, and was associated with decreases in physical activity levels.

When considered as such, glycemic index can also impact substrate metabolism as part of exercise. A study of nine healthy male recreational runners was used to investigate the impact of glycemic index on substrate utilization (Wu et al. 2003); each subject completed three trials: a high-glycemic-index meal, a low-glycemic-index meal, and a fasting condition. In each trial, subjects consumed the test meal three hours before performing a 60-minute run at 65% VO$_2$Max on a treadmill. As expected, when either form of carbohydrate was ingested, increases in glucose and insulin were seen during the postprandial period, but the increases in glucose levels were twofold greater during exercise when a high-glycemic-index meal was ingested in comparison to a low-glycemic-index meal. During exercise, when a higher-glycemic-index food is ingested, fat oxidation was found to be significantly lower in comparison to when a lower-glycemic-index food was ingested (Wu et al. 2003).

The results of this study are in agreement with other previously published studies. Eight endurance-trained men ingested a high-glycemic-index, low-glycemic-index, or a placebo meal 45 minutes before exercise and then cycled for 50 minutes at 67% VO$_2$Max (Sparks et al. 1998). As expected, ingestion of a high-glycemic-index meal resulted in the smallest increase in free fatty acid levels in the blood (a marker of fat breakdown) both before and after the exercise bout. When a placebo or lower-glycemic-index foods were ingested, respiratory exchange ratio and carbohydrate oxidation were higher throughout completion of a submaximal bout of exercise.

A final study used women to investigate the same research question (Stevenson et al. 2006). In this study, the authors completed similar measurements and concluded that a low-glycemic-index preexercise meal resulted in a higher rate of fat oxidation during exercise than did a high-glycemic-index meal.

In addition to glycemic index, many people feel that the overall glycemic load (Glycemic load = Glycemic index of food × Gram amount of carbohydrate food consumed) may be a more important factor when determining changes in substrate oxidation (Galgani et al. 2006; Wolever and Bolognesi 1996). Indeed, when five different meals were ingested containing varying amounts of carbohydrates, fats, and proteins, the source and amount of carbohydrate (i.e., glycemic load) accounted for the greatest amount of variation regarding glucose and insulin responses (Wolever and Bolognesi 1996). Ten years later and in support of these initial findings, Galgani and colleagues gave obese women combinations of large and small meals containing both high- and low-glycemic-index foods, which effectively created meals ranging from low to high glycemic loads. They concluded that glycemic load was useful in predicting the acute impact on glucose and insulin changes in mixed meals (Galgani et al. 2006).

In summary, the impact of glycemic index and glycemic load has been closely considered for their ability to influence glycemic as well as insulinemic changes. While a lack of data currently exists specifically examining timed administration of varying carbohydrates for changes in weight, body composition, and energy expenditure, the foundation for such research to explore these areas is certainly warranted.

16.5 TIME OF DAY

Another important consideration regarding the timing of nutrients in association with weight loss and changes in body composition is what time of day the feedings are taking place. Certainly, this is an area that has been discussed, both anecdotally and scientifically. The previous chapters have highlighted the importance of consuming certain nutrients at opportune times and how that may have an impact on athletic performance, but the focus of this chapter and section are centered on influences related to weight loss, body composition, and appetite. Countless anecdotal reports exist regarding the importance of breakfast as well as the impact of eating late in the evening on these endpoints. Scientific evidence also exists outlining this relationship and is an area of focus for this section.

16.5.1 BREAKFAST

Many people are proponents of eating breakfast to increase or sustain metabolic rate. Physiologically, an overnight sleep is likened to a prolonged period of fasting; thus, it is thought and often verbalized that eating breakfast helps to control metabolic rate, while helping a person to control appetite and facilitate weight loss goals. Review articles on the topic have reported and begun to explain what physiological mechanism may be responsible to explain why breakfast skipping leads to an upregulation of appetite and likely increases in weight gain, as well as changes in risk factors for diabetes and cardiovascular disease (Rampersaud et al. 2005; Timlin and Pereira 2007). Additional observational studies have suggested that breakfast skipping is linked to poorer diet quality, while daily breakfast consumption is associated with higher fiber intake and related prevention of obesity and various cardiovascular diseases (Pereira et al. 2002, 2011; Rampersaud et al. 2005; Timlin and Pereira 2007).

Pereira and colleagues, in a 2011 review, reported that several cross-sectional, observational studies have indicated an inverse association between breakfast consumption and BMI, even after adjustments were made for potential confounding variables (Cho et al. 2003; Song et al. 2005; Summerbell et al. 1996; Wyatt et al. 2002). Cross-sectional evidence supports this notion; researchers at the University of Massachusetts Medical School (Ma et al. 2003) investigated the association between eating patterns and obesity. Three 24-hour dietary recalls and a body weight measurement were collected at five equally spaced time points over a one-year period from 499 participants. Data were averaged for five time periods, and a cross-sectional analysis was conducted. Skipping breakfast was associated with a significantly higher risk of obesity. Subjects who regularly skipped breakfast (i.e., 75% of days measured by 24-hour recall) had a 4.5 times greater risk for obesity than those who regularly consumed breakfast. Also using a cross-sectional approach of over 2,500 subjects, Wyatt and colleagues (2002) determined that subjects who ate breakfast were more successful at losing weight.

Finally, Alexander and colleagues (2009) sought to determine whether breakfast consumption is associated with adiposity, specifically intra-abdominal adipose tissue, and insulin dynamics in overweight Latino youth. Over a two-day period, all participants provided 24-hour dietary recalls and completed an assessment of intra-abdominal adipose tissue and insulin dynamics. Participants were divided into three breakfast consumption categories: (1) those who reported not eating breakfast on either day, (2) those who reported eating breakfast on one of two days, and (3) those who ate breakfast on both days. The authors concluded that eating breakfast is associated with lower visceral adiposity in overweight Latino youth.

These longitudinal studies in free-living subjects suggest that a pattern of eating breakfast can aid in weight loss or weight maintenance. However, authors of both studies (Ma et al. 2003 and Alexander et al. 2009) indicate caution related to their interpretation as significant error is regularly introduced when using diet logs and questionnaires (Black et al. 1993; Lichtman et al. 1992; Prentice et al. 1986). In this respect, further studies using this approach have reported that breakfast eaters consume less dietary fat and cholesterol (Morgan et al. 1986; Song et al. 2005; Stanton and Keast 1989) and more fiber when compared to breakfast skippers.

Using an experimental approach to investigate the effects of eating or abstaining from breakfast on metabolism, researchers conducted a randomized crossover trial on 10 women who underwent two 14-day trials of eating or abstaining from breakfast separated by a two-week interval (Farshchi et al. 2005b). Glucose, lipid, and insulin concentrations and resting energy expenditure measurements were made before and after meal ingestion of each two-week study interval. The researchers found that abstaining from breakfast negatively impacted fasting lipids and postprandial insulin sensitivity. In addition, those abstaining from breakfast ate more calories throughout the day, suggesting that eating breakfast helps satiety throughout the day. While no impact of energy expenditure was noted in this study, a reduction in energy intake favorably tilts the energy balance equation toward weight loss.

Regardless of the lack of metabolic data on this issue, there does appear to be a metabolic advantage to eating breakfast. A 2010 review concluded that the breakfast meal and the frequency with which it is eaten may influence appetite control, overall quality of the diet, dietary intake and composition, and chronic disease risk. Breakfast skipping may lead to an upregulation of appetite, possibly leading to weight gain over time and deleterious changes in risk factors for diabetes and cardiovascular disease (Giovannini et al. 2010).

16.5.2 EVENING

John de Castro has done extensive work regarding eating behaviors. He and colleagues have determined that circadian and diurnal rhythms affect food intake, meal sizes, and satiety (de Castro 1991, 1998). In a 2004 study, de Castro (2004) investigated whether time of day of food intake would be related to total food intake. It was hypothesized that food intake early in the day would tend to reduce overall food intake, whereas food intake later in the day would tend to increase food intake over the entire day. Thus, the food intakes of 375 male and 492 female free-living individuals, previously obtained via seven-day diet diaries, were analyzed. The proportion of food intake in the morning was negatively correlated with overall food intake, whereas the proportion of food ingested late in the evening was positively correlated with overall food intake. It was concluded that food intake in the morning can reduce the total amount of calories ingested for the day, and that food intake later in the evening can result in greater overall daily food intake.

In a tightly controlled clinical trial, inpatient healthy subjects were used to evaluate the impact of nighttime eating (Gluck et al. 2008). After consuming a standardized diet for three days, participants ate ad libitum from a computer-operated vending machine that recorded the time of food selection. Energy intake was calculated as mean calories per day. The nighttime eaters consumed more calories per day than did nonnighttime eaters, but the percentage of calories from macronutrients did not differ. The authors found that nighttime eating was common and predictive of weight gain, providing support to the notion that nighttime eating can lead to an increase in body weight.

A possible explanation for this phenomenon was described by Qin et al. (2003). These researchers observed the 24-hour endocrine patterns of medical students who lived either a diurnal life or nocturnal life. Nocturnal life was designed by skipping their breakfast but consuming a majority of their food (>50% of their daily food intake) in the evening and at night, with sleep from 1:30 a.m. to 8:30 a.m. the next morning. After three weeks of following each plan, 24-hour plasma concentrations of melatonin, leptin, glucose, and insulin were measured every three hours. Both plasma melatonin and leptin showed peaks at 3:00 a.m. in the diurnal lifestyle group, and the night peaks decreased in the nocturnal lifestyle group. The changes in the patterns of melatonin and leptin were highly consistent with that of night-eating syndrome. Plasma glucose increased after all meals and maintained a high level in the nocturnal lifestyle group between midnight and early morning, while insulin secretion decreased markedly during this period. Researchers concluded that a nocturnal life leads to impairment of the insulin response to glucose. Less research is available outlining the impact of eating late at night when compared to breakfast eating.

Until further experimental approaches become available controlling for total dietary intake, conclusions should be viewed with caution. It is quite possible that any effect associated with eating late at night and changes in body mass and adiposity are linked entirely to total caloric intake rather than the time of day food is consumed. However, when considering the health implications of eating later at night and the impact it may have on glucose, insulin, and cholesterol changes in the blood, it is prudent to recommend not eating food right before bedtime; however, this suggestion at best is anecdotal until scientific evidence becomes available to support or refute the suggestion.

16.6 CONCLUSIONS AND RECOMMENDATIONS

Nutrient timing has proven to be a critically important factor in the application of sports nutrition. The timing of carbohydrates to enhance glycogen uptake and replenishment and the timing of proteins to optimize muscle protein synthesis have been well defined, but the extent to which this concept may have an impact on weight loss or body fat loss remains to be determined. The popularity of this topic is widespread as most individuals who are interested in their health, weight loss, or weight maintenance have likely been advised to alter their meal frequency in some capacity.

A review article published by La Bounty and colleagues (2011) provides a nice summary of the available literature discussed in this chapter. In this review, the authors concluded that an increased meal frequency does not have a favorable impact on body composition in sedentary populations or enhance metabolic rates but may favorably improve health markers found in the blood and help to control hunger. In accordance with these recommendations, three predominant areas exist for which the scientific literature has provided information: meal frequency, the thermic effect of food, and meal timing. A summary of these findings is as follows:

- Eating meals more frequently (greater than three meals per day vs. less than three meals per day) does not appear to promote greater weight loss when energy intake is balanced.
- The thermic effect or overall metabolic activity of protein ingestion is greatest, a value reported to be four times greater than the thermic effect seen from carbohydrate ingestion.
- Ingestion of lower-glycemic-index carbohydrate sources promotes greater fat oxidation during exercise, an effect that could potentially be exploited for weight loss pursuits; however, studies have yet to investigate this suggestion.
- A more consistent or regular schedule of eating appears to be more advantageous than an unstructured eating pattern.
- Eating breakfast correlates strongly with weight loss, body weight, cognitive function, decreased dietary fat and cholesterol intake, increased dietary fiber intake, and exercise patterns. However, there is limited evidence that eating breakfast increases metabolism.
- Eating late at night also correlates with increases in body weight and obesity. However, there is little evidence that eating at night causes increased fat storage, especially when total caloric intake is controlled.

References

Abete, I., D. Parra, and J.A. Martinez. 2008. Energy-Restricted Diets Based on a Distinct Food Selection Affecting the Glycemic Index Induce Different Weight Loss and Oxidative Response. *Clin Nutr* 27(4):545–51.

Abiru, N., E. Kawasaki, and K. Eguch. 2002. Current Knowledge of Japanese Type 1 Diabetic Syndrome. *Diabetes Metab Res Rev* 18(5):357–66.

Alexander, K.E., E.E. Ventura, D. Spruijt-Metz, M.J. Weigensberg, M.I. Goran, and J.N. Davis. 2009. Association of Breakfast Skipping with Visceral Fat and Insulin Indices in Overweight Latino Youth. *Obesity (Silver Spring)* 17(8):1528–33.

Ali, A., C. Williams, C.W. Nicholas, and A. Foskett. 2007. The Influence of Carbohydrate-Electrolyte Ingestion on Soccer Skill Performance. *Med Sci Sports Exerc* 39(11):1969–76.

Ammon, H.P., and M.A. Wahl. 1991. Pharmacology of *Curcuma longa*. *Planta Med* 57(1):1–7.

Anastasiou, C.A., S.A. Kavouras, G. Arnaoutis, A. Gioxari, M. Kollia, E. Botoula, and L.S. Sidossis. 2009. Sodium Replacement and Plasma Sodium Drop During Exercise in the Heat When Fluid Intake Matches Fluid Loss. *J Athl Train* 44(2):117–23.

Andersen, L.L., G. Tufekovic, M.K. Zebis, R.M. Crameri, G. Verlaan, M. Kjaer, C. Suetta, P. Magnusson, and P. Aagaard. 2005. The Effect of Resistance Training Combined with Timed Ingestion of Protein on Muscle Fiber Size and Muscle Strength. *Metabolism* 54(2):151–56.

Andrade, P.M., B.G. Ribeiro, M.T. Bozza, L.F. Costa Rosa, and M.G. Tavares Do Carmo. 2007. Effects of Fish Oil Supplementation on the Immuno Inflammatory Responses in Elite Swimmers. *Prostaglandins Leukot Essent Fatty Acids* 77:139–45.

Angus, D.J., M. Hargreaves, J. Dancey, and M.A. Febbraio. 2000. Effect of Carbohydrate or Carbohydrate Plus Medium-Chain Triglyceride Ingestion on Cycling Time Trial Performance. *J Appl Physiol* 88(1):113–19.

Angus, R.G., R.J. Heslegrave, and W.S. Myles. 1985. Effects of Prolonged Sleep Deprivation, with and without Chronic Physical Exercise, on Mood and Performance. *Psychophysiology* 22(3):276–82.

Anthony, J.C., T.G. Anthony, S.R. Kimball, T.C. Vary, and L.S. Jefferson. 2000. Orally Administered Leucine Stimulates Protein Synthesis in Skeletal Muscle of Postabsorptive Rats in Association with Increased EIF4F Formation. *J Nutr* 130(2):139–45.

Anthony, J.C., C.H. Lang, S.J. Crozier, T.G. Anthony, D.A. Maclean, S.R. Kimball, and L.S. Jefferson. 2002. Contribution of Insulin to the Translational Control of Protein Synthesis in Skeletal Muscle by Leucine. *Am J Physiol Endocrinol Metab* 282(5):E1092–101.

Antonio, J., and J.R. Stout. 2004. *Fit Kids for Life: A Parent's Guide to Optimal Nutrition and Training for Young Athletes*. New York: Basic Health Media.

Applegate, E.A., and L.E. Grivetti. 1997. Search for the Competitive Edge: A History of Dietary Fads and Supplements. *J Nutr* 127(5 Suppl):869S–73S.

Archer, D.T., and S.M. Shirreffs. 2001. Effect of Fluid Ingestion Rate on Post-Exercise Rehydration in Human Subjects. *Proc Nutr Soc* 60(4 special issue 3):200A.

Askew, E.W., I. Munro, M.A. Sharp, S. Siegel, R. Popper, M.S. Rose, R.W. Hoyt, J.W. Martin, K. Reynolds, H.R. Lieberman, D. Engell, and C.P. Shaw. 1987. Nutritional Status and Physical and Mental Performance of Special Operations Soldiers Consuming the Ration, Lightweight, or the Meal, Ready-to-Eat Military Field Ration during a 30-Day Field Exercise. (T787) U.S. Army Research Institute of Environmental Medicine.

Atherton, P.J., K. Smith, T. Etheridge, D. Rankin, and M.J. Rennie. 2010. Distinct Anabolic Signalling Responses to Amino Acids in C2C12 Skeletal Muscle Cells. *Amino Acids* 38(5):1533–39.

Aubert, A., F. Beckers, and B. Seps. 2002. Non-Linear Dynamics of Heart Rate Variability in Athletes: Effect of Training. *Comput Cardiol* 29:441–44.

Austin, K., and B. Seebohar (2011). Performance Nutrition: Applying the Science of Nutrient Timing. Human Kinetics: Champaign, IL.

Bach, A.C., and V.K. Babayan. 1982. Medium-Chain Triglycerides: An Update. *Am J Clin Nutr* 36(5):950–62.

Backhouse, S.H., A. Ali, S.J. Biddle, and C. Williams. 2007. Carbohydrate Ingestion During Prolonged High-Intensity Intermittent Exercise: Impact on Affect and Perceived Exertion. *Scand J Med Sci Sports* 17(5):605–10.

Backhouse, S.H., N.C. Bishop, S.J. Biddle, and C. Williams. 2005. Effect of Carbohydrate and Prolonged Exercise on Affect and Perceived Exertion. *Med Sci Sports Exerc* 37(10):1768–73.

Bailey, D.A., A.D. Martin, H.A. Mckay, S. Whiting, and R. Mirwald. 2000. Calcium Accretion in Girls and Boys During Puberty: A Longitudinal Analysis. *J Bone Miner Res* 15(11):2245–50.

Banister, E.W., and B.J. Cameron. 1990. Exercise-Induced Hyperammonemia: Peripheral and Central Effects. *Int J Sports Med* 11(Suppl 2):S129–42.

Barnet, A. 2006. Using Training Recovery Modalities between Training Sessions in Elite Athletes. *Sports Med* 36(9):781–96.

Bar-Or, O. 2001. Nutritional Considerations for the Child Athlete. *Can J Appl Physiol* 26 Suppl:S186–91.

Barr, K., and S. McGee. 2008. Optimising Training Adaptations by Manipulating Glycogen. *Eur J Sport Sci* 8:97–106.

Bates, G.P., and V.S. Miller. 2008. Sweat Rate and Sodium Loss During Work in the Heat. *J Occup Med Toxicol* 3:4.

Battram, D.S., J. Shearer, D. Robinson, and T.E. Graham. 2004. Caffeine Ingestion Does Not Impede the Resynthesis of Proglycogen and Macroglycogen after Prolonged Exercise and Carbohydrate Supplementation in Humans. *J Appl Physiol* 96(3):943–50.

Bechet, D., A. Tassa, D. Taillandier, L. Combaret, and D. Attaix. 2005. Lysosomal Proteolysis in Skeletal Muscle. *Int J Biochem Cell Biol* 37(10):2098–114.

Bechet, D.M., C. Deval, J. Robelin, M.J. Ferrara, and A. Obled. 1996. Developmental Control of Cathepsin B Expression in Bovine Fetal Muscles. *Arch Biochem Biophys* 334(2):362–68.

Beelen, M., J. Berghuis, B. Bonaparte, S.B. Ballak, A.E. Jeukendrup, and L.J. Van Loon. 2009. Carbohydrate Mouth Rinsing in the Fed State: Lack of Enhancement of Time-Trial Performance. *Int J Sport Nutr Exerc Metab* 19(4):400–9.

Beelen, M., R. Koopman, A.P. Gijsen, H. Vandereyt, A.K. Kies, H. Kuipers, W.H. Saris, and L.J. Van Loon. 2008. Protein Coingestion Stimulates Muscle Protein Synthesis During Resistance-Type Exercise. *Am J Physiol Endocrinol Metab* 295(1):E70–77.

Beelen, M., M. Tieland, A.P. Gijsen, H. Vandereyt, A.K. Kies, H. Kuipers, W.H. Saris, R. Koopman, and L.J. Van Loon. 2008. Coingestion of Carbohydrate and Protein Hydrolysate Stimulates Muscle Protein Synthesis During Exercise in Young Men, with No Further Increase During Subsequent Overnight Recovery. *J Nutr* 138(11):2198–204.

Belko, A.Z., E. Obarzanek, H.J. Kalkwarf, M.A. Rotter, S. Bogusz, D. Miller, J.D. Haas, and D.A. Roe. 1983. Effects of Exercise on Riboflavin Requirements of Young Women. *Am J Clin Nutr* 37(4):509–17.

Bellisle, F., R. Mcdevitt, and A.M. Prentice. 1997. Meal Frequency and Energy Balance. *Br J Nutr* 77(Suppl 1):S57–S70.

Below, P.R., R. Mora-Rodriguez, J. Gonzalez-Alonso, and E.F. Coyle. 1995. Fluid and Carbohydrate Ingestion Independently Improve Performance During 1 h of Intense Exercise. *Med Sci Sports Exerc* 27(2):200–210.

Berardi, J.M., E.E. Noreen, and P.W. Lemon. 2008. Recovery from a Cycling Time Trial Is Enhanced with Carbohydrate-Protein Supplementation vs. Isoenergetic Carbohydrate Supplementation. *J Int Soc Sports Nutr* 5:24.

Berardi, J.M., T.B. Price, E.E. Noreen, and P.W. Lemon. 2006. Postexercise Muscle Glycogen Recovery Enhanced with a Carbohydrate-Protein Supplement. *Med Sci Sports Exerc* 38(6):1106–13.

Bergstrom, J., L. Hermansen, E. Hultman, and B. Saltin. 1967. Diet, Muscle Glycogen and Physical Performance. *Acta Physiol Scand* 71(2):140–50.

Bergstrom, J., and E. Hultman. 1966. Muscle Glycogen Synthesis after Exercise: An Enhancing Factor Localized to the Muscle Cells in Man. *Nature* 210(5033):309–10.

Bergstrom, J., and E. Hultman. 1967. A Study of the Glycogen Metabolism During Exercise in Man. *Scand J Clin Lab Invest* 19(3):218–28.

Berneis, K., R. Ninnis, D. Haussinger, and U. Keller. 1999. Effects of Hyper- and Hypoosmolality on Whole Body Protein and Glucose Kinetics in Humans. *Am J Physiol* 276(1 Pt 1):E188–95.

Betts, J.A., E. Stevenson, C. Williams, C. Sheppard, E. Grey, and J. Griffin. 2005. Recovery of Endurance Running Capacity: Effect of Carbohydrate-Protein Mixtures. *Int J Sport Nutr Exerc Metab* 15(6):590–609.

Bilsborough, S., and N. Mann. 2006. A Review of Issues of Dietary Protein Intake in Humans. *Int J Sport Nutr Exerc Metab* 16(2):129–52.

Binnert, C., C. Pachiaudi, M. Beylot, M. Croset, R. Cohen, J.P. Riou, and M. Laville. 1996. Metabolic Fate of an Oral Long-Chain Triglyceride Load in Humans. *Am J Physiol* 270(3 Pt 1):E445–50.

Biolo, G., S.P. Maggi, B.D. Williams, K.D. Tipton, and R.R. Wolfe. 1995. Increased Rates of Muscle Protein Turnover and Amino Acid Transport after Resistance Exercise in Humans. *Am J Physiol* 268(3 Pt 1):E514–20.

Biolo, G., K.D. Tipton, S. Klein, and R.R. Wolfe. 1997. An Abundant Supply of Amino Acids Enhances the Metabolic Effect of Exercise on Muscle Protein. *Am J Physiol* 273(1 Pt 1):E122–29.

Biolo, G., B.D. Williams, R.Y. Fleming, and R.R. Wolfe. 1999. Insulin Action on Muscle Protein Kinetics and Amino Acid Transport During Recovery after Resistance Exercise. *Diabetes* 48(5):949–57.

Bird, S.P., K.M. Tarpenning, and F.E. Marino. 2006a. Effects of Liquid Carbohydrate/Essential Amino Acid Ingestion on Acute Hormonal Response During a Single Bout of Resistance Exercise in Untrained Men. *Nutrition* 22(4):367–75.

Bird, S.P., K.M. Tarpenning, and F.E. Marino. 2006b. Independent and Combined Effects of Liquid Carbohydrate/Essential Amino Acid Ingestion on Hormonal and Muscular Adaptations Following Resistance Training in Untrained Men. *Eur J Appl Physiol* 97(2):225–38.

Bird, S.P., K.M. Tarpenning, and F.E. Marino. 2006c. Liquid Carbohydrate/Essential Amino Acid Ingestion during a Short-Term Bout of Resistance Exercise Suppresses Myofibrillar Protein Degradation. *Metabolism* 55(5):570–77.

Bishai, D., and R. Nalubola. 2002. The History of Food Fortification in the United States: Its Relevance for Current Fortification Efforts in Developing Countries. *Econ Dev Cultural Change* 51(1):37–53.

Bishop, P., E. Jones, and K. Woods. 2008. Recovery from Training: A Brief Review. *J Strength Cond Res* 22(3):1015–24.

Bjorkman, O., K. Sahlin, L. Hagenfeldt, and J. Wahren. 1984. Influence of Glucose and Fructose Ingestion on the Capacity for Long-Term Exercise in Well-Trained Men. *Clin Physiol* 4(6):483–94.

Black, A.E., A.M. Prentice, G.R. Goldberg, S.A. Jebb, S.A. Bingham, M.B. Livingstone, and W.A. Coward. 1993. Measurements of Total Energy Expenditure Provide Insights into the Validity of Dietary Measurements of Energy Intake. *J Am Diet Assoc* 93(5):572–79.

Bleakley, C., S. McDonough, and D. Macauley. 2004. The Use of Ice in the Treatment of Acute Soft-Tissue Injury: A Systematic Review of Randomized Controlled Trials. *Am J Sports Med* 32(1):251–61.

Blom, P.C., A.T. Hostmark, O. Vaage, K.R. Kardel, and S. Maehlum. 1987. Effect of Different Post-Exercise Sugar Diets on the Rate of Muscle Glycogen Synthesis. *Med Sci Sports Exerc* 19(5):491–96.

Blom, P.C., N.K. Vollestad, and D.L. Costill. 1986. Factors Affecting Changes in Muscle Glycogen Concentration During and after Prolonged Exercise. *Acta Physiol Scand Suppl* 556:67–74.

Blomstrand, E., F. Celsing, and E.A. Newsholme. 1988. Changes in Plasma Concentrations of Aromatic and Branched-Chain Amino Acids During Sustained Exercise in Man and Their Possible Role in Fatigue. *Acta Physiol Scand* 133(1):115–21.

Blomstrand, E., P. Hassmen, S. Ek, B. Ekblom, and E.A. Newsholme. 1997. Influence of Ingesting a Solution of Branched-Chain Amino Acids on Perceived Exertion During Exercise. *Acta Physiol Scand* 159(1):41–49.

Blomstrand, E., P. Hassmen, B. Ekblom, and E.A. Newsholme. 1991. Administration of Branched-Chain Amino Acids During Sustained Exercise—Effects on Performance and on Plasma Concentration of Some Amino Acids. *Eur J Appl Physiol Occup Physiol* 63(2):83–88.

Blomstrand, E., P. Hassmen, and E.A. Newsholme. 1991. Effect of Branched-Chain Amino Acid Supplementation on Mental Performance. *Acta Physiol Scand* 143(2):225–26.

Bohe, J., A. Low, R.R. Wolfe, and M.J. Rennie. 2003. Human Muscle Protein Synthesis Is Modulated by Extracellular, Not Intramuscular Amino Acid Availability: A Dose-Response Study. *J Physiol* 552(Pt 1):315–24.

Bohe, J., J.F. Low, R.R. Wolfe, and M.J. Rennie. 2001. Latency and Duration of Stimulation of Human Muscle Protein Synthesis During Continuous Infusion of Amino Acids. *J Physiol* 532(Pt 2):575–79.

Boirie, Y., M. Dangin, P. Gachon, M.P. Vasson, J.L. Maubois, and B. Beaufrere. 1997. Slow and Fast Dietary Proteins Differently Modulate Postprandial Protein Accretion. *Proc Natl Acad Sci USA* 94(26):14930–35.

Boisseau, N., M. Vermorel, M. Rance, P. Duche, and P. Patureau-Mirand. 2007. Protein Requirements in Male Adolescent Soccer Players. *Eur J Appl Physiol* 100(1):27–33.

Borsheim, E., Q.U. Bui, S. Tissier, H. Kobayashi, A.A. Ferrando, and R.R. Wolfe. 2008. Effect of Amino Acid Supplementation on Muscle Mass, Strength and Physical Function in Elderly. *Clin Nutr* 27(2):189–95.

Borsheim, E., M.G. Cree, K.D. Tipton, T.A. Elliott, A. Aarsland, and R.R. Wolfe. 2004. Effect of Carbohydrate Intake on Net Muscle Protein Synthesis During Recovery from Resistance Exercise. *J Appl Physiol* 96(2):674–78.

Bos, C., C. Gaudichon, and D. Tome. 2000. Nutritional and Physiological Criteria in the Assessment of Milk Protein Quality for Humans. *J Am Coll Nutr* 19(2 Suppl):191S–205S.

Bos, C., C.C. Metges, C. Gaudichon, K.J. Petzke, M.E. Pueyo, C. Morens, J. Everwand, R. Benamouzig, and D. Tome. 2003. Postprandial Kinetics of Dietary Amino Acids Are the Main Determinant of Their Metabolism after Soy or Milk Protein Ingestion in Humans. *J Nutr* 133(5):1308–15.

Bosch, A.N., S.C. Dennis, and T.D. Noakes. 1994. Influence of Carbohydrate Ingestion on Fuel Substrate Turnover and Oxidation During Prolonged Exercise. *J Appl Physiol* 76(6):2364–72.

Brand-Miller, J.C., S.H. Holt, D.B. Pawlak, and J. McMillan. 2002. Glycemic Index and Obesity. *Am J Clin Nutr* 76(1):281S–85S.

Bray, G.A., and B.M. Popkin. 1998. Dietary Fat Intake Does Affect Obesity! *Am J Clin Nutr* 68(6):1157–73.

Bray, M.S., J.M. Hagberg, L. Perusse, T. Rankinen, S.M. Roth, B. Wolfarth, and C. Bouchard. 2009. The Human Gene Map for Performance and Health-Related Fitness Phenotypes: The 2006–2007 Update. *Med Sci Sports Exerc* 41(1):35–73.

Breen, L., K.D. Tipton, and A.E. Jeukendrup. 2010. No Effect of Carbohydrate-Protein on Cycling Performance and Indices of Recovery. *Med Sci Sports Exerc* 42(6):1140–48.

Brooks, G. 2002. Lactate Shuttles in Nature. *Biochem Soc Trans* 30:258–64.

Brooks, G.A., Fahey, T.D., White, T.P., Baldwin, K.M. 2000. *Exercise Physiology.* 3rd ed. *Human Bioenergetics and Its Application.* Mountain View, CA: Mayfield.

Brose, A., G. Parise, and M.A. Tarnopolsky. 2003. Creatine Supplementation Enhances Isometric Strength and Body Composition Improvements Following Strength Exercise Training in Older Adults. *J Gerontol* 58(1):11–19.

Brouns, F., and E. Beckers. 1993. Is the Gut an Athletic Organ? Digestion, Absorption and Exercise. *Sports Med* 15(4):242–57.

Brown, E.C., R.A. Disilvestro, A. Babaknia, and S.T. Devor. 2004. Soy versus Whey Protein Bars: Effects on Exercise Training Impact on Lean Body Mass and Antioxidant Status. *Nutr J* 3:22.

Brozek, J., F. Grande, H.L. Taylor, J.T. Anderson, E.R. Buskirk, and A. Keys. 1957. Changes in Body Weight and Body Dimensions in Men Performing Work on a Low Calorie Carbohydrate Diet. *J Appl Physiol* 10(3):412–20.

Buckley, C., D. Pilling, J. Lord, A. Akbar, D. Sheel-Toeller, and M. Salmon. 2001. Fibroblasts Regulate the Switch from Acute Resolving to Chronic Persistent Inflammation. *Trends Immunol* 22:191–204.

Buford, T.W., R.B. Kreider, J.R. Stout, M. Greenwood, B. Campbell, M. Spano, T. Ziegenfuss, H. Lopez, J. Landis, and J. Antonio. 2007. International Society of Sports Nutrition Position Stand: Creatine Supplementation and Exercise. *J Int Soc Sports Nutr* 4:6.

Burd, N.A., A.W. Staples, D.W.D. West, D.R. Moore, A.M. Holwerda, S.K. Baker, and S.M. Phillips. 2009. Latent Increases in Fasting and Fed-State Muscle Protein Turnover with Resistance Exercise Irrespective of Intensity. *Appl Physiol Nutr Metab* 34:1122.

Burd, N.A., J.E. Tang, D.R. Moore, and S.M. Phillips. 2009. Exercise Training and Protein Metabolism: Influences of Contraction, Protein Intake, and Sex-Based Differences. *J Appl Physiol* 106(5):1692–701.

Burd, N.A., D.W. West, A.W. Staples, P.J. Atherton, J.M. Baker, D.R. Moore, A.M. Holwerda, G. Parise, M.J. Rennie, S.K. Baker, and S.M. Phillips. 2010. Low-Load High Volume Resistance Exercise Stimulates Muscle Protein Synthesis More Than High-Load Low Volume Resistance Exercise in Young Men. *PLoS One* 5(8):e12033.

Burk, A., S. Timpmann, L. Medijainen, M. Vahi, and V. Oopik. 2009. Time-Divided Ingestion Pattern of Casein-Based Protein Supplement Stimulates an Increase in Fat-Free Body Mass during Resistance Training in Young Untrained Men. *Nutr Res* 29(6):405–13.

Burke, D.G., P.D. Chilibeck, K.S. Davidson, D.G. Candow, J. Farthing, and T. Smith-Palmer. 2001. The Effect of Whey Protein Supplementation with and without Creatine Monohydrate Combined with Resistance Training on Lean Tissue Mass and Muscle Strength. *Int J Sport Nutr Exerc Metab* 11(3):349–64.

Burke, L. 2010a. Fasting and Recovery from Exercise. *Br J Sports Med* 44(7):502–8.

Burke, L., G. Cox, N. Cummings, and B. Desbrow. 2001. Guidelines for Daily Carbohydrate Intake: Do Athletes Achieve Them? *Sports Med* 31:267–99.

Burke, L.M. 2001. Energy Needs of Athletes. *Can J Appl Physiol* 26 Suppl:S202–19.

Burke, L.M. 2010b. Fueling Strategies to Optimise Performance—Training High or Training Low? *Scand J Med Sci Sports* 20(Suppl 2):48–58.

Burke, L.M.. 2007. Training and Competition Nutrition. In *Practical Sports Nutrition*, edited by L.M. Burke. Champaign, IL: Human Kinetics, pp. 1–26.

Burke, L.M., D.J. Angus, G.R. Cox, N.K. Cummings, M.A. Febbraio, K. Gawthorn, J.A. Hawley, M. Minehan, D.T. Martin, and M. Hargreaves. 2000. Effect of Fat Adaptation and Carbohydrate Restoration on Metabolism and Performance during Prolonged Cycling. *J Appl Physiol* 89(6):2413–21.

Burke, L.M., G.R. Collier, S.K. Beasley, P.G. Davis, P.A. Fricker, P. Heeley, K. Walder, and M. Hargreaves. 1995. Effect of Coingestion of Fat and Protein with Carbohydrate Feedings on Muscle Glycogen Storage. *J Appl Physiol* 78(6):2187–92.

Burke, L.M., G.R. Collier, P.G. Davis, P.A. Fricker, A.J. Sanigorski, and M. Hargreaves. 1996. Muscle Glycogen Storage after Prolonged Exercise: Effect of the Frequency of Carbohydrate Feedings. *Am J Clin Nutr* 64(1):115–19.

Burke, L.M., G.R. Collier, and M. Hargreaves. 1993. Muscle Glycogen Storage after Prolonged Exercise: Effect of the Glycemic Index of Carbohydrate Feedings. *J Appl Physiol* 75(2):1019–23.

Burke, L.M., J.A. Hawley, D.J. Angus, G.R. Cox, S.A. Clark, N.K. Cummings, B. Desbrow, and M. Hargreaves. 2002. Adaptations to Short-Term High-Fat Diet Persist during Exercise Despite High Carbohydrate Availability. *Med Sci Sports Exerc* 34(1):83–91.

Burke, L.M., and B. Kiens. 2006. "Fat Adaptation" for Athletic Performance: The Nail in the Coffin? *J Appl Physiol* 100(1):7–8.

Burke, L.M., B. Kiens, and J.L. Ivy. 2004. Carbohydrates and Fat for Training and Recovery. *J Sports Sci* 22(1):15–30.

Burke, L.M., G. Slater, E.M. Broad, J. Haukka, S. Modulon, and W.G. Hopkins. 2003. Eating Patterns and Meal Frequency of Elite Australian Athletes. *Int J Sport Nutr Exerc Metab* 13(4):521–38.

Buskirk, E.R., P.F. Iampietro, and D.E. Bass. 1958. Work Performance after Dehydration: Effects of Physical Conditioning and Heat Acclimatization. *J Appl Physiol* 12(2):189–94.

Bussau, V.A., T.J. Fairchild, A. Rao, P. Steele, and P.A. Fournier. 2002. Carbohydrate Loading in Human Muscle: An Improved 1 Day Protocol. *Eur J Appl Physiol* 87(3):290–95.

Calder, A. 1995. Accelerating Adaptation to Training. Paper presented at the Australian Strength and Conditioning Association National Conference and Trade Show, Gold Coast, Australia.

Camera, D.M., J. Edge, M.J. Short, J.A. Hawley, and V.G. Coffey. 2010. Early Time-Course of Akt Phosphorylation Following Endurance and Resistance Exercise. *Med Sci Sports Exerc* 42(10):1843–52.

Cameron, J.D., M.J. Cyr, and E. Doucet. 2010. Increased Meal Frequency Does Not Promote Greater Weight Loss in Subjects Who Were Prescribed an 8-Week Equi-Energetic Energy-Restricted Diet. *Br J Nutr* 103(8):1098–101.

Campbell, B., R.B. Kreider, T. Ziegenfuss, P. La Bounty, M. Roberts, D. Burke, J. Landis, H. Lopez, and J. Antonio. 2007. International Society of Sports Nutrition Position Stand: Protein and Exercise. *J Int Soc Sports Nutr* 4:8.

Campbell, W.W., T.A. Trappe, R.R. Wolfe, and W.J. Evans. 2001. The Recommended Dietary Allowance for Protein May Not Be Adequate for Older People to Maintain Skeletal Muscle. *J Gerontol* 56(6):M373–80.

Candow, D.G., N.C. Burke, T. Smith-Palmer, and D.G. Burke. 2006. Effect of Whey and Soy Protein Supplementation Combined with Resistance Training in Young Adults. *Int J Sport Nutr Exerc Metab* 16(3):233–44.

Candow, D.G., P.D. Chilibeck, M. Facci, S. Abeysekara, and G.A. Zello. 2006. Protein Supplementation Before and After Resistance Training in Older Men. *Eur J Appl Physiol* 97(5):548–56.

Candow, D.G., J.P. Little, P.D. Chilibeck, S. Abeysekara, G.A. Zello, M. Kazachkov, S.M. Cornish, and P.H. Yu. 2008. Low-Dose Creatine Combined with Protein During Resistance Training in Older Men. *Med Sci Sports Exerc* 40(9):1645–52.

Cardinale, M., R. Soiza, J. Leiper, A. Gibson, and W. Primrose. 2010. Hormonal Responses to a Single Session of Whole Body Vibration Exercise in Older Individuals. *Br J Sports Med* 44:284–88.

Carpenter, K.J., A.E. Harper, and R.E. Olson. 1997. Experiments that Changed Nutritional Thinking. *J. Nutr* 127:1017S–53S.

Cartee, G.D., D.A. Young, M.D. Sleeper, J. Zierath, H. Wallberg-Henriksson, and J.O. Holloszy. 1989. Prolonged Increase in Insulin-Stimulated Glucose Transport in Muscle after Exercise. *Am J Physiol* 256(4 Pt 1):E494–99.

Carter, J.M., A.E. Jeukendrup, and D.A. Jones. 2004. The Effect of Carbohydrate Mouth Rinse on 1-h Cycle Time Trial Performance. *Med Sci Sports Exerc* 36(12):2107–11.

Carter, J.M., A.E. Jeukendrup, C.H. Mann, and D.A. Jones. 2004. The Effect of Glucose Infusion on Glucose Kinetics During a 1-h Time Trial. *Med Sci Sports Exerc* 36(9):1543–50.

Casa, D., L. Armstrong, S. Hilllman, S. Montain, R. Reiff, B. Rich, W. Roberts, and J. Stone. 2000. National Athletic Trainers' Association Position Statement: Fluid Replacement for Athletes. *J Athl Train* 35(2):212–224.

Casey, A., D. Constantin-Teodosiu, S. Howell, E. Hultman, and P.L. Greenhaff. 1996. Creatine Ingestion Favorably Affects Performance and Muscle Metabolism During Maximal Exercise in Humans. *Am J Physiol* 271(1 Pt 1):E31–37.

Casey, A., A.H. Short, E. Hultman, and P.L. Greenhaff. 1995. Glycogen Resynthesis in Human Muscle Fibre Types Following Exercise-Induced Glycogen Depletion. *J Physiol* 483(Pt 1):265–71.

Castaneda, T.R., H. Jurgens, P. Wiedmer, P. Pfluger, S. Diano, T.L. Horvath, M. Tang-Christensen, and M.H. Tschop. 2005. Obesity and the Neuroendocrine Control of Energy Homeostasis: The Role of Spontaneous Locomotor Activity. *J Nutr* 135(5):1314–19.

Castellanos, V.H., M.D. Litchford, and W.W. Campbell. 2006. Modular Protein Supplements and Their Application to Long-Term Care. *Nutr Clin Pract* 21(5):485–504.

Cermak, N.M., A.S. Solheim, M.S. Gardner, M.A. Tarnopolsky, and M.J. Gibala. 2009. Muscle Metabolism during Exercise with Carbohydrate or Protein-Carbohydrate Ingestion. *Med Sci Sports Exerc* 41(12):2158–64.

Chambers, E.S., M.W. Bridge, and D.A. Jones. 2009. Carbohydrate Sensing in the Human Mouth: Effects on Exercise Performance and Brain Activity. *J Physiol* 587(Pt 8):1779–94.

Chaouachi, A., J.B. Leiper, N. Souissi, A.J. Coutts, and K. Chamari. 2009. Effects of Ramadan Intermittent Fasting on Sports Performance and Training: A Review. *Int J Sports Physiol Perform* 4(4):419–34.

Chaouloff, F., D. Laude, D. Merino, B. Serrurrier, Y. Guezennec, and J.L. Elghozi. 1987. Amphetamine and Alpha-Methyl-P-Tyrosine Affect the Exercise-Induced Imbalance between the Availability of Tryptophan and Synthesis of Serotonin in the Brain of the Rat. *Neuropharmacology* 26(8):1099–106.

Chattington, M. 2007. Sleep Deprivation Affects Eye-Steering Coordination When Driving. Paper presented at the 21st annual meeting of the Associated Professional Sleep Societies. Minneapolis, MN. June 11, 2007.

Chaveau, A. 1896. Source Et Nature Du Potentiel Directement Utilisé Dans Le Travail Musculaire, D'après Les Échanges Respiratoires, Chez L'homme En État D'abstience. *Acad Sci (Paris)* 122:1163–69.

Cheetham, M.E., L.H. Boobis, S. Brooks, and C. Williams. 1986. Human Muscle Metabolism During Sprint Running. *J Appl Physiol* 61(1):54–60.

Chesley, A., J.D. Macdougall, M.A. Tarnopolsky, S.A. Atkinson, and K. Smith. 1992. Changes in Human Muscle Protein Synthesis after Resistance Exercise. *J Appl Physiol* 73(4):1383–88.

Cheuvront, S.N., R. Carter III, and M.N. Sawka. 2003. Fluid Balance and Endurance Exercise Performance. *Curr Sports Med Rep* 2(4):202–8.

Chinevere, T.D., R.D. Sawyer, A.R. Creer, R.K. Conlee, and A.C. Parcell. 2002. Effects of L-Tyrosine and Carbohydrate Ingestion on Endurance Exercise Performance. *J Appl Physiol* 93(5):1590–97.

Chiu, L., and J. Barnes. 2003. The Fitness-Fatigue Model Revisted: Implications for Planning Short- and Long-Term Training. *J Strength Cond Res* 25(6):42–51.

Chiu, L., L. Weiss, and A. Fry. 2001. Post-Training Massage: A Review for Strength and Power Athletes. *Strength Cond J* 23(4):65–159.

Cho, S., M. Dietrich, C.J. Brown, C.A. Clark, and G. Block. 2003. The Effect of Breakfast Type on Total Daily Energy Intake and Body Mass Index: Results from the Third National Health and Nutrition Examination Survey (NHANES III). *J Am Coll Nutr* 22(4):296–302.

Christensen, E.H., and O. Hanson. 1939. Arbeitsfahigkeit Und Ehrnahrung. *Skand Arch Physiol* 81:160–71.

Chromiak, J.A., B. Smedley, W. Carpenter, R. Brown, Y.S. Koh, J.G. Lamberth, L.A. Joe, B.R. Abadie, and G. Altorfer. 2004. Effect of a 10-Week Strength Training Program and Recovery Drink on Body Composition, Muscular Strength and Endurance, and Anaerobic Power and Capacity. *Nutrition* 20(5):420–27.

Chrusch, M.J., P.D. Chilibeck, K.E. Chad, K.S. Davison, and D.G. Burke. 2001. Creatine Supplementation Combined with Resistance Training in Older Men. *Med Sci Sports Exerc* 33(12):2111–17.

Chryssanthopoulos, C., and C. Williams. 1997. Pre-Exercise Carbohydrate Meal and Endurance Running Capacity When Carbohydrates Are Ingested During Exercise. *Int J Sports Med* 18(7):543–48.

Churchley, E.G., V.G. Coffey, D.J. Pedersen, A. Shield, K.A. Carey, D. Cameron-Smith, and J.A. Hawley. 2007. Influence of Preexercise Muscle Glycogen Content on Transcriptional Activity of Metabolic and Myogenic Genes in Well-Trained Humans. *J Appl Physiol* 102(4):1604–11.

Clark, M., S. Rattigan, L. Clerk, M. Vincent, J. Clark, J. Youd, and J. Newman. 2000. Nutritive and Non-Nutritive Blood Flow: Rest and Exercise. *Acta Physiol Scand* 168:519–30.

Coburn, J.W., D.J. Housh, T.J. Housh, M.H. Malek, T.W. Beck, J.T. Cramer, G.O. Johnson, and P.E. Donlin. 2006. Effects of Leucine and Whey Protein Supplementation During Eight Weeks of Unilateral Resistance Training. *J Strength Cond Res* 20(2):284–91.

Cochrane, D.J. 2004. Alternating Hot and Cold Water Immersion for Athlete Recovery: A Review. *Phys Ther Sport* 5:26–32.

Coffey, V.G., A. Shield, B.J. Canny, K.A. Carey, D. Cameron-Smith, and J.A. Hawley. 2006. Interaction of Contractile Activity and Training History on mRNA Abundance in Skeletal Muscle from Trained Athletes. *Am J Physiol Endocrinol Metab* 290(5):E849–55.

Coggan, A.R., and E.F. Coyle. 1987. Reversal of Fatigue During Prolonged Exercise by Carbohydrate Infusion or Ingestion. *J Appl Physiol* 63(6):2388–95.

Coggan, A.R., and E.F. Coyle. 1991. Carbohydrate Ingestion during Prolonged Exercise: Effects on Metabolism and Performance. *Exerc Sport Sci Rev* 19:1–40.

Cole, K.J., P.W. Grandjean, R.J. Sobszak, and J.B. Mitchell. 1993. Effect of Carbohydrate Composition on Fluid Balance, Gastric Emptying, and Exercise Performance. *Int J Sport Nutr* 3(4):408–17.

Colombani, P.C., E. Kovacs, P. Frey-Rindova, W. Frey, W. Langhans, M. Arnold, and C. Wenk. 1999. Metabolic Effects of a Protein-Supplemented Carbohydrate Drink in Marathon Runners. *Int J Sport Nutr* 9(2):181–201.

Combaret, L., D. Dardevet, I. Rieu, M.N. Pouch, D. Bechet, D. Taillandier, J. Grizard, and D. Attaix. 2005. A Leucine-Supplemented Diet Restores the Defective Postprandial Inhibition of Proteasome-Dependent Proteolysis in Aged Rat Skeletal Muscle. *J Physiol* 569(Pt 2):489–99.

Copeland, K.C., R.B. Colletti, J.T. Devlin, and T.L. McAuliffe. 1990. The Relationship between Insulin-Like Growth Factor-I, Adiposity, and Aging. *Metabolism* 39(6):584–87.

Corsi, A., M. Midrio, and A.L. Granata. 1969. In Situ Utilization of Glycogen and Blood Glucose by Skeletal Muscle During Tetanus. *Am J Physiol* 216(6):1534–41.

Costill, D.L., A. Bennett, G. Branam, and D. Eddy. 1973. Glucose Ingestion at Rest and During Prolonged Exercise. *J Appl Physiol* 34(6):764–69.

Costill, D.L., R. Bowers, G. Branam, and K. Sparks. 1971. Muscle Glycogen Utilization During Prolonged Exercise on Successive Days. *J Appl Physiol* 31(6):834–38.

Costill, D.L., E. Coyle, G. Dalsky, W. Evans, W. Fink, and D. Hoopes. 1977. Effects of Elevated Plasma FFA and Insulin on Muscle Glycogen Usage during Exercise. *J Appl Physiol* 43(4):695–99.

Costill, D.L., and J.M. Miller. 1980. Nutrition for Endurance Sport: Carbohydrate and Fluid Balance. *Int J Sports Med* 1:2–14.

Costill, D.L., and B. Saltin. 1974. Factors Limiting Gastric Emptying during Rest and Exercise. *J Appl Physiol* 37(5):679–83.

Costill, D.L., W.M. Sherman, W.J. Fink, C. Maresh, M. Witten, and J.M. Miller. 1981. The Role of Dietary Carbohydrates in Muscle Glycogen Resynthesis after Strenuous Running. *Am J Clin Nutr* 34(9):1831–36.

Courtney-Martin, G., M. Rafii, L.J. Wykes, R.O. Ball, and P.B. Pencharz. 2008. Methionine-Adequate Cysteine-Free Diet Does Not Limit Erythrocyte Glutathione Synthesis in Young Healthy Adult Men. *J Nutr* 138(11):2172–78.

Cox, G.R., S.A. Clark, A.J. Cox, S.L. Halson, M. Hargreaves, J.A. Hawley, N. Jeacocke, R.J. Snow, W.K. Yeo, and L.M. Burke. 2010. Daily Training with High Carbohydrate Availability Increases Exogenous Carbohydrate Oxidation during Endurance Cycling. *J Appl Physiol* 109(1):126–34.

Coyle, E.F. 1992. Carbohydrate Supplementation During Exercise. *J Nutr* 122(3 Suppl):788–95.

Coyle, E.F. 2004. Fluid and Fuel Intake During Exercise. *J Sports Sci* 22(1):39–55.

Coyle, E.F., A.R. Coggan, M.K. Hemmert, and J.L. Ivy. 1986. Muscle Glycogen Utilization during Prolonged Strenuous Exercise When Fed Carbohydrate. *J Appl Physiol* 61(1):165–72.

Coyle, E.F., A.R. Coggan, M.K. Hemmert, R.C. Lowe, and T.J. Walters. 1985. Substrate Usage During Prolonged Exercise Following a Preexercise Meal. *J Appl Physiol* 59(2):429–33.

Coyle, E.F., D.L. Costill, W.J. Fink, and D.G. Hoopes. 1978. Gastric Emptying Rates for Selected Athletic Drinks. *Res Q* 49(2):119–24.

Coyle, E.F., J.M. Hagberg, B.F. Hurley, W.H. Martin, A.A. Ehsani, and J.O. Holloszy. 1983. Carbohydrate Feeding during Prolonged Strenuous Exercise Can Delay Fatigue. *J Appl Physiol* 55(1 Pt 1):230–5.

Coyle, E.F., M.T. Hamilton, J.G. Alonso, S.J. Montain, and J.L. Ivy. 1991. Carbohydrate Metabolism during Intense Exercise When Hyperglycemic. *J Appl Physiol* 70(2):834–40.

Craig, B.W., R. Brown, and J. Everhart. 1989. Effects of Progressive Resistance Training on Growth Hormone and Testosterone Levels in Young and Elderly Subjects. *Mech Ageing Dev* 49(2):159–69.

Cramp, T., E. Broad, D. Martin, and B.J. Meyer. 2004. Effects of Preexercise Carbohydrate Ingestion on Mountain Bike Performance. *Med Sci Sports Exerc* 36(9):1602–9.

Creer, A., P. Gallagher, D. Slivka, B. Jemiolo, W. Fink, and S. Trappe. 2005. Influence of Muscle Glycogen Availability on ERK1/2 and Akt Signaling after Resistance Exercise in Human Skeletal Muscle. *J Appl Physiol* 99(3):950–56.

Cribb, P.J., and A. Hayes. 2006. Effects of Supplement Timing and Resistance Exercise on Skeletal Muscle Hypertrophy. *Med Sci Sports Exerc.* 38(11):1918–1925.

Cribb, P.J., A.D. Williams, M.F. Carey, and A. Hayes. 2006. The Effect of Whey Isolate and Resistance Training on Strength, Body Composition, and Plasma Glutamine. *Int J Sport Nutr Exerc Metab* 16(5):494–509.

Cribb, P.J., A.D. Williams, and A. Hayes. 2007. A Creatine-Protein-Carbohydrate Supplement Enhances Responses to Resistance Training. *Med Sci Sports Exerc* 39(11):1960–8.

Cribb, P.J., A.D. Williams, C.G. Stathis, M.F. Carey, and A. Hayes. 2007. Effects of Whey Isolate, Creatine, and Resistance Training on Muscle Hypertrophy. *Med Sci Sports Exerc* 39(2):298–307.

Crozier, S.J., S.R. Kimball, S.W. Emmert, J.C. Anthony, and L.S. Jefferson. 2005. Oral Leucine Administration Stimulates Protein Synthesis in Rat Skeletal Muscle. *J Nutr* 135(3):376–82.

Cummings, N., F. Pelly, V. Dang, R. Crawford, and M. Cort, Eds. 2010. Providing Meals for Athletic Groups. In *Clinical Sports Nutrition*, edited by L. Burke and V. Deakin. Sydney: McGraw-Hill, pp. 727–43.

Currell, K., S. Conway, and A.E. Jeukendrup. 2009. Carbohydrate Ingestion Improves Performance of a New Reliable Test of Soccer Performance. *Int J Sport Nutr Exerc Metab* 19(1):34–46.

Currell, K., and A.E. Jeukendrup. 2008. Superior Endurance Performance with Ingestion of Multiple Transportable Carbohydrates. *Med Sci Sports Exerc* 40(2):275–81.

Cuthbertson, D., K. Smith, J. Babraj, G. Leese, T. Waddell, P. Atherton, H. Wackerhage, P.M. Taylor, and M.J. Rennie. 2005. Anabolic Signaling Deficits Underlie Amino Acid Resistance of Wasting, Aging Muscle. *FASEB J* 19(3):422–24.

Dalbo, V.J., M.D. Roberts, J.R. Stout, and C.M. Kerksick. 2008. Putting to Rest the Myth of Creatine Supplementation Leading to Muscle Cramps and Dehydration. *Br J Sports Med* 42(7):567–73.

Dallosso, H.M., P.R. Murgatroyd, and W.P. James. 1982. Feeding Frequency and Energy Balance in Adult Males. *Hum Nutr Clin Nutr* 36C(1):25–39.

Daneman, D. 2006. Type 1 Diabetes. *Lancet* 367(9513):847–58.

Dangin, M., Y. Boirie, C. Garcia-Rodenas, P. Gachon, J. Fauquant, P. Callier, O. Ballevre, and B. Beaufrere. 2001. The Digestion Rate of Protein Is an Independent Regulating Factor of Postprandial Protein Retention. *Am J Physiol Endocrinol Metab* 280(2):E340–48.

Dangin, M., C. Guillet, C. Garcia-Rodenas, P. Gachon, C. Bouteloup-Demange, K. Reiffers-Magnani, J. Fauquant, O. Ballevre, and B. Beaufrere. 2003. The Rate of Protein Digestion Affects Protein Gain Differently during Aging in Humans. *J Physiol* 549(Pt 2):635–44.

Dangott, B., E. Schultz, and P.E. Mozdziak. 2000. Dietary Creatine Monohydrate Supplementation Increases Satellite Cell Mitotic Activity during Compensatory Hypertrophy. *Int J Sports Med* 21(1):13–16.

Dardevet, D., C. Sornet, M. Balage, and J. Grizard. 2000. Stimulation of In Vitro Rat Muscle Protein Synthesis by Leucine Decreases with Age. *J Nutr* 130(11):2630–35.

Davis, J.M. 2000. Nutrition, Neurotransmitters and Central Nervous System Fatigue. In *Nutrition in Sport*, edited by R.J. Maughan Oxford, UK: Blackwell Science, 171–183.

Davis, J.M., W.A. Burgess, C.A. Slentz, W.P. Bartoli, and R.R. Pate. 1988. Effects of Ingesting 6% and 12% Glucose/Electrolyte Beverages during Prolonged Intermittent Cycling in the Heat. *Eur J Appl Physiol Occup Physiol* 57(5):563–69.

Davis, J.M., E.A. Murphy, M.D. Carmichael, and B. Davis. 2009. Quercetin Increases Brain and Muscle Mitochondrial Biogenesis and Exercise Tolerance. *Am J Physiol Regul Integ Compar Phys* 296(4):R1071.

Davis, J.M., E.A. Murphy, M.D. Carmichael, M.R. Zielinski, C.M. Groschwitz, A.S. Brown, J.D. Gangemi, A. Ghaffar, and E.P. Mayer. 2007. Curcumin Effects on Inflammation and Performance Recovery Following Eccentric Exercise-Induced Muscle Damage. *Am J Physiol Regul Integr Comp Physiol* 292(6):R2168.

Davis, S.N., P. Galassetti, D.H. Wasserman, and D. Tate. 2000. Effects of Antecedent Hypoglycemia on Subsequent Counterregulatory Responses to Exercise. *Diabetes* 49(1):73–81.

Dayton, W.R., J.V. Schollmeyer, A.C. Chan, and C.E. Allen. 1979. Elevated Levels of a Calcium-Activated Muscle Protease in Rapidly Atrophying Muscles from Vitamin E-Deficient Rabbits. *Biochim Biophys Acta* 584(2):216–30.

De Bock, K., W. Derave, M. Ramaekers, E.A. Richter, and P. Hespel. 2007. Fiber Type-Specific Muscle Glycogen Sparing Due to Carbohydrate Intake before and during Exercise. *J Appl Physiol* 102(1):183–88.

De Castro, J.M. 1991. Weekly Rhythms of Spontaneous Nutrient Intake and Meal Pattern of Humans. *Physiol Behav* 50(4):729–38.

De Castro, J.M. 1998. Genes and Environment Have Gender-Independent Influences on the Eating and Drinking of Free-Living Humans. *Physiol Behav* 63(3):385–95.

De Castro, J.M. 2004. The Time of Day of Food Intake Influences Overall Intake in Humans. *J Nutr* 134(1):104–11.

Decombaz, J., M.J. Arnaud, H. Milon, H. Moesch, G. Philippossian, A.L. Thelin, and H. Howald. 1983. Energy Metabolism of Medium-Chain Triglycerides Versus Carbohydrates during Exercise. *Eur J Appl Physiol Occup Physiol* 52(1):9–14.

DeMarco, H.M., K.P. Sucher, C.J. Cisar, and G.E. Butterfield. 1999. Pre-Exercise Carbohydrate Meals: Application of Glycemic Index. *Med Sci Sports Exerc* 31(1):164–70.

Demling, R.H., and L. Desanti. 2000. Effect of a Hypocaloric Diet, Increased Protein Intake and Resistance Training on Lean Mass Gains and Fat Mass Loss in Overweight Police Officers. *Ann Nutr Metab* 44(1):21–29.

Deutz, R.C., D. Benardot, D.E. Martin, and M.M. Cody. 2000. Relationship between Energy Deficits and Body Composition in Elite Female Gymnasts and Runners. *Med Sci Sports Exerc* 32(3):659–68.

Devadoss, M., L. Kennedy, and N. Herbold. 2011. Endurance Athletes and Type 1 Diabetes. *Diabetes Educ* 37(2):193–207.

Devendra, D., E. Liu, and G.S. Eisenbarth. 2004. Type 1 Diabetes: Recent Developments. *BMJ* 328(7442):750–54.

Dietary Reference Intakes for Energy, Carbohydrate, Fiber, Fat, Fatty Acids, Cholesterol, Protein, and Amino Acids. 2005. Institute of Medicine. The National Academics Press, Washington, DC.

Dill, D.B., H.T. Edwards, and J.H. Talbott. 1932. Studies in Muscular Activity: VII. Factors Limiting the Capacity for Work. *J Physiol* 77(1):49–62.

Dillon, E.L., M. Sheffield-Moore, D. Paddon-Jones, C. Gilkison, A.P. Sanford, S.L. Casperson, J. Jiang, D.L. Chinkes, and R.J. Urban. 2009. Amino Acid Supplementation Increases Lean Body Mass, Basal Muscle Protein Synthesis, and Insulin-Like Growth Factor-I Expression in Older Women. *J Clin Endocrinol Metab* 94(5):1630–37.

DiPietro, L. 1995. Physical Activity, Body Weight, and Adiposity: An Epidemiologic Perspective. *Exerc Sport Sci Rev* 23:275–303.

Dohm, G.L. 1986. Protein as a Fuel for Endurance Exercise. *Exerc Sport Sci Rev* 14:143–73.

Donaldson, C.M., T.L. Perry, and M.C. Rose. 2010. Glycemic Index and Endurance Performance. *Int J Sport Nutr Exerc Metab* 20(2):154–65.

Dreyer, H.C., S. Fujita, J.G. Cadenas, D.L. Chinkes, E. Volpi, and B.B. Rasmussen. 2006. Resistance Exercise Increases AMPK Activity and Reduces 4E-BP1 Phosphorylation and Protein Synthesis in Human Skeletal Muscle. *J Physiol* 576(Pt 2):613–24.

Drummond, S.E., N.E. Crombie, M.C. Cursiter, and T.R. Kirk. 1998. Evidence that Eating Frequency Is Inversely Related to Body Weight Status in Male, but Not Female, Non-Obese Adults Reporting Valid Dietary Intakes. *Int J Obes Relat Metab Disord* 22(2):105–12.

Du, J., X. Wang, C. Miereles, J.L. Bailey, R. Debigare, B. Zheng, S.R. Price, and W.E. Mitch. 2004. Activation of Caspase-3 Is an Initial Step Triggering Accelerated Muscle Proteolysis in Catabolic Conditions. *J Clin Invest* 113(1):115–23.

Duthie, G.G., J.D. Robertson, R.J. Maughan, and P.C. Morrice. 1990. Blood Antioxidant Status and Erythrocyte Lipid Peroxidation Following Distance Running. *Arch Biochem Biophys* 282(1):78–83.

Easton, C., S. Turner, and Y.P. Pitsiladis. 2007. Creatine and Glycerol Hyperhydration in Trained Subjects before Exercise in the Heat. *Int J Sport Nutr Exerc Metab* 17(1):70–91.

Ebashi, S.O., and E.O. Ozawa. 1983. *Muscular Dystrophy: Biomedical Aspects.* Tokyo: Japan Scientific Societies Press.

Economos, C.D., S.S. Bortz, and M.E. Nelson. 1993. Nutritional Practices of Elite Athletes. Practical Recommendations. *Sports Med* 16(6):381–99.

Edirisinghe, I., B. Burton-Freeman, and C. Tissa Kappagoda. 2008. Mechanism of the Endothelium-Dependent Relaxation Evoked by a Grape Seed Extract. *Clin Sci (Lond)* 114(4):331–37.

Ekmekcioglu, C., and Y. Touitou. 2011. Chronobiological Aspects of Food Intake and Metabolism and Their Relevance on Energy Balance and Weight Regulation. *Obes Rev* 12(1):14–25.

Elder, J.H., M. Shankar, J. Shuster, D. Theriaque, S. Burns, and L. Sherrill. 2006. The Gluten-Free, Casein-Free Diet in Autism: Results of a Preliminary Double Blind Clinical Trial. *J Autism Dev Disord* 36(3):413–20.

Elliot, T.A., M.G. Cree, A.P. Sanford, R.R. Wolfe, and K.D. Tipton. 2006. Milk Ingestion Stimulates Net Muscle Protein Synthesis Following Resistance Exercise. *Med Sci Sports Exerc* 38(4):667–74.

Enoka, R. 1995. Central Factors and Task Dependency. *J Electromyog Kinesiol* 5:141–49.

Enwemeka, C., C. Allen, P. Avila, J. Bina, J. Konrade, and S. Munns. 2002. Soft Tissue Thermodynamics before, during and after Cold Pack Therapy. *Med Sci Sports Exerc* 34(1):45–50.

Ernst, E. 1998. Does Post-Exercise Massage Treatment Reduce Delayed Onset Muscle Soreness? A Systematic Review. *Brit J Sports Med* 32:212–14.

Esmarck, B., J.L. Andersen, S. Olsen, E.A. Richter, M. Mizuno, and M. Kjaer. 2001. Timing of Postexercise Protein Intake Is Important for Muscle Hypertrophy with Resistance Training in Elderly Humans. *J Physiol* 535(Pt 1):301–11.

Evans, W. 1997. Functional and Metabolic Consequences of Sarcopenia. *J Nutr* 127(5 Suppl):998S–1003S.

Evans, W.J. 2000. Vitamin E, Vitamin C, and Exercise. *Am J Clin Nutr* 72(2 Suppl):647S–52S.

Ewing, R. 2009. Vitamin D and Endurance Exercise. 2009. Available from http://running.competitor.com/2009/11/features/vitamin-d-and-endurance-exercise_6776.

Fabry, P., S. Hejda, K. Cerny, K. Osancova, and J. Pechar. 1966. Effect of Meal Frequency in Schoolchildren: Changes in Weight-Height Proportion and Skinfold Thickness. *Am J Clin Nutr* 18(5):358–61.

Fabry, P., Z. Hejl, J. Fodor, T. Braun, and K. Zvolankova. 1964. The Frequency of Meals: Its Relation to Overweight, Hypercholesterolaemia, and Decreased Glucose-Tolerance. *Lancet* 2(7360):614–15.

Farshchi, H.R., M.A. Taylor, and I.A. Macdonald. 2005a. Beneficial Metabolic Effects of Regular Meal Frequency on Dietary Thermogenesis, Insulin Sensitivity, and Fasting Lipid Profiles in Healthy Obese Women. *Am J Clin Nutr* 81(1):16–24.

Farshchi, H.R., M.A. Taylor, and I.A. Macdonald. 2005b. Deleterious Effects of Omitting Breakfast on Insulin Sensitivity and Fasting Lipid Profiles in Healthy Lean Women. *Am J Clin Nutr* 81(2):388–96.

Feasson, L., D. Stockholm, D. Freyssenet, I. Richard, S. Duguez, J.S. Beckmann, and C. Denis. 2002. Molecular Adaptations of Neuromuscular Disease-Associated Proteins in Response to Eccentric Exercise in Human Skeletal Muscle. *J Physiol* 543 (Pt 1):297–306.

Febbraio, M.A., J. Keenan, D.J. Angus, S.E. Campbell, and A.P. Garnham. 2000. Preexercise Carbohydrate Ingestion, Glucose Kinetics, and Muscle Glycogen Use: Effect of the Glycemic Index. *J Appl Physiol* 89(5):1845–51.

Febbraio, M.A., and C. Martin. 2010. Nutritional Issues for Special Environments: Training and Competing at Altitude and in Hot Climates. In *Clinical Sports Nutrition*, edited by L. Burke and V. Deakin. Sydney: McGraw-Hill.

Febbraio, M.A., and K.L. Stewart. 1996. CHO Feeding before Prolonged Exercise: Effect of Glycemic Index on Muscle Glycogenolysis and Exercise Performance. *J Appl Physiol* 81(3):1115–20.

Felig, P., A. Cherif, A. Minagawa, and J. Wahren. 1982. Hypoglycemia during Prolonged Exercise in Normal Men. *N Engl J Med* 306(15):895–900.

Felig, P., and J. Wahren. 1975. Fuel Homeostasis in Exercise. *N Engl J Med* 293(21):1078–84.

Fiatarone, M.A., E.C. Marks, N.D. Ryan, C.N. Meredith, L.A. Lipsitz, and W.J. Evans. 1990. High-Intensity Strength Training in Nonagenarians: Effects on Skeletal Muscle. *JAMA* 263(22):3029–34.

Fick, A., and Wislicenus, J. 1866. On the Origin of Muscular Power. *Phil Mag Lond (4th ser.)* 31:485–503.

Fielding, R.A., D.L. Costill, W.J. Fink, D.S. King, M. Hargreaves, and J.E. Kovaleski. 1985. Effect of Carbohydrate Feeding Frequencies and Dosage on Muscle Glycogen Use during Exercise. *Med Sci Sports Exerc* 17(4):472–76.

Fink, W.J., D.L. Costill, and P.J. Van Handel. 1975. Leg Muscle Metabolism during Exercise in the Heat and Cold. *Eur J Appl Physiol Occup Physiol* 34(3):183–90.

Fisher, B.M., J.G. Cleland, H.J. Dargie, and B.M. Frier. 1989. Non-Invasive Evaluation of Cardiac Function in Young Patients with Type 1 Diabetes. *Diabet Med* 6(8):677–81.

Fisher-Wellman, K., and R.J. Bloomer. 2009. Acute Exercise and Oxidative Stress: A 30 Year History. *Dyn Med* 8:1.

Flegal, K.M., M.D. Carroll, C.L. Ogden, and L.R. Curtin. 2010. Prevalence and Trends in Obesity among US Adults, 1999–2008. *JAMA* 303(3):235–41.

Fleming, K.H., and J.T. Heimbach. 1994. Consumption of Calcium in the U.S.: Food Sources and Intake Levels. *J Nutr* 124(8 Suppl):1426S–30S.

Flynn, M.G., D.L. Costill, J.A. Hawley, W.J. Fink, P.D. Neufer, R.A. Fielding, and M.D. Sleeper. 1987. Influence of Selected Carbohydrate Drinks on Cycling Performance and Glycogen Use. *Med Sci Sports Exerc* 19(1):37–40.

Flynn, M.G., T.J. Michaud, J. Rodriguez-Zayas, C.P. Lambert, J.B. Boone, and R.W. Moleski. 1989. Effects of 4- and 8-h Preexercise Feedings on Substrate Use and Performance. *J Appl Physiol* 67(5):2066–71.

Food and Drug Administration (FDA). 2008. Department of Health and Human Services (US FDA). Guidance for Industry: Substantiation for Dietary Supplement Claims Made under Section 403(R)(6) of the Federal Food, Drug, and Cosmetic Act. *Federal Register* 74(2):304–5.

Foote, J.A., A.R. Giuliano, and R.B. Harris. 2000. Older Adults Need Guidance to Meet Nutritional Recommendations. *J Am Coll Nutr* 19(5):628–40.

Forshee, R.A., M.L. Storey, D.B. Allison, W.H. Glinsmann, G.L. Hein, D.R. Lineback, S.A. Miller, T.A. Nicklas, G.A. Weaver, and J.S. White. 2007. A Critical Examination of the Evidence Relating High Fructose Corn Syrup and Weight Gain. *Crit Rev Food Sci Nutr* 47(6):561–82.

Foster, C., D.L. Costill, and W.J. Fink. 1979. Effects of Preexercise Feedings on Endurance Performance. *Med Sci Sports* 11(1):1–5.

Foster-Powell, K., S.H. Holt, and J.C. Brand-Miller. 2002. International Table of Glycemic Index and Glycemic Load Values. *Am J Clin Nutr* 76(1):5–56.

Fouillet, H., F. Mariotti, C. Gaudichon, C. Bos, and D. Tome. 2002. Peripheral and Splanchnic Metabolism of Dietary Nitrogen Are Differently Affected by the Protein Source in Humans as Assessed by Compartmental Modeling. *J Nutr* 132(1):125–33.

Frankland, E. 1866. On the Source of Muscular Power. *R Institution Proc* 4:661–85.

Frontera, W.R., C.N. Meredith, K.P. O'reilly, H.G. Knuttgen, and W.J. Evans. 1988. Strength Conditioning in Older Men: Skeletal Muscle Hypertrophy and Improved Function. *J Appl Physiol* 64(3):1038–44.

Frosig, C., M.P. Sajan, S.J. Maarbjerg, N. Brandt, C. Roepstorff, J.F. Wojtaszewski, B. Kiens, R.V. Farese, and E.A. Richter. 2007. Exercise Improves Phosphatidylinositol-3,4,5-Trisphosphate Responsiveness of Atypical Protein Kinase C and Interacts with Insulin Signalling to Peptide Elongation in Human Skeletal Muscle. *J Physiol* 582(Pt 3):1289–1301.

Fujita, S., H.C. Dreyer, M.J. Drummond, E.L. Glynn, J.G. Cadenas, F. Yoshizawa, E. Volpi, and B.B. Rasmussen. 2007. Nutrient Signalling in the Regulation of Human Muscle Protein Synthesis. *J Physiol* 582(Pt 2):813–23.

Fujita, S., H.C. Dreyer, M.J. Drummond, E.L. Glynn, E. Volpi, and B.B. Rasmussen. 2009. Essential Amino Acid and Carbohydrate Ingestion before Resistance Exercise Does Not Enhance Postexercise Muscle Protein Synthesis. *J Appl Physiol* 106(5):1730–39.

Galgani, J., C. Aguirre, and E. Diaz. 2006. Acute Effect of Meal Glycemic Index and Glycemic Load on Blood Glucose and Insulin Responses in Humans. *Nutr J* 5:22.

Gallen, I.W., C. Hume, and A. Lumb. 2011. Fuelling the Athlete with Type 1 Diabetes. *Diabetes Obes Metab* 13(2):130–36.

Galloway, S.D., S.A. Wootton, J.L. Murphy, and R.J. Maughan. 2001. Exogenous Carbohydrate Oxidation from Drinks Ingested during Prolonged Exercise in a Cold Environment in Humans. *J Appl Physiol* 91(2):654–60.

Gandevia, S. 1998. Neural Control in Human Muscle Fatigue: Changes I Muscle Afferents, Moto Neurons, and Moto Cortical Drive. *Acta Physiol Scand* 162:275–83.

Gardner, G.W., V.R. Edgerton, R.J. Barnard, and E.M. Bernauer. 1975. Cardiorespiratory, Hematological and Physical Performance Responses of Anemic Subjects to Iron Treatment. *Am J Clin Nutr* 28(9):982–88.

Garrett, A.T., N.G. Goossens, N.J. Rehrer, M.J. Patterson, and J.D. Cotter. 2004. The Role of Dehydration in Short-Term Heat Acclimation (Abstract). *Med Sci Sports Exerc* 36(5):S83.

Gerich, J.E. 2010. Role of the Kidney in Normal Glucose Homeostasis and in the Hyperglycaemia of Diabetes Mellitus: Therapeutic Implications. *Diabet Med* 27(2):136–42.

Gidding, S.S., B.A. Dennison, L.L. Birch, S.R. Daniels, M.W. Gillman, A.H. Lichtenstein, K.T. Rattay, J. Steinberger, N. Stettler, and L. Van Horn. 2005. Dietary Recommendations for Children and Adolescents: A Guide for Practitioners: Consensus Statement from the American Heart Association. *Circulation* 112(13):2061–75.

Gill, N., C. Beaven, and C. Cook. 2006. Effectiveness of Post Match Recovery Strategies in Rugby Players. *Br J Sports Med* 40:260–63.

Giovannini, M., C. Agostoni, and R. Shamir. 2010. Symposium Overview: Do We All Eat Breakfast and Is It Important? *Crit Rev Food Sci Nutr* 50(2):97–99.

Giresi, P.G., E.J. Stevenson, J. Theilhaber, A. Koncarevic, J. Parkington, R.A. Fielding, and S.C. Kandarian. 2005. Identification of a Molecular Signature of Sarcopenia. *Physiol Genomics* 21(2):253–63.

Gleeson, M. 2007. Immune Function in Sport and Exercise. *J Appl Physiol* 103(2):693–99.

Gleeson, M., and B. Nicolette. 2000. Modification of Immune Responses to Exercise by Carbohydrate, Glutamine, and Anti-Oxidant Supplements. *Immunol Cell Biol* 78:554–61.

Gluck, M.E., C.A. Venti, A.D. Salbe, and J. Krakoff. 2008. Nighttime Eating: Commonly Observed and Related to Weight Gain in an Inpatient Food Intake Study. *Am J Clin Nutr* 88(4):900–905.

Goedecke, J.H., V.R. Clark, T.D. Noakes, and E.V. Lambert. 2005. The Effects of Medium-Chain Triacylglycerol and Carbohydrate Ingestion on Ultra-Endurance Exercise Performance. *Int J Sport Nutr Exerc Metab* 15(1):15–27.

Goldberg, A.L. 1969. Protein Turnover in Skeletal Muscle. II. Effects of Denervation and Cortisone on Protein Catabolism in Skeletal Muscle. *J Biol Chem* 244(12):3223–29.

Goldfarb, A.H., R.J. Bloomer, and M.J. Mckenzie. 2005. Combined Antioxidant Treatment Effects on Blood Oxidative Stress after Eccentric Exercise. *Med Sci Sports Exerc* 37(2):234–39.

Gollnick, P.D., K. Piehl, and B. Saltin. 1974. Selective Glycogen Depletion Pattern in Human Muscle Fibres after Exercise of Varying Intensity and at Varying Pedalling Rates. *J Physiol* 241(1):45–57.

Gomez-Cabrera, M.C., E. Domenech, M. Romagnoli, A. Arduini, C. Borras, F.V. Pallardo, J. Sastre, and J. Vina. 2008. Oral Administration of Vitamin C Decreases Muscle Mitochondrial Biogenesis and Hampers Training-Induced Adaptations in Endurance Performance. *Am J Clin Nutr* 87(1):142–49.

Goodpaster, B.H., D.L. Costill, W.J. Fink, T.A. Trappe, A.C. Jozsi, R.D. Starling, and S.W. Trappe. 1996. The Effects of Pre-Exercise Starch Ingestion on Endurance Performance. *Int J Sports Med* 17(5):366–72.

Gotshalk, L.A., W.J. Kraemer, M.A. Mendonca, J.L. Vingren, A.M. Kenny, B.A. Spiering, D.L. Hatfield, M.S. Fragala, and J.S. Volek. 2008. Creatine Supplementation Improves Muscular Performance in Older Women. *Eur J Appl Physiol* 102(2):223–31.

Gotshalk, L.A., J.S. Volek, R.S. Staron, C.R. Denegar, F.C. Hagerman, and W.J. Kraemer. 2002. Creatine Supplementation Improves Muscular Performance in Older Men. *Med Sci Sports Exerc* 34(3):537–43.

Gray, A., H.A. Feldman, J.B. McKinlay, and C. Longcope. 1991. Age, Disease, and Changing Sex Hormone Levels in Middle-Aged Men: Results of the Massachusetts Male Aging Study. *J Clin Endocrinol Metab* 73(5):1016–25.

Greenwood, J.D., G.E. Moses, F.M. Bernardino, G.A. Gaesser, and A. Weltman. 2008. Intensity of Exercise Recovery, Blood Lactate Disappearance, and Subsequent Swimming Performance. *J Sports Sci* 26(1):29–34.

Grivetti, L.E., and E.A. Applegate. 1997. From Olympia to Atlanta: A Cultural-Historical Perspective on Diet and Athletic Training. *J Nutr* 127(5 Suppl):860S–68S.

Guelfi, K.J., T.W. Jones, and P.A. Fournier. 2007. New Insights into Managing the Risk of Hypoglycaemia Associated with Intermittent High-Intensity Exercise in Individuals with Type 1 Diabetes Mellitus: Implications for Existing Guidelines. *Sports Med* 37(11):937–46.

Guezennec, C.Y., P. Satabin, H. Legrand, and A.X. Bigard. 1994. Physical Performance and Metabolic Changes Induced by Combined Prolonged Exercise and Different Energy Intakes in Humans. *Eur J Appl Physiol Occup Physiol* 68(6):525–30.

Gupta, S., A. Goswami, A. Sadhukkan, and D. Mathur. 1996. Comparative Study of Lactate Removal in Short Term Massage of Extremities, Active Recovery, and Apassive Recovery Period after Supramaximal Exercise Sessions. *Int J Sports Med* 17:106–10.

Haase, L., B. Cerf-Ducastel, and C. Murphy. 2009. Cortical Activation in Response to Pure Taste Stimuli during the Physiological States of Hunger and Satiety. *Neuroimage* 44(3):1008–21.

Hackney, K.J., A.J. Bruenger, and J.T. Lemmer. 2010. Timing Protein Intake Increases Energy Expenditure 24 h after Resistance Training. *Med Sci Sports Exerc* 42(5):998–1003.

Haff, G. 2004. Roundtable Discussion: Periodization of Training—Part 1. *Strength Cond J* 26(1):50–69.

Haff, G.G., M.J. Lehmkuhl, L.B. McCoy, and M.H. Stone. 2003. Carbohydrate Supplementation and Resistance Training. *J Strength Cond Res* 17(1):187–96.

Haff, G.G., and A. Whitley. 2002. Low-Carbohydrate Diets and High-Intensity Anaerobic Exercise. *Strength Cond J* 24(4):42–53.

Hakkinen, K., and A. Pakarinen. 1995. Acute Hormonal Responses to Heavy Resistance Exercise in Men and Women at Different Ages. *Int J Sports Med* 16(8):507–13.

Halson, S., and A. Jeukendrup. 2004. Does Overtraining Exist? An Analysis of Overreaching and Overtraining Research. *Sports Med* 34(14):967–81.

Halton, T.L., and F.B. Hu. 2004. The Effects of High Protein Diets on Thermogenesis, Satiety and Weight Loss: A Critical Review. *J Am Coll Nutr* 23(5):373–85.

Harber, M.P., J.D. Crane, J.M. Dickinson, B. Jemiolo, U. Raue, T.A. Trappe, and S.W. Trappe. 2009. Protein Synthesis and the Expression of Growth-Related Genes Are Altered by Running in Human Vastus Lateralis and Soleus Muscles. *Am J Physiol Regul Integr Comp Physiol* 296(3):R708–14.

Hargreaves, M., and C.A. Briggs. 1988. Effect of Carbohydrate Ingestion on Exercise Metabolism. *J Appl Physiol* 65(4):1553–55.

Hargreaves, M., D.L. Costill, A. Coggan, W.J. Fink, and I. Nishibata. 1984. Effect of Carbohydrate Feedings on Muscle Glycogen Utilization and Exercise Performance. *Med Sci Sports Exerc* 16(3):219–22.

Harmon, J.H., J.R. Burckhard, and J.G. Seifert. 2007. Ingestion of a Carbohydrate-Protein Supplement Improves Performance during Repeated Bouts of High Intensity Cycling (Abstract). *Med Sci Sports Exerc* 39(5):S363.

Harper, A.E. 2003. Contributions of women scientists in the U.S. to the development of Recommended Daily Allowances. *J Nutr* 133(11):3698–702.

Harris, R.C., M.J. Tallon, M. Dunnett, L. Boobis, J. Coakley, H.J. Kim, J.L. Fallowfield, C.A. Hill, C. Sale, and J.A. Wise. 2006. The Absorption of Orally Supplied Beta-Alanine and Its Effect on Muscle Carnosine Synthesis in Human Vastus Lateralis. *Amino Acids* 30(3):279–89.

Hartman, J.W., J.E. Tang, S.B. Wilkinson, M.A. Tarnopolsky, R.L. Lawrence, A.V. Fullerton, and S.M. Phillips. 2007. Consumption of Fat-Free Fluid Milk after Resistance Exercise Promotes Greater Lean Mass Accretion than Does Consumption of Soy or Carbohydrate in Young, Novice, Male Weightlifters. *Am J Clin Nutr* 86(2):373–81.

Harvey, K.A., T. Arnold, T. Rasool, C. Antalis, S.J. Miller, and R.A. Siddiqui. 2008. Trans-Fatty Acids Induce Pro-Inflammatory Responses and Endothelial Cell Dysfunction. *Br J Nutr* 99(4):723–31.

Havemann, L., S.J. West, J.H. Goedecke, I.A. Macdonald, A. St. Clair Gibson, T.D. Noakes, and E.V. Lambert. 2006. Fat Adaptation Followed by Carbohydrate Loading Compromises High-Intensity Sprint Performance. *J Appl Physiol* 100(1):194–202.

Hawley, J.A., and L.M. Burke. 1997. Effect of Meal Frequency and Timing on Physical Performance. *Br J Nutr* 77(Suppl 1):S91–S103.

Hawley, J.A., G.S. Palmer, and T.D. Noakes. 1997. Effects of 3 Days of Carbohydrate Supplementation on Muscle Glycogen Content and Utilisation during a 1-h Cycling Performance. *Eur J Appl Physiol Occup Physiol* 75(5):407–12.

Hawley, J.A., E.J. Schabort, T.D. Noakes, and S.C. Dennis. 1997. Carbohydrate-Loading and Exercise Performance: An Update. *Sports Med* 24(2):73–81.

Hawley, J.A., K.D. Tipton, and M.L. Millard-Stafford. 2006. Promoting Training Adaptations through Nutritional Interventions. *J Sports Sci* 24(7):709–21.

Hayes, A., and P.J. Cribb. 2008. Effect of Whey Protein Isolate on Strength, Body Composition and Muscle Hypertrophy during Resistance Training. *Curr Opin Clin Nutr Metab Care* 11(1):40–44.

Heath, E.M., A.R. Wilcox, and C.M. Quinn. 1993. Effects of Nicotinic Acid on Respiratory Exchange Ratio and Substrate Levels during Exercise. *Med Sci Sports Exerc* 25(9):1018–23.

Heinemeyer, W., M. Fischer, T. Krimmer, U. Stachon, and D.H. Wolf. 1997. The Active Sites of the Eukaryotic 20 S Proteasome and Their Involvement in Subunit Precursor Processing. *J Biol Chem* 272(40):25200–209.

Heitmann, B.L., and L. Lissner. 1995. Dietary Underreporting by Obese Individuals—Is It Specific or Non-Specific? *BMJ* 311(7011):986–89.

Hejda, S., and P. Fabry. 1964. Frequency of Food Intake in Relation to Some Parameters of the Nutritional Status. *Nutr Dieta Eur Rev Nutr Diet* 64:216–28.

Hemmings, B., M. Smith, J. Graydon, and R. Dyson. 2000. Effects of Massage on Physiological Restoration, Perceived Recovery, and Repeated Sports Performance. *Br J Sports Med* 34:109–15.

Hermansen, L., E. Hultman, and B. Saltin. 1967. Muscle Glycogen during Prolonged Severe Exercise. *Acta Physiol Scand* 71(2):129–39.

Hermsdorff, H.H., A.C. Volp, and J. Bressan. 2007. Macronutrient Profile Affects Diet-Induced Thermogenesis and Energy Intake. *Arch Latinoam Nutr* 57(1):33–42.

Hespel, P., B. Op't Eijnde, M. Van Leemputte, B. Urso, P.L. Greenhaff, V. Labarque, S. Dymarkowski, P. Van Hecke, and E.A. Richter. 2001. Oral Creatine Supplementation Facilitates the Rehabilitation of Disuse Atrophy and Alters the Expression of Muscle Myogenic Factors in Humans. *J Physiol* 536(Pt 2):625–33.

Hickner, R.C., J.S. Fisher, P.A. Hansen, S.B. Racette, C.M. Mier, M.J. Turner, and J.O. Holloszy. 1997. Muscle Glycogen Accumulation after Endurance Exercise in Trained and Untrained Individuals. *J Appl Physiol* 83(3):897.

Hickson, R.C., M.J. Rennie, R.K. Conlee, W.W. Winder, and J.O. Holloszy. 1977. Effects of Increased Plasma Fatty Acids on Glycogen Utilization and Endurance. *J Appl Physiol* 43(5):829–33.

Hightower, L. 2000. Osteoporosis: Pediatric Disease with Geriatric Consequences. *Orthop Nurs* 19(5):59–62.

Hill, C.A., R.C. Harris, H.J. Kim, B.D. Harris, C. Sale, L.H. Boobis, C.K. Kim, and J.A. Wise. 2007. Influence of Beta-Alanine Supplementation on Skeletal Muscle Carnosine Concentrations and High Intensity Cycling Capacity. *Amino Acids* 32(2):225–33.

Hinton, P.S., C. Giordano, T. Brownlie, and J.D. Haas. 2000. Iron Supplementation Improves Endurance after Training in Iron-Depleted, Nonanemic Women. *J Appl Physiol* 88(3):1103–11.

Ho, J.Y., W.J. Kraemer, J.S. Volek, M.S. Fragala, G.A. Thomas, C. Dunn-Lewis, M. Coday, K. Hakkinen, and C.M. Maresh. 2010. L-Carnitine L-Tartrate Supplementation Favorably Affects Biochemical Markers of Recovery from Physical Exertion in Middle-Aged Men and Women. *Metabolism* 59(8):1190–99.

Hoffman, J.R., N.A. Ratamess, C.P. Tranchina, S.L. Rashti, J. Kang, and A.D. Faigenbaum. 2009. Effect of Protein-Supplement Timing on Strength, Power, and Body-Composition Changes in Resistance-Trained Men. *Int J Sport Nutr Exerc Metab* 19(2):172–85.

Hoffman, J.R., N.A. Ratamess, C.P. Tranchina, S.L. Rashti, J. Kang, and A.D. Faigenbaum. 2010. Effect of a Proprietary Protein Supplement on Recovery Indices Following Resistance Exercise in Strength/Power Athletes. *Amino Acids* 38(3):771–78.

Holloszy, J.O. 1973. Biochemical Adaptations to Exercise: Aerobic Metabolism. *Exerc Sport Sci Rev* 1:45–71.

Holmback, U., A. Lowden, T. Akerfeldt, M. Lennernas, L. Hambraeus, J. Forslund, T. Akerstedt, M. Stridsberg, and A. Forslund. 2003. The Human Body May Buffer Small Differences in Meal Size and Timing during a 24-h Wake Period Provided Energy Balance Is Maintained. *J Nutr* 133(9):2748–55.

Honein, M.A., L.J. Paulozzi, T.J. Mathews, J.D. Erickson, and L.Y. Wong. 2001. Impact of Folic Acid Fortification of the U.S. Food Supply on the Occurrence of Neural Tube Defects. *JAMA* 285(23):2981–86.

Horowitz, J.F., and S. Klein. 2000. Lipid Metabolism during Endurance Exercise. *Am J Clin Nutr* 72(2 Suppl):558S–63S.

Houston, D.K., B.J. Nicklas, J. Ding, T.B. Harris, F.A. Tylavsky, A.B. Newman, J.S. Lee, N.R. Sahyoun, M. Visser, and S.B. Kritchevsky. 2008. Dietary Protein Intake Is Associated with Lean Mass Change in Older, Community-Dwelling Adults: The Health, Aging, and Body Composition (Health ABC) Study. *Am J Clin Nutr* 87(1):150–55.

Houston, M. 2006. *Biochemistry Primer for Exercise Science*. 3rd Ed. Champaign, IL: Human Kinetics.

Hu, F.B., M.J. Stampfer, J.E. Manson, E. Rimm, G.A. Colditz, B.A. Rosner, C.H. Hennekens, and W.C. Willett. 1997. Dietary Fat Intake and the Risk of Coronary Heart Disease in Women. *N Engl J Med* 337(21):1491–99.

Hulmi, J.J., V. Kovanen, H. Selanne, W.J. Kraemer, K. Hakkinen, and A.A. Mero. 2009. Acute and Long-Term Effects of Resistance Exercise with or without Protein Ingestion on Muscle Hypertrophy and Gene Expression. *Amino Acids* 37(2):297–308.

Hulmi, J.J., J.S. Volek, H. Selanne, and A.A. Mero. 2005. Protein Ingestion Prior to Strength Exercise Affects Blood Hormones and Metabolism. *Med Sci Sports Exerc* 37(11):1990–97.

Hulston, C.J., M.C. Venables, C.H. Mann, C. Martin, A. Philp, K. Baar, and A.E. Jeukendrup. 2010. Training with Low Muscle Glycogen Enhances Fat Metabolism in Well-Trained Cyclists. *Med Sci Sports Exerc* 42(11):2046–55.

Hultman, E. 1995. Fuel Selection, Muscle Fibre. *Proc Nutr Soc* 54(1):107–21.

Hunding, A., R. Jordal, and P.E. Paulev. 1981. Runner's Anemia and Iron Deficiency. *Acta Med Scand* 209(4):315–18.

Imoberdorf, R., P.J. Garlick, M.A. Mcnurlan, G.A. Casella, J.C. Marini, M. Turgay, P. Bartsch, and P.E. Ballmer. 2006. Skeletal Muscle Protein Synthesis after Active or Passive Ascent to High Altitude. *Med Sci Sports Exerc* 38(6):1082–87.

Ingram, J., B. Dawson, C. Goodman, K. Wallman, and J. Beibly. 2009. Effect of Water Immersion Methods on Post-Exercise Recovery from Simulated Team Sport Exercise. *J Sci Med Sport* 12:417–21.

Ingwall, J.S. 1976. Creatine and the Control of Muscle-Specific Protein Synthesis in Cardiac and Skeletal Muscle. *Circ Res* 38(5 Suppl 1):I115–23.

Institute of Medicine. 2005. Dietary Reference Intakes for Energy, Carbohydrate, Fiber, Fat, Fatty Acids, Cholesterol, Protein, and Amino Acids. Washington, DC: National Academies Press.

IOC Consensus Statement on Sports Nutrition. 2010. www.olympic.org/Document/Reports/EN/CONSENSUS-Final-V8-en.pdf.

Ivy, J., and R. Portman. 2007. *The Future of Sports Nutrition: Nutrient Timing*. Basic Health Publications: Laguna Beach, CA.

Ivy, J.L. 1998. Glycogen Resynthesis after Exercise: Effect of Carbohydrate Intake. *Int J Sports Med* 19(Suppl 2):S142–45.

Ivy, J.L., H.W. Goforth, Jr., B.M. Damon, T.R. McCauley, E.C. Parsons, and T.B. Price. 2002. Early Postexercise Muscle Glycogen Recovery Is Enhanced with a Carbohydrate-Protein Supplement. *J Appl Physiol* 93(4):1337–44.

Ivy, J.L., A.L. Katz, C.L. Cutler, W.M. Sherman, and E.F. Coyle. 1988. Muscle Glycogen Synthesis after Exercise: Effect of Time of Carbohydrate Ingestion. *J Appl Physiol* 64(4):1480–85.

Ivy, J.L., M.C. Lee, J.T. Brozinick, Jr., and M.J. Reed. 1988. Muscle Glycogen Storage after Different Amounts of Carbohydrate Ingestion. *J Appl Physiol* 65(5):2018–23.

Ivy, J.L., P.T. Res, R.C. Sprague, and M.O. Widzer. 2003. Effect of a Carbohydrate-Protein Supplement on Endurance Performance during Exercise of Varying Intensity. *Int J Sport Nutr Exerc Metab* 13(3):382–95.

Jackman, R.W., and S.C. Kandarian. 2004. The Molecular Basis of Skeletal Muscle Atrophy. *Am J Physiol* 287(4):C834–43.

Jagoe, R.T., and A.L. Goldberg. 2001. What Do We Really Know About the Ubiquitin-Proteasome Pathway in Muscle Atrophy? *Curr Opin Clin Nutr Metab Care* 4(3):183–90.

Janssen, I., D.S. Shepard, P.T. Katzmarzyk, and R. Roubenoff. 2004. The Healthcare Costs of Sarcopenia in the United States. *J Am Geriatr Soc* 52(1):80–85.

Jay Cutler (American Football). 2010. http://en.wikipedia.org/wiki/Jay_Cutler_(American _football).

Jenkins, D.J., T.M. Wolever, A.L. Jenkins, R.G. Josse, and G.S. Wong. 1984. The Glycaemic Response to Carbohydrate Foods. *Lancet* 2(8399):388–91.

Jenkins, D.J., T.M. Wolever, R.H. Taylor, H. Barker, H. Fielden, J.M. Baldwin, A.C. Bowling, H.C. Newman, A.L. Jenkins, and D.V. Goff. 1981. Glycemic Index of Foods: A Physiological Basis for Carbohydrate Exchange. *Am J Clin Nutr* 34(3):362–66.

Jentjens, R., and A. Jeukendrup. 2003. Determinants of Post-Exercise Glycogen Synthesis during Short-Term Recovery. *Sports Med* 33(2):117–44.

Jentjens, R.L., and A.E. Jeukendrup. 2005. High Rates of Exogenous Carbohydrate Oxidation from a Mixture of Glucose and Fructose Ingested during Prolonged Cycling Exercise. *Br J Nutr* 93(4):485–92.

Jentjens, R.L., L. Moseley, R.H. Waring, L.K. Harding, and A.E. Jeukendrup. 2004. Oxidation of Combined Ingestion of Glucose and Fructose during Exercise. *J Appl Physiol* 96(4):1277–84.

Jentjens, R.L., M.C. Venables, and A.E. Jeukendrup. 2004. Oxidation of Exogenous Glucose, Sucrose, and Maltose during Prolonged Cycling Exercise. *J Appl Physiol* 96(4):1285–91.

Jeukendrup, A., F. Brouns, A.J. Wagenmakers, and W.H. Saris. 1997. Carbohydrate-Electrolyte Feedings Improve 1 h Time Trial Cycling Performance. *Int J Sports Med* 18(2):125–29.

Jeukendrup, A.E. 2004. Carbohydrate Intake during Exercise and Performance. *Nutrition* 20(7–8):669–77.

Jeukendrup, A.E. 2008. Carbohydrate Feeding during Exercise. *Eur J Sport Sci* 8(2):77–86.

Jeukendrup, A.E., and R. Jentjens. 2000. Oxidation of Carbohydrate Feedings during Prolonged Exercise: Current Thoughts, Guidelines and Directions for Future Research. *Sports Med* 29(6):407–24.

Jeukendrup, A.E., and L. Moseley. 2008. Multiple Transportable Carbohydrates Enhance Gastric Emptying and Fluid Delivery. *Scand J Med Sci Sports* 20(1):112–21.

Jeukendrup, A.E., L. Moseley, G.I. Mainwaring, S. Samuels, S. Perry, and C.H. Mann. 2006. Exogenous Carbohydrate Oxidation during Ultraendurance Exercise. *J Appl Physiol* 100(4):1134–41.

Jeukendrup, A.E., W.H. Saris, F. Brouns, D. Halliday, and J.M. Wagenmakers. 1996. Effects of Carbohydrate (CHO) and Fat Supplementation on CHO Metabolism during Prolonged Exercise. *Metabolism* 45(7):915–21.

Jeukendrup, A.E., W.H. Saris, P. Schrauwen, F. Brouns, and A.J. Wagenmakers. 1995. Metabolic Availability of Medium-Chain Triglycerides Coingested with Carbohydrates during Prolonged Exercise. *J Appl Physiol* 79(3):756–62.

Jeukendrup, A.E., J.J. Thielen, A.J. Wagenmakers, F. Brouns, and W.H. Saris. 1998. Effect of Medium-Chain Triacylglycerol and Carbohydrate Ingestion during Exercise on Substrate Utilization and Subsequent Cycling Performance. *Am J Clin Nutr* 67(3):397–404.

Jeukendrup, A.E., K. Vet-Joop, A. Sturk, J.H. Stegen, J. Senden, W.H. Saris, and A.J. Wagenmakers. 2000. Relationship between Gastro-Intestinal Complaints and Endotoxaemia, Cytokine Release and the Acute-Phase Reaction during and after a Long-Distance Triathlon in Highly Trained Men. *Clin Sci (Lond)* 98(1):47–55.

Jeukendrup, A.E., A.J. Wagenmakers, J.H. Stegen, A.P. Gijsen, F. Brouns, and W.H. Saris. 1999. Carbohydrate Ingestion Can Completely Suppress Endogenous Glucose Production during Exercise. *Am J Physiol* 276(4 Pt 1):E672–83.

Johnson, H.L., C.F. Consolazio, H.J. Krzywicki, G.J. Isaac, and N.F. Witt. 1971. Metabolic Aspects of Caloric Restriction: Nutrient Balances with 500-Kilocalorie Intakes. *Am J Clin Nutr* 24(8):913–23.

Johnson, J.J., and H. Mukhtar. 2007. Curcumin for Chemoprevention of Colon Cancer. *Cancer Lett* 255(2):170–81.

Johnston, C.S., C.S. Day, and P.D. Swan. 2002. Postprandial Thermogenesis Is Increased 100% on a High-Protein, Low-Fat Diet Versus a High-Carbohydrate, Low-Fat Diet in Healthy, Young Women. *J Am Coll Nutr* 21(1):55–61.

Josse, A.R., J.E. Tang, M.A. Tarnopolsky, and S.M. Phillips. 2010. Body Composition and Strength Changes in Women with Milk and Resistance Exercise. *Med Sci Sports Exerc* 42(6):1122–30.

Judelson, D.A., C.M. Maresh, J.M. Anderson, L.E. Armstrong, D.J. Casa, W.J. Kraemer, and J.S. Volek. 2007. Hydration and Muscular Performance: Does Fluid Balance Affect Strength, Power and High-Intensity Endurance? *Sports Med* 37(10):907–21.

Kaastra, B., R.J. Manders, E. Van Breda, A. Kies, A.E. Jeukendrup, H.A. Keizer, H. Kuipers, and L.J. Van Loon. 2006. Effects of Increasing Insulin Secretion on Acute Postexercise Blood Glucose Disposal. *Med Sci Sports Exerc* 38(2):268–75.

Kandarian, S.C., and R.W. Jackman. 2006. Intracellular Signaling during Skeletal Muscle Atrophy. *Muscle Nerve* 33(2):155–65.

Kant, A.K., A. Schatzkin, B.I. Graubard, and R. Ballard-Barbash. 1995. Frequency of Eating Occasions and Weight Change in the NHANES I Epidemiologic Follow-up Study. *Int J Obes Relat Metab Disord* 19(7):468–74.

Karlsson, J., and B. Saltin. 1971. Diet, Muscle Glycogen, and Endurance Performance. *J Appl Physiol* 31(2):203–6.

Karp, J.R., J.D. Johnston, S. Tecklenburg, T.D. Mickleborough, A.D. Fly, and J.M. Stager. 2006. Chocolate Milk as a Post-Exercise Recovery Aid. *Int J Sport Nutr Exerc Metab* 16(1):78–91.

Kato, H., J. Tillotson, M.Z. Nichaman, G.G. Rhoads, and H.B. Hamilton. 1973. Epidemiologic Studies of Coronary Heart Disease and Stroke in Japanese Men Living in Japan, Hawaii and California. *Am J Epidemiol* 97(6):372–85.

Katsanos, C.S., D.L. Chinkes, D. Paddon-Jones, X.J. Zhang, A. Aarsland, and R.R. Wolfe. 2008. Whey Protein Ingestion in Elderly Persons Results in Greater Muscle Protein Accrual than Ingestion of Its Constituent Essential Amino Acid Content. *Nutr Res* 28(10):651–58.

Katsanos, C.S., H. Kobayashi, M. Sheffield-Moore, A. Aarsland, and R.R. Wolfe. 2005. Aging Is Associated with Diminished Accretion of Muscle Proteins after the Ingestion of a Small Bolus of Essential Amino Acids. *Am J Clin Nutr* 82(5):1065–73.

Katsanos, C.S., H. Kobayashi, M. Sheffield-Moore, A. Aarsland, and R.R. Wolfe. 2006. A High Proportion of Leucine Is Required for Optimal Stimulation of the Rate of Muscle Protein Synthesis by Essential Amino Acids in the Elderly. *Am J Physiol Endocrinol Metab* 291(2):E381–87.

Kay, D., F. Marino, J. Cannon, A. St. Clair Gibson, M. Lambert, and T. Noakes. 2001. Evidence for Neuromuscular Fatigue during High-Intensity Cycling in Warm, Humid Conditions. *Eur J Appl Physiol* 84:115–21.

Keizer, H.A., H. Kuipers, K.G. Van, and P. Geurten. 1987. Influence of Liquid and Solid Meals on Muscle Glycogen Resynthesis, Plasma Fuel Hormone Response, and Maximal Physical Working Capacity. *Int J Sports Med* 8(2):99–104.

Kerksick, C., T. Harvey, J. Stout, B. Campbell, C. Wilborn, R. Kreider, D. Kalman, T. Ziegenfuss, H. Lopez, J. Landis, J.L. Ivy, and J. Antonio. 2008. International Society of Sports Nutrition Position Stand: Nutrient Timing. *J Int Soc Sports Nutr* 5:17.

Kerksick, C., A. Thomas, B. Campbell, L. Taylor, C. Wilborn, B. Marcello, M. Roberts, E. Pfau, M. Grimstvedt, J. Opusunju, T. Magrans-Courtney, C. Rasmussen, R. Wilson, and R.B. Kreider. 2009. Effects of a Popular Exercise and Weight Loss Program on Weight Loss, Body Composition, Energy Expenditure and Health in Obese Women. *Nutr Metab (Lond)* 6:23.

Kerksick, C.M., C. Rasmussen, S. Lancaster, M. Starks, P. Smith, C. Melton, M. Greenwood, A. Almada, and R. Kreider. 2007. Impact of Differing Protein Sources and a Creatine Containing Nutritional Formula after 12 Weeks of Resistance Training. *Nutrition* 23(9):647–56.

Kerksick, C.M., C.J. Rasmussen, S.L. Lancaster, B. Magu, P. Smith, C. Melton, M. Greenwood, A.L. Almada, C.P. Earnest, and R.B. Kreider. 2006. The Effects of Protein and Amino Acid Supplementation on Performance and Training Adaptations during Ten Weeks of Resistance Training. *J Strength Cond Res* 20(3):643–53.

Kerksick, C.M., J. Wismann-Bunn, D. Fogt, A.R. Thomas, L. Taylor, B.I. Campbell, C.D. Wilborn, T. Harvey, M.D. Roberts, P. La Bounty, M. Galbreath, B. Marcello, C.J. Rasmussen, and R.B. Kreider. 2010. Changes in Weight Loss, Body Composition and Cardiovascular Disease Risk after Altering Macronutrient Distributions during a Regular Exercise Program in Obese Women. *Nutr J* 9:59.

Kern, W., C. Dodt, J. Born, and H.L. Fehm. 1996. Changes in Cortisol and Growth Hormone Secretion during Nocturnal Sleep in the Course of Aging. *J Gerontol* 51(1):M3–M9.

Keys, A., C. Aravanis, H.W. Blackburn, F.S. Van Buchem, R. Buzina, B.D. Djordjevic, A.S. Dontas, F. Fidanza, M.J. Karvonen, N. Kimura, D. Lekos, M. Monti, V. Puddu, and H.L. Taylor. 1966. Epidemiological Studies Related to Coronary Heart Disease: Characteristics of Men Aged 40–59 in Seven Countries. *Acta Med Scand Suppl* 460:1–392.

Kiens, B., and J.A. Hawley. 2011. Fat Metabolism. In *Nutrition Society Textbook on Sport and Exercise Nutrition*, edited by S. Stear and S. Shirreffs. New York: Wiley-Blackwell.

Kimball, S.R., L.M. Shantz, R.L. Horetsky, and L.S. Jefferson. 1999. Leucine Regulates Translation of Specific mRNAs in L6 Myoblasts through Motor-Mediated Changes in Availability of EIF4e and Phosphorylation of Ribosomal Protein S6. *J Biol Chem* 274(17):11647–52.

Kinabo, J.L., and J.V. Durnin. 1990. Effect of Meal Frequency on the Thermic Effect of Food in Women. *Eur J Clin Nutr* 44(5):389–95.

Kipps, C., S. Sharma, and D. Tunstall Pedoe. 2009. The Incidence of Exercise-Associated Hyponatraemia in the London Marathon. *Br J Sports Med* 45(1):14–19.

Kirby, C.R., and V.A. Convertino. 1986. Plasma Aldosterone and Sweat Sodium Concentrations after Exercise and Heat Acclimation. *J Appl Physiol* 61(3):967.

Kirwan, J.P., D.L. Costill, J.B. Mitchell, J.A. Houmard, M.G. Flynn, W.J. Fink, and J.D. Beltz. 1988. Carbohydrate Balance in Competitive Runners during Successive Days of Intense Training. *J Appl Physiol* 65(6):2601–6.

Kirwan, J.P., D.J. O'Gorman, D. Cyr-Campbell, W.W. Campbell, K.E. Yarasheski, and W.J. Evans. 2001. Effects of a Moderate Glycemic Meal on Exercise Duration and Substrate Utilization. *Med Sci Sports Exerc* 33(9):1517–23.

Klein, J., W.L. Nyhan, and M. Kern. 2009. The Effects of Alanine Ingestion on Metabolic Responses to Exercise in Cyclists. *Amino Acids* 37(4):673–80.

Klein, S., E.F. Coyle, and R.R. Wolfe. 1994. Fat Metabolism during Low-Intensity Exercise in Endurance-Trained and Untrained Men. *Am J Physiol* 267(6 Pt 1):E934–40.

Koopman, R., M. Beelen, T. Stellingwerff, B. Pennings, W.H. Saris, A.K. Kies, H. Kuipers, and L.J. Van Loon. 2007. Coingestion of Carbohydrate with Protein Does Not Further Augment Postexercise Muscle Protein Synthesis. *Am J Physiol Endocrinol Metab* 293(3):E833–42.

Koopman, R., N. Crombach, A.P. Gijsen, S. Walrand, J. Fauquant, A.K. Kies, S. Lemosquet, W.H. Saris, Y. Boirie, and L.J. Van Loon. 2009. Ingestion of a Protein Hydrolysate Is Accompanied by an Accelerated in Vivo Digestion and Absorption Rate When Compared with Its Intact Protein. *Am J Clin Nutr* 90(1):106–15.

Koopman, R., R.J. Manders, R.A. Jonkers, G.B. Hul, H. Kuipers, and L.J. Van Loon. 2006. Intramyocellular Lipid and Glycogen Content Are Reduced Following Resistance Exercise in Untrained Healthy Males. *Eur J Appl Physiol* 96(5):525–34.

Koopman, R., D.L. Pannemans, A.E. Jeukendrup, A.P. Gijsen, J.M. Senden, D. Halliday, W.H. Saris, L.J. Van Loon, and A.J. Wagenmakers. 2004. Combined Ingestion of Protein and Carbohydrate Improves Protein Balance during Ultra-Endurance Exercise. *Am J Physiol Endocrinol Metab* 287(4):E712–20.

Koopman, R., A.J. Wagenmakers, R.J. Manders, A.H. Zorenc, J.M. Senden, M. Gorselink, H.A. Keizer, and L.J. Van Loon. 2005. Combined Ingestion of Protein and Free Leucine with Carbohydrate Increases Postexercise Muscle Protein Synthesis In Vivo in Male Subjects. *Am J Physiol Endocrinol Metab* 288(4):E645–53.

Kopelman, P.G. 2000. Obesity as a Medical Problem. *Nature* 404(6778):635–43.

Korach-Andre, M., Y. Burelle, F. Peronnet, D. Massicotte, C. Lavoie, and C. Hillaire-Marcel. 2002. Differential Metabolic Fate of the Carbon Skeleton and Amino-N of [13C]Alanine and [15N]Alanine Ingested during Prolonged Exercise. *J Appl Physiol* 93(2):499–504.

Koro, C.E., S.J. Bowlin, N. Bourgeois, and D.O. Fedder. 2004. Glycemic Control from 1988 to 2000 among U.S. Adults Diagnosed with Type 2 Diabetes: A Preliminary Report. *Diabetes Care* 27(1):17–20.

Kovacs, E.M., R.M. Schmahl, J.M. Senden, and F. Brouns. 2002. Effect of High and Low Rates of Fluid Intake on Post-Exercise Rehydration. *Int J Sport Nutr Exerc Metab* 12(1):14–23.

Kraemer, W.J., K. Hakkinen, R.U. Newton, B.C. Nindl, J.S. Volek, M. Mccormick, L.A. Gotshalk, S.E. Gordon, S.J. Fleck, W.W. Campbell, M. Putukian, and W.J. Evans. 1999. Effects of Heavy-Resistance Training on Hormonal Response Patterns in Younger vs. Older Men. *J Appl Physiol* 87(3):982–92.

Kraemer, W.J., D.L. Hatfield, B.A. Spiering, J.L. Vingren, M.S. Fragala, J.Y. Ho, J.S. Volek, J.M. Anderson, and C.M. Maresh. 2007. Effects of a Multi-Nutrient Supplement on Exercise Performance and Hormonal Responses to Resistance Exercise. *Eur J Appl Physiol* 101(5):637–46.

Kraemer, W.J., and N.A. Ratamess. 2005. Hormonal Responses and Adaptations to Resistance Exercise and Training. *Sports Med* 35(4):339–61.

Kreider, R.B. 2003. Effects of Creatine Supplementation on Performance and Training Adaptations. *Mol Cell Biochem* 244(1–2):89–94.

Kreider, R.B., C.D. Wilborn, L. Taylor, B. Campbell, A.L. Almada, R. Collins, M. Cooke, C.P. Earnest, M. Greenwood, D.S. Kalman, C.M. Kerksick, S.M. Kleiner, B. Leutholtz, H. Lopez, L.M. Lowery, R. Mendel, A. Smith, M. Spano, R. Wildman, D.S. Willoughby, T.N. Ziegenfuss, and J. Antonio. 2010. ISSN Exercise and Sport Nutrition Review: Research and Recommendations. *J Int Soc Sports Nutr* 7:7.

Krogh, A., and J. Lindhard. 1920. The Relative Value of Fat and Carbohydrate as Sources of Muscular Energy: With Appendices on the Correlation between Standard Metabolism and the Respiratory Quotient during Rest and Work. *Biochem J* 14(3–4):290–363.

Kuipers, H., D.L. Costill, D.A. Porter, W.J. Fink, and W.M. Morse. 1986. Glucose Feeding and Exercise in Trained Rats: Mechanisms for Glycogen Sparing. *J Appl Physiol* 61(3):859–63.

Kuipers, H., E.J. Fransen, and H.A. Keizer. 1999. Pre-Exercise Ingestion of Carbohydrate and Transient Hypoglycemia during Exercise. *Int J Sports Med* 20(4):227–31.

Kuipers, H., and H. Keizer. 1988. Overtraining in Elite Athletes: Review and Directions for the Future. *Sports Medicine* 6:79–92.

Kuipers, H., H.A. Keizer, F. Brouns, and W.H. Saris. 1987. Carbohydrate Feeding and Glycogen Synthesis during Exercise in Man. *Pflugers Arch* 410(6):652–56.

Kvorning, T., M. Bagger, P. Caserotti, and K. Madsen. 2006. Effects of Vibration and Resistance Training on Neuromuscular and Hormonal Measures. *Eur J Appl Physiol* 96:615–25.

La Bounty, P.M., B.I. Campbell, J. Wilson, E. Galvan, J. Berardi, S.M. Kleiner, R.B. Kreider, J.R. Stout, T. Ziegenfuss, M. Spano, A. Smith, and J. Antonio. 2011. International Society of Sports Nutrition Position Stand: Meal Frequency. *J Int Soc Sports Nutr* 8(1):4.

Laidlaw, S.A., and J.D. Kopple. 1987. Newer Concepts of the Indispensable Amino Acids. *Am J Clin Nutr* 46(4):593–605.

Lainer, A. 2003. Use of Nonsterodial Anti-Inflammatory Drugs Following Exercise Induced Muscle Injury. *Sports Med* 33:177–186.

Lambert, G.P., J. Lang, A. Bull, J. Eckerson, S. Lanspa, and J. O'Brien. 2008. Fluid Tolerance While Running: Effect of Repeated Trials. *Int J Sports Med* 29(11):878–82.

Lamberts, S.W., A.W. Van Den Beld, and A.J. Van Der Lely. 1997. The Endocrinology of Aging. *Science* 278(5337):419–24.

Lancaster, G.I., R.L. Jentjens, L. Moseley, A.E. Jeukendrup, and M. Gleeson. 2003. Effect of Pre-Exercise Carbohydrate Ingestion on Plasma Cytokine, Stress Hormone, and Neutrophil Degranulation Responses to Continuous, High-Intensity Exercise. *Int J Sport Nutr Exerc Metab* 13(4):436–53.

Layman, D.K. 2002. Role of Leucine in Protein Metabolism during Exercise and Recovery. *Can J Appl Physiol* 27(6):646–63.

Layman, D.K., R.A. Boileau, D.J. Erickson, J.E. Painter, H. Shiue, C. Sather, and D.D. Christou. 2003. A Reduced Ratio of Dietary Carbohydrate to Protein Improves Body Composition and Blood Lipid Profiles during Weight Loss in Adult Women. *J Nutr* 133(2):411–17.

Layman, D.K., E. Evans, J.I. Baum, J. Seyler, D.J. Erickson, and R.A. Boileau. 2005. Dietary Protein and Exercise Have Additive Effects on Body Composition during Weight Loss in Adult Women. *J Nutr* 135(8):1903–10.

Lee, W.T., S.S. Leung, S.H. Wang, Y.C. Xu, W.P. Zeng, J. Lau, S.J. Oppenheimer, and J.C. Cheng. 1994. Double-Blind, Controlled Calcium Supplementation and Bone Mineral Accretion in Children Accustomed to a Low-Calcium Diet. *Am J Clin Nutr* 60(5):744–50.

Lehman, M., C. Foster, and H. Dickhuth. 1998. Autonomic Imbalance Hypothesis and Overtraining Syndrome. *Med Sci Sports Exerc* 30(7):1140–45.

Lehmann, M., C. Foster, U. Gastmann, H. Keizer, and J. Steinacker. 1999. Definition, Types, Symptoms, Findings, Underlying Mechanisms, and Frequency of Overtraining and Overtraining Syndrome. In *Overload, Fatigue, Performance Incompetence, and Regeneration in Sport*, edited by M. Lehmann, C. Foster, U. Gastmann, H. Keizer, and J. Steinacker. New York: Plenum.

Leidy, H.J., C.L. Armstrong, M. Tang, R.D. Mattes, and W.W. Campbell. 2010. The Influence of Higher Protein Intake and Greater Eating Frequency on Appetite Control in Overweight and Obese Men. *Obesity (Silver Spring)* 18(9):1725–32.

Leidy, H.J., and W.W. Campbell. 2011. The Effect of Eating Frequency on Appetite Control and Food Intake: Brief Synopsis of Controlled Feeding Studies. *J Nutr* 141(1):154–57.

Leiper, J.B. 2001. Gastric Emptying and Intestinal Absorption of Fluids, Carbohydrates, and Electrolytes. In *Sports Drinks: Basic Science and Practical Aspects*, edited by R. J. Maughan and R. Murray. Boca Raton, FL: CRC Press, 89–128.

Leiper, J.B., K.P. Aulin, and K. Soderlund. 2000. Improved Gastric Emptying Rate in Humans of a Unique Glucose Polymer with Gel-Forming Properties. *Scand J Gastroenterol* 35(11):1143–49.

Lemaitre, R.N., I.B. King, D. Mozaffarian, N. Sotoodehnia, T.D. Rea, L.H. Kuller, R.P. Tracy, and D.S. Siscovick. 2006. Plasma Phospholipid Trans Fatty Acids, Fatal Ischemic Heart Disease, and Sudden Cardiac Death in Older Adults: The Cardiovascular Health Study. *Circulation* 114(3):209–15.

Lemon, P.W., J.M. Berardi, and E.E. Noreen. 2002. The Role of Protein and Amino Acid Supplements in the Athlete's Diet: Does Type or Timing of Ingestion Matter? *Curr Sports Med Rep* 1(4):214–21.

Lemon, P.W., and J.P. Mullin. 1980. Effect of Initial Muscle Glycogen Levels on Protein Catabolism during Exercise. *J Appl Physiol* 48(4):624–29.

Levenhagen, D.K., J.D. Gresham, M.G. Carlson, D.J. Maron, M.J. Borel, and P.J. Flakoll. 2001. Postexercise Nutrient Intake Timing in Humans Is Critical to Recovery of Leg Glucose and Protein Homeostasis. *Am J Physiol Endocrinol Metab* 280(6):E982–93.

Levine, S.A., B. Gordon, and C.L. Derick. 1924. Some Changes in the Chemical Constituents of the Blood Following a Marathon Race. *JAMA* 82(22):1778–79.

Lewis, J.S., and F.M. Sandford. 2009. Rotator Cuff Tendinopathy: Is There a Role for Polyunsaturated Fatty Acids and Antioxidants? *J Hand Ther*:49–55.

Lexell, J., and D.Y. Downham. 1991. The Occurrence of Fibre-Type Grouping in Healthy Human Muscle: A Quantitative Study of Cross-Sections of Whole Vastus Lateralis from Men between 15 and 83 Years. *Acta Neuropathol* 81(4):377–81.

Li, Y., S. Gazdoiu, Z.Q. Pan, and S.Y. Fuchs. 2004. Stability of Homologue of Slimb F-Box Protein Is Regulated by Availability of Its Substrate. *J Biol Chem* 279(12):11074–80.

Lichtman, S.W., K. Pisarska, E.R. Berman, M. Pestone, H. Dowling, E. Offenbacher, H. Weisel, S. Heshka, D.E. Matthews, and S.B. Heymsfield. 1992. Discrepancy between Self-Reported and Actual Caloric Intake and Exercise in Obese Subjects. *N Engl J Med* 327(27):1893–98.

Lieberman, H.R., W.J. Tharion, B. Shukitt-Hale, K.L. Speckman, and R. Tulley. 2002. Effects of Caffeine, Sleep Loss, and Stress on Cognitive Performance and Mood during U.S. Navy Seal Training. Sea-Air-Land. *Psychopharmacology (Berl)* 164(3):250–61.

Little, J.P., and S.M. Phillips. 2009. Resistance Exercise and Nutrition to Counteract Muscle Wasting. *Appl Physiol Nutr Metab* 34(5):817–28.

Liu, K. 1997. *Soybeans: Chemistry, Technology, and Utilization.* New York: Chapman & Hall.

Livingstone, M.B., A.M. Prentice, J.J. Strain, W.A. Coward, A.E. Black, M.E. Barker, P.G. Mckenna, and R.G. Whitehead. 1990. Accuracy of Weighed Dietary Records in Studies of Diet and Health. *BMJ* 300(6726):708–12.

Lockwood, C.M., J.R. Moon, A.E. Smith, S.E. Tobkin, K.L. Kendall, J.L. Graef, J.T. Cramer, and J.R. Stout. 2010. Low-Calorie Energy Drink Improves Physiological Response to Exercise in Previously Sedentary Men: A Placebo-Controlled Efficacy and Safety Study. *J Strength Cond Res* 24(8):2227–38.

Loucks, A.B. 2004. Energy Balance and Body Composition in Sports and Exercise. *J Sports Sci* 22(1):1–14.

Louis, E., U. Raue, Y. Yang, B. Jemiolo, and S. Trappe. 2007. Time Course of Proteolytic, Cytokine, and Myostatin Gene Expression after Acute Exercise in Human Skeletal Muscle. *J Appl Physiol* 103(5):1744–51.

Low, S.Y., M.J. Rennie, and P.M. Taylor. 1996. Modulation of Glycogen Synthesis in Rat Skeletal Muscle by Changes in Cell Volume. *J Physiol* 495(Pt 2):299–303.

Lowe, J., D. Stock, B. Jap, P. Zwickl, W. Baumeister, and R. Huber. 1995. Crystal Structure of the 20s Proteasome from the Archaeon T. Acidophilum at 3.4 205 Resolution. *Science* 268(5210):533–39.

Lowery, L., and C. Forsythe. 2006. Protein and Overtraining: Potential Applications for Free Living Athletes. *J Int Soc Sports Nutr* 3(1):42–50.

Ludwig, D.S., J.A. Majzoub, A. Al-Zahrani, G.E. Dallal, I. Blanco, and S.B. Roberts. 1999. High Glycemic Index Foods, Overeating, and Obesity. *Pediatrics* 103(3):E26.

Lugo, M., W.M. Sherman, G.S. Wimer, and K. Garleb. 1993. Metabolic Responses When Different Forms of Carbohydrate Energy Are Consumed during Cycling. *Int J Sport Nutr* 3(4):398–407.

Luiking, Y.C., M.P. Engelen, and N.E. Deutz. 2010. Regulation of Nitric Oxide Production in Health and Disease. *Curr Opin Clin Nutr Metab Care* 13(1):97–104.

Lukaski, H.C. 2004. Vitamin and Mineral Status: Effects on Physical Performance. *Nutrition* 20(7–8):632–44.

Lukaski, H.C., and F.H. Nielsen. 2002. Dietary Magnesium Depletion Affects Metabolic Responses during Submaximal Exercise in Postmenopausal Women. *J Nutr* 132(5):930–35.

Ma, Y., E.R. Bertone, E.J. Stanek, 3rd, G.W. Reed, J.R. Hebert, N.L. Cohen, P.A. Merriam, and I.S. Ockene. 2003. Association between Eating Patterns and Obesity in a Free-Living U.S. Adult Population. *Am J Epidemiol* 158(1):85–92.

MacArthur, D.G., and K.N. North. 2005. Genes and Human Elite Athletic Performance. *Human Genetics* 116(5):331–39.

Machefer, G., C. Groussard, F. Rannou-Bekono, H. Zouhal, H. Faure, S. Vincent, J. Cillard, and A. Gratas-Delamarche. 2004. Extreme Running Competition Decreases Blood Antioxidant Defense Capacity. *J Am Coll Nutr* 23(4):358–64.

Machefer, G., C. Groussard, S. Vincent, H. Zouhal, H. Faure, J. Cillard, Z. Radak, and A. Gratas-Delamarche. 2007. Multivitamin-Mineral Supplementation Prevents Lipid Peroxidation during "the Marathon Des Sables." *J Am Coll Nutr* 26(2):111–20.

MacLean, D.A., and T.E. Graham. 1993. Branched-Chain Amino Acid Supplementation Augments Plasma Ammonia Responses during Exercise in Humans. *J Appl Physiol* 74(6):2711–17.

MacLean, D.A., T.E. Graham, and B. Saltin. 1994. Branched-Chain Amino Acids Augment Ammonia Metabolism While Attenuating Protein Breakdown during Exercise. *Am J Physiol* 267(6 Pt 1):E1010–22.

MacRae, H.S., and K.M. Mefferd. 2006. Dietary Antioxidant Supplementation Combined with Quercetin Improves Cycling Time Trial Performance. *Int J Sport Nutr Exerc Metab* 16(4):405.

Madsen, K., D.A. Maclean, B. Kiens, and D. Christensen. 1996. Effects of Glucose, Glucose Plus Branched-Chain Amino Acids, or Placebo on Bike Performance over 100 km. *J Appl Physiol* 81(6):2644–50.

Maesta, N., E.A. Nahas, J. Nahas-Neto, F.L. Orsatti, C.E. Fernandes, P. Traiman, and R.C. Burini. 2007. Effects of Soy Protein and Resistance Exercise on Body Composition and Blood Lipids in Postmenopausal Women. *Maturitas* 56(4):350–58.

Maffucci, D.M., and R.G. McMurray. 2000. Towards Optimizing the Timing of the Pre-Exercise Meal. *Int J Sport Nutr Exerc Metab* 10(2):103–13.

Mahoney, D.J., G. Parise, S. Melov, A. Safdar, and M.A. Tarnopolsky. 2005. Analysis of Global mRNA Expression in Human Skeletal Muscle during Recovery from Endurance Exercise. *FASEB J* 19(11):1498–500.

Maier, S., and L. Watkins. 1998. Cytokines for Psychologists: Implications for Bidirectional Immune to Brain Communication for Understanding Behavior, Mood, Cognition. *Clin Psychol Rev* 105:83–107.

Major, G.C., J.P. Chaput, M. Ledoux, S. St-Pierre, G.H. Anderson, M.B. Zemel, and A. Tremblay. 2008. Recent Developments in Calcium-Related Obesity Research. *Obes Rev* 9(5):428–45.

Manore, M., S. Bar, and G. Butterfield. 2000. Position of the American Dietetic Association, Dietitians of Canada, and the American College of Sports Medicine: Nutrition and Physical Performance. *Med Sci Sports Exerc* 32(12):2130–45.

Manore, M.M. 2000. Effect of Physical Activity on Thiamine, Riboflavin, and Vitamin B-6 Requirements. *Am J Clin Nutr* 72(2 Suppl):598S–606S.

Marin, P.J., and M.R. Rhea. 2010a. Effects of Vibration Training on Muscle Power: A Meta-Analysis. *J Strength Cond Res* 24(3):871–78.

Marin, P., and M. Rhea. 2010b. Effects of Vibration Training on Muscle Strength: A Meta Analysis. *J Strength Cond Res* 24(2):548–56.

Marlett, J.A., M.I. Mcburney, and J.L. Slavin. 2002. Position of the American Dietetic Association: Health Implications of Dietary Fiber. *J Am Diet Assoc* 102(7):993–1000.

Marriott, B.M. 1995. *Not Eating Enough: Overcoming Underconsumption of Military Operational Rations*. Washington, DC: National Academy Press.

Martin, B.J. 1981. Effect of Sleep Deprivation on Tolerance of Prolonged Exercise. *Eur J Appl Physiol Occup Physiol* 47(4):345–54.

Martin, N.A., R.F. Zoeller, R.J. Robertson, and S.M. Lephart. 1998. The Comparative Effects of Sports Massage, Active Recovery, and Rest in Promoting Blood Lactate Clearance after Supramaximal Leg Exercise. *J Athl Train* 33(1):30–35.

Martinez-Lagunas, V., Z. Ding, J.R. Bernard, B. Wang, and J.L. Ivy. 2010. Added Protein Maintains Efficacy of a Low-Carbohydrate Sports Drink. *J Strength Cond Res* 24(1):48–59.

Mascher, H., H. Andersson, P.A. Nilsson, B. Ekblom, and E. Blomstrand. 2007. Changes in Signalling Pathways Regulating Protein Synthesis in Human Muscle in the Recovery Period after Endurance Exercise. *Acta Physiol* 191(1):67–75.

Mascher, H., J. Tannerstedt, T. Brink-Elfegoun, B. Ekblom, T. Gustafsson, and E. Blomstrand. 2008. Repeated Resistance Exercise Training Induces Different Changes in mRNA Expression of MAFbx and MuRF-1 in Human Skeletal Muscle. *Am J Physiol Endocrinol Metab* 294(1):E43–E51.

Mashima, T., M. Naito, K. Noguchi, D.K. Miller, D.W. Nicholson, and T. Tsuruo. 1997. Actin Cleavage by Cpp-32/Apopain during the Development of Apoptosis. *Oncogene* 14(9):1007–12.

Massicotte, D., F. Peronnet, G.R. Brisson, and C. Hillaire-Marcel. 1992. Oxidation of Exogenous Medium-Chain Free Fatty Acids during Prolonged Exercise: Comparison with Glucose. *J Appl Physiol* 73(4):1334–39.

Matsukura, U., A. Okitani, T. Nishimuro, and H. Kato. 1981. Mode of Degradation of Myofibrillar Proteins by an Endogenous Protease, Cathepsin L. *Biochim Biophys Acta* 662(1):41–47.

Maughan, R.J. 1991. Fluid and Electrolyte Loss and Replacement in Exercise. *J Sports Sci* 9:117–42.

Maughan, R.J., L.R. Bethell, and J.B. Leiper. 1996. Effects of Ingested Fluids on Exercise Capacity and on Cardiovascular and Metabolic Responses to Prolonged Exercise in Man. *Exp Physiol* 81(5):847–59.

Maughan, R.J., J. Fallah, and E.F. Coyle. 2010. The Effects of Fasting on Metabolism and Performance. *Br J Sports Med* 44(7):490–94.

Maughan, R.J., C.E. Fenn, and J.B. Leiper. 1989. Effects of Fluid, Electrolyte and Substrate Ingestion on Endurance Capacity. *Eur J Appl Physiol Occup Physiol* 58(5):481–86.

Mauvais-Jarvis, F., E. Sobngwi, R. Porcher, J.P. Garnier, P. Vexiau, A. Duvallet, and J.F. Gautier. 2003. Glucose Response to Intense Aerobic Exercise in Type 1 Diabetes: Maintenance of Near Euglycemia Despite a Drastic Decrease in Insulin Dose. *Diabetes Care* 26(4):1316–17.

Mavrogenis, S., E. Johannessen, P. Jansen, and C. Sindberg. 2004. The Effect of Essential Fatty Acids and Antioxidants Compined with Physiotherapy Treatment in Recreational Athletes with Chronic Tendon Disorders: A Randomised, Double-Blind, Placebo-Controlled Study. *Physical Ther Sport* 5:194–99.

Mayhew, D.L., J.S. Kim, J.M. Cross, A.A. Ferrando, and M.M. Bamman. 2009. Translational Signaling Responses Preceding Resistance Training-Mediated Myofiber Hypertrophy in Young and Old Humans. *J Appl Physiol* 107(5):1655–62.

McAnulty, S.R., D.C. Nieman, M.F. Rabnovick, V. Duran, L.S. McAnulty, D.A. Henson, F. Jin, and M. Landram. 2010. Effect of N-3 Fatty Acids and Antioxidants on Oxidative Stress after Exercise. *Med Sci Sports Exerc* 42(9):1704–11.

McArdle, W., F. Katch, and V. Katch. 2001. *Energy, Nutrition and Human Performance*. 5th ed. Philadelphia: Lippincott Williams and Wilkins.

McArdle, W.D., F.I. Katch, and V.L. Katch. 2007. *Exercise Physiology: Energy, Nutrition, and Human Performance*. 6th ed. Baltimore: Lippincott Williams & Wilkins.

McConell, G., K. Kloot, and M. Hargreaves. 1996. Effect of Timing of Carbohydrate Ingestion on Endurance Exercise Performance. *Med Sci Sports Exerc* 28(10):1300–4.

McConell, G.K., B.J. Canny, M.C. Daddo, M.J. Nance, and R.J. Snow. 2000. Effect of Carbohydrate Ingestion on Glucose Kinetics and Muscle Metabolism during Intense Endurance Exercise. *J Appl Physiol* 89(5):1690–98.

McKewen, M.W., N.J. Rehrer, C. Cox, and J. Mann. 1999. Glycaemic Control, Muscle Glycogen and Exercise Performance in IDDM Athletes on Diets of Varying Carbohydrate Content. *Int J Sports Med* 20(6):349–53.

McLellan, T.M., G.H. Kamimori, D.G. Bell, I.F. Smith, D. Johnson, and G. Belenky. 2005. Caffeine Maintains Vigilance and Marksmanship in Simulated Urban Operations with Sleep Deprivation. *Aviat Space Environ Med* 76(1):39–45.

McLellan, T.M., G.H. Kamimori, D.M. Voss, D.G. Bell, K.G. Cole, and D. Johnson. 2005. Caffeine Maintains Vigilance and Improves Run Times during Night Operations for Special Forces. *Aviat Space Environ Med* 76(7):647–54.

McMorris, T., R.C. Harris, A.N. Howard, G. Langridge, B. Hall, J. Corbett, M. Dicks, and C. Hodgson. 2007. Creatine Supplementation, Sleep Deprivation, Cortisol, Melatonin and Behavior. *Physiol Behav* 90(1):21–28.

McMorris, T., R.C. Harris, J. Swain, J. Corbett, K. Collard, R.J. Dyson, L. Dye, C. Hodgson, and N. Draper. 2006. Effect of Creatine Supplementation and Sleep Deprivation, with Mild Exercise, on Cognitive and Psychomotor Performance, Mood State, and Plasma Concentrations of Catecholamines and Cortisol. *Psychopharmacology (Berl)* 185(1):93–103.

Meeusen, R., and P. Lievens. 1986. The Use of Cryotherapy in Sports Injuries. *Sports Med* 3(6):398–414.

Menzies, P., C. Menzies, L. Mcintyre, P. Paterson, J. Wilson, and O.J. Kemi. 2010. Blood Lactate Clearance during Active Recovery after an Intense Running Bout Depends on the Intensity of the Active Recovery. *J Sports Sci* 28(9):975–82.

Metzner, H.L., D.E. Lamphiear, N.C. Wheeler, and F.A. Larkin. 1977. The Relationship between Frequency of Eating and Adiposity in Adult Men and Women in the Tecumseh Community Health Study. *Am J Clin Nutr* 30(5):712–15.

Millard-Stafford, M., W.L. Childers, S.A. Conger, A.J. Kampfer, and J.A. Rahnert. 2008. Recovery Nutrition: Timing and Composition after Endurance Exercise. *Curr Sports Med Rep* 7(4):193–201.

Millard-Stafford, M., P.B. Sparling, L.B. Rosskopf, B.T. Hinson, and L.J. Dicarlo. 1990. Carbohydrate-Electrolyte Replacement during a Simulated Triathlon in the Heat. *Med Sci Sports Exerc* 22(5):621–28.

Millard-Stafford, M., G.L. Warren, L.M. Thomas, J.A. Doyle, T. Snow, and K. Hitchcock. 2005. Recovery from Run Training: Efficacy of a Carbohydrate-Protein Beverage? *Int J Sport Nutr Exerc Metab* 15(6):610–24.

Millard-Stafford, M.L., P.B. Sparling, L.B. Rosskopf, and L.J. Dicarlo. 1992. Carbohydrate-Electrolyte Replacement Improves Distance Running Performance in the Heat. *Med Sci Sports Exerc* 24(8):934–40.

Miller, G.D., Jarvis, J.K., and McBean, L.D. 2006. *Handbook of Dairy Foods and Nutrition*. CRC Press: Boca Raton, FL.

Miller, S.L., K.D. Tipton, D.L. Chinkes, S.E. Wolf, and R.R. Wolfe. 2003. Independent and Combined Effects of Amino Acids and Glucose after Resistance Exercise. *Med Sci Sports Exerc* 35(3):449–55.

Millward, D.J. 1999. Optimal Intakes of Protein in the Human Diet. *Proc Nutr Soc* 58(2):403–13.

Millward, D.J., A. Fereday, N. Gibson, and P.J. Pacy. 1997. Aging, Protein Requirements, and Protein Turnover. *Am J Clin Nutr* 66(4):774–86.

Mitchell, J.B., D.L. Costill, J.A. Houmard, W.J. Fink, D.D. Pascoe, and D.R. Pearson. 1989. Influence of Carbohydrate Dosage on Exercise Performance and Glycogen Metabolism. *J Appl Physiol* 67(5):1843–49.

Mitchell, J.B., D.L. Costill, J.A. Houmard, M.G. Flynn, W.J. Fink, and J.D. Beltz. 1988. Effects of Carbohydrate Ingestion on Gastric Emptying and Exercise Performance. *Med Sci Sports Exerc* 20(2):110–15.

Mitchell, J.B., M.D. Phillips, S.P. Mercer, H.L. Baylies, and F.X. Pizza. 2000. Postexercise Rehydration: Effect of Na(+) and Volume on Restoration of Fluid Spaces and Cardiovascular Function. *J Appl Physiol* 89(4):1302–9.

Moore, D.R., M.J. Robinson, J.L. Fry, J.E. Tang, E.I. Glover, S.B. Wilkinson, T. Prior, M.A. Tarnopolsky, and S.M. Phillips. 2009. Ingested Protein Dose Response of Muscle and Albumin Protein Synthesis after Resistance Exercise in Young Men. *Am J Clin Nutr* 89(1):161–68.

Moore, D.R., J.E. Tang, N.A. Burd, T. Rerecich, M.A. Tarnopolsky, and S.M. Phillips. 2009. Differential Stimulation of Myofibrillar and Sarcoplasmic Protein Synthesis with Protein Ingestion at Rest and after Resistance Exercise. *J Physiol* 587(Pt 4):897–904.

Moore, L.J., A.W. Midgley, S. Thurlow, G. Thomas, and L.R. McNaughton. 2010. Effect of the Glycaemic Index of a Pre-Exercise Meal on Metabolism and Cycling Time Trial Performance. *J Sci Med Sport* 13(1):182–88.

Morais, J.A., S. Chevalier, and R. Gougeon. 2006. Protein Turnover and Requirements in the Healthy and Frail Elderly. *J Nutr Health Aging* 10(4):272–83.

Morens, C., C. Bos, M.E. Pueyo, R. Benamouzig, N. Gausseres, C. Luengo, D. Tome, and C. Gaudichon. 2003. Increasing Habitual Protein Intake Accentuates Differences in Postprandial Dietary Nitrogen Utilization between Protein Sources in Humans. *J Nutr* 133(9):2733–40.

Morgan, K.J., M.E. Zabik, and G.L. Stampley. 1986. The Role of Breakfast in Diet Adequacy of the U.S. Adult Population. *J Am Coll Nutr* 5(6):551–63.

Moseley, L., G.I. Lancaster, and A.E. Jeukendrup. 2003. Effects of Timing of Pre-Exercise Ingestion of Carbohydrate on Subsequent Metabolism and Cycling Performance. *Eur J Appl Physiol* 88(4–5):453–58.

Moughan, P.J. 2005. Dietary Protein Quality in Humans—An Overview. *J AOAC Int* 88(3):874–76.

Moyer, C.A., T. Dryden, and S. Shipwright. 2009. Directions and Dilemmas in Massage Therapy Research: A Workshop Report from the 2009 North Amaerican Research Conference on Complementary and Integratve Medicine. *Int J Ther Massage Bodywork* 2(2):15–27.

Mudambo, K.S., G.P. Leese, and M.J. Rennie. 1997. Dehydration in Soldiers during Walking/ Running Exercise in the Heat and the Effects of Fluid Ingestion during and after Exercise. *Eur J Appl Physiol Occup Physiol* 76(6):517–24.

Murdoch, S.D., T.L. Bazzarre, I.P. Snider, and A.H. Goldfarb. 1993. Differences in the Effects of Carbohydrate Food Form on Endurance Performance to Exhaustion. *Int J Sport Nutr* 3(1):41–54.

Murray, R., G.L. Paul, J.G. Seifert, D.E. Eddy, and G.A. Halaby. 1989. The Effects of Glucose, Fructose, and Sucrose Ingestion during Exercise. *Med Sci Sports Exerc* 21(3):275–82.

National Nutrition Conference for Defense. 1941. Proceedings of the National Nutrition Conference for Defense. Federal Security Agency, Washington, DC.

Nelson, A.G., D.A. Arnall, J. Kokkonen, R. Day, and J. Evans. 2001. Muscle Glycogen Supercompensation Is Enhanced by Prior Creatine Supplementation. *Med Sci Sports Exerc* 33(7):1096–1100.

Neufer, P.D., D.L. Costill, M.G. Flynn, J.P. Kirwan, J.B. Mitchell, and J. Houmard. 1987. Improvements in Exercise Performance: Effects of Carbohydrate Feedings and Diet. *J Appl Physiol* 62(3):983–88.

Neufer, P.D., A.J. Young, and M.N. Sawka. 1989. Gastric Emptying during Exercise: Effects of Heat Stress and Hypohydration. *Eur J Appl Physiol Occup Physiol* 58(4):433–39.

Newhouse, I.J., and E.W. Finstad. 2000. The Effects of Magnesium Supplementation on Exercise Performance. *Clin J Sport Med* 10(3):195–200.

Nicholas, C.W., K. Tsintzas, L. Boobis, and C. Williams. 1999. Carbohydrate-Electrolyte Ingestion during Intermittent High-Intensity Running. *Med Sci Sports Exerc* 31(9):1280–86.

Nicklas, B.J., A.J. Ryan, M.M. Treuth, S.M. Harman, M.R. Blackman, B.F. Hurley, and M.A. Rogers. 1995. Testosterone, Growth Hormone and IGF-1 Responses to Acute and Chronic Resistive Exercise in Men Aged 55–70 Years. *Int J Sports Med* 16(7):445–50.

Nielsen, J.N., W. Derave, S. Kristiansen, E. Ralston, T. Ploug, and E.A. Richter. 2001. Glycogen Synthase Localization and Activity in Rat Skeletal Muscle Is Strongly Dependent on Glycogen Content. *J Physiol* 531(Pt 3):757–69.

Nielsen, S.J., A.M. Siega-Riz, and B.M. Popkin. 2002. Trends in Food Locations and Sources among Adolescents and Young Adults. *Prev Med* 35(2):107–13.

Nieman, D.C. 1998. Influence of Carbohydrate on the Immune Response to Intensive, Prolonged Exercise. *Exerc Immunol Rev* 4:64–76.

Nieman, D.C. 2008. Immunonutrition Support for Athletes. *Nutr Rev* 66(6):310–20.

Nieman, D.C., C.L. Dumke, D.A. Henson, S.R. Mcanulty, S.J. Gross, and R.H. Lind. 2005. Muscle Damage Is Linked to Cytokine Changes Following a 160-km Race. *Brain, Behav Immun* 19(5):398–403.

Nieman, D.C., D.A. Henson, S.J. Gross, D.P. Jenkins, J. Davis, E.A. Murphy, M.D. Carmichael, C.L. Dumke, A.C. Utter, and S.R. McAnulty. 2007. Quercetin Reduces Illness but Not Immune Perturbations after Intensive Exercise. *Med Sci Sports Exerc* 39(9):1561.

Nieman, D.C., D.A. Henson, L.L. Smith, A.C. Utter, D.M. Vinci, J.M. Davis, D.E. Kaminsky, and M. Shute. 2001. Cytokine Changes after a Marathon Race. *J Appl Physiol* 91(1):109–14.

Nieman, D.C., L.M. Johanssen, J.W. Lee, and K. Arabatzis. 1990. Infectious Episodes in Runners before and after the Los Angeles Marathon. *J Sports Med Phys Fitness* 30(3):316.

Noakes, M., J.B. Keogh, P.R. Foster, and P.M. Clifton. 2005. Effect of an Energy-Restricted, High-Protein, Low-Fat Diet Relative to a Conventional High-Carbohydrate, Low-Fat Diet on Weight Loss, Body Composition, Nutritional Status, and Markers of Cardiovascular Health in Obese Women. *Am J Clin Nutr* 81(6):1298–1306.

Noakes, T.D. 1993. Fluid Replacement during Exercise. *Exerc Sport Sci Rev* 21:297–330.

Noda, T., K. Isogai, H. Hayashi, and N. Katunuma. 1981. Susceptibilities of Various Myofibrillar Proteins to Cathepsin B and Morphological Alteration of Isolated Myofibrils by This Enzyme. *J Biochemistry* 90(2):371–79.

Nugent, A.M., I.C. Steele, F. Al-Modaris, S. Vallely, A. Moore, N.P. Campbell, P.M. Bell, K.D. Buchanan, E.R. Trimble, and D.P. Nicholls. 1997. Exercise Responses in Patients with IDDM. *Diabetes Care* 20(12):1814–21.

Nunez, G., M.A. Benedict, Y. Hu, and N. Inohara. 1998. Caspases: The Proteases of the Apoptotic Pathway. *Oncogene* 17(25):3237–45.

Nybo, L., M.K. Dalsgaard, A. Steensberg, K. Moller, and N.H. Secher. 2005. Cerebral Ammonia Uptake and Accumulation during Prolonged Exercise in Humans. *J Physiol* 563(Pt 1):285–90.

Okano, G., Y. Sato, Y. Takumi, and M. Sugawara. 1996. Effect of 4h Preexercise High Carbohydrate and High Fat Meal Ingestion on Endurance Performance and Metabolism. *Int J Sports Med* 17(7):530–34.

Olsen, S., P. Aagaard, F. Kadi, G. Tufekovic, J. Verney, J.L. Olesen, C. Suetta, and M. Kjaer. 2006. Creatine Supplementation Augments the Increase in Satellite Cell and Myonuclei Number in Human Skeletal Muscle Induced by Strength Training. *J Physiol* 573(Pt 2):525–34.

Olsson, K.E., and B. Saltin. 1970. Variation in Total Body Water with Muscle Glycogen Changes in Man. *Acta Physiol Scand* 80(1):11–18.

Osterberg, K.L., J.J. Zachwieja, and J.W. Smith. 2008. Carbohydrate and Carbohydrate + Protein for Cycling Time-Trial Performance. *J Sports Sci* 26(3):227–33.

Ostojic, S.M., and S. Mazic. 2002. Effects of a Carbohydrate-Electrolyte Drink on Specific Soccer Tests and Performance. *J Sports Sci Med* 1:47–53.

Paddon-Jones, D. 2006. Interplay of Stress and Physical Inactivity on Muscle Loss: Nutritional Countermeasures. *J Nutr* 136(8):2123–26.

Paddon-Jones, D., and B.B. Rasmussen. 2009. Dietary Protein Recommendations and the Prevention of Sarcopenia. *Curr Opin Clin Nutr Metab Care* 12(1):86–90.

Paddon-Jones, D., M. Sheffield-Moore, X.J. Zhang, E. Volpi, S.E. Wolf, A. Aarsland, A.A. Ferrando, and R.R. Wolfe. 2004. Amino Acid Ingestion Improves Muscle Protein Synthesis in the Young and Elderly. *Am J Physiol Endocrinol Metab* 286(3):E321–28.

Paddon-Jones, D., K.R. Short, W.W. Campbell, E. Volpi, and R.R. Wolfe. 2008. Role of Dietary Protein in the Sarcopenia of Aging. *Am J Clin Nutr* 87(5):1562S–66S.

Paik, I.Y., C.H. Jin, H.E. Jin, Y.I. Kim, S.Y. Cho, H.T. Roh, A.R. Suh, and S.H. Suh. 2009. Effects of the NADPH Oxidase p22phox C242T Polymorphism on Endurance Exercise Performance and Oxidative DNA Damage in Response to Aerobic Exercise Training. *Mol Cells* 27(5):557–62.

Panel on Macronutrients et al., Food and Nutrition Board, Institute of Medicine. 2005. *Dietary Reference Intakes for Energy, Carbohydrate, Fiber, Fat, Fatty Acids, Cholesterol, Protein, and Amino Acids*. Washington, DC: National Academies Press.

Parkin, J.A., M.F. Carey, I.K. Martin, L. Stojanovska, and M.A. Febbraio. 1997. Muscle Glycogen Storage Following Prolonged Exercise: Effect of Timing of Ingestion of High Glycemic Index Food. *Med Sci Sports Exerc* 29(2):220–24.

Pascoe, D.D., D.L. Costill, W.J. Fink, R.A. Robergs, and J.J. Zachwieja. 1993. Glycogen Resynthesis in Skeletal Muscle Following Resistive Exercise. *Med Sci Sports Exerc* 25(3):349–54.

Passe, D.H. 2001. Physiological and Psychological Determinants of Fluid Intake. In *Sports Drinks: Basic Science and Practical Aspects*, edited by R.J. Maughan and R. Murray. Boca Raton, FL: CRC Press, 45–88.

Pedersen, D.J., S.J. Lessard, V.G. Coffey, E.G. Churchley, A.M. Wootton, T. Ng, M.J. Watt, and J.A. Hawley. 2008. High Rates of Muscle Glycogen Resynthesis after Exhaustive Exercise When Carbohydrate Is Coingested with Caffeine. *J Appl Physiol* 105(1):7–13.

Pereira, M.A., E. Erickson, P. McKee, K. Schrankler, S.K. Raatz, L.A. Lytle, and A.D. Pellegrini. 2011. Breakfast Frequency and Quality May Affect Glycemia and Appetite in Adults and Children. *J Nutr* 141(1):163–68.

Pereira, M.A., D.R. Jacobs, Jr., J.J. Pins, S.K. Raatz, M.D. Gross, J.L. Slavin, and E.R. Seaquist. 2002. Effect of Whole Grains on Insulin Sensitivity in Overweight Hyperinsulinemic Adults. *Am J Clin Nutr* 75(5):848–55.

Peters, E.M., J.M. Goetzsche, B. Grobbelaar, and T.D. Noakes. 1993. Vitamin C Supplementation Reduces the Incidence of Postrace Symptoms of Upper-Respiratory-Tract Infection in Ultramarathon Runners. *Am J Clin Nutr* 57(2):170.

Peters, H.P., M. Bos, L. Seebregts, L.M. Akkermans, G.P. Van Berge Henegouwen, E. Bol, W.L. Mosterd, and W.R. De Vries. 1999. Gastrointestinal Symptoms in Long-Distance Runners, Cyclists, and Triathletes: Prevalence, Medication, and Etiology. *Am J Gastroenterol* 94(6):1570–81.

Peters, H.P., F.W. Van Schelven, P.A. Verstappen, R.W. De Boer, E. Bol, W.B. Erich, C.R. Van Der Togt, and W.R. De Vries. 1993. Gastrointestinal Problems as a Function of Carbohydrate Supplements and Mode of Exercise. *Med Sci Sports Exerc* 25(11):1211–24.

Pfeiffer, B., A. Cotterill, D. Grathwohl, T. Stellingwerff, and A.E. Jeukendrup. 2009. The Effect of Carbohydrate Gels on Gastrointestinal Tolerance during a 16-km Run. *Int J Sport Nutr Exerc Metab* 19(5):485–503.

Pfeiffer, B., T. Stellingwerff, E. Zaltas, and A.E. Jeukendrup. 2010a. CHO Oxidation from a CHO Gel Compared with a Drink during Exercise. *Med Sci Sports Exerc* 42(11):2038–45.

Pfeiffer, B., T. Stellingwerff, E. Zaltas, and A.E. Jeukendrup. 2010b. Oxidation of Solid Versus Liquid CHO Sources during Exercise. *Med Sci Sports Exerc* 42(11):2030–37.

Phillips, S., 2006. Dietary Protein for Athletes. *Appl Physiol Nutr Metab* 31:647–54.

Phillips, S.M. 2004. Protein Requirements and Supplementation in Strength Sports. *Nutrition* 20(7–8):689–95.

Phillips, S.M., G. Parise, B.D. Roy, K.D. Tipton, R.R. Wolfe, and M.A. Tamopolsky. 2002. Resistance-Training-Induced Adaptations in Skeletal Muscle Protein Turnover in the Fed State. *Can J Physiol Pharmacol* 80(11):1045–53.

Phillips, S.M., J.E. Tang, and D.R. Moore. 2009. The Role of Milk- and Soy-Based Protein in Support of Muscle Protein Synthesis and Muscle Protein Accretion in Young and Elderly Persons. *J Am Coll Nutr* 28(4):343–54.

Phillips, S.M., K.D. Tipton, A. Aarsland, S.E. Wolf, and R.R. Wolfe. 1997. Mixed Muscle Protein Synthesis and Breakdown after Resistance Exercise in Humans. *Am J Physiol* 273(1 Pt 1):E99–E107.

Phillips, S.M., K.D. Tipton, A.A. Ferrando, and R.R. Wolfe. 1999. Resistance Training Reduces the Acute Exercise-Induced Increase in Muscle Protein Turnover. *Am J Physiol* 276(1 Pt 1):E118–24.

Phillips, S.M., A.P. Turner, S. Gray, M.F. Sanderson, and J. Sproule. 2010. Ingesting a 6% Carbohydrate-Electrolyte Solution Improves Endurance Capacity, but Not Sprint Performance, during Intermittent, High-Intensity Shuttle Running in Adolescent Team Games Players Aged 12–14 Years. *Eur J Appl Physiol* 109(5):811–21.

Piehl Aulin, K., K. Soderlund, and E. Hultman. 2000. Muscle Glycogen Resynthesis Rate in Humans after Supplementation of Drinks Containing Carbohydrates with Low and High Molecular Masses. *Eur J Appl Physiol* 81(4):346–51.

Pikosky, M.A., P.C. Gaine, W.F. Martin, K.C. Grabarz, A.A. Ferrando, R.R. Wolfe, and N.R. Rodriguez. 2006. Aerobic Exercise Training Increases Skeletal Muscle Protein Turnover in Healthy Adults at Rest. *J Nutr* 136(2):379–83.

Pitsiladis, Y.P., I. Smith, and R.J. Maughan. 1999. Increased Fat Availability Enhances the Capacity of Trained Individuals to Perform Prolonged Exercise. *Med Sci Sports Exerc* 31(11):1570–79.

Platz, E.A. 2009. Selenium, Genetic Variation, and Prostate Cancer Risk: Epidemiology Reflects Back on Selenium and Vitamin E Cancer Prevention Trial. *J Clin Oncol* 27(22):3569–72.

Plyley, M.J., R.J. Shephard, G.M. Davis, and R.C. Goode. 1987. Sleep Deprivation and Cardiorespiratory Function. Influence of Intermittent Submaximal Exercise. *Eur J Appl Physiol Occup Physiol* 56(3):338–44.

Pottier, A., J. Bouckaert, W. Gilis, T. Roels, and W. Derave. 2010. Mouth Rinse but Not Ingestion of a Carbohydrate Solution Improves 1-h Cycle Time Trial Performance. *Scand J Med Sci Sports* 20(1):105–11.

Prentice, A.M., A.E. Black, W.A. Coward, H.L. Davies, G.R. Goldberg, P.R. Murgatroyd, J. Ashford, M. Sawyer, and R.G. Whitehead. 1986. High Levels of Energy Expenditure in Obese Women. *Br Med J (Clin Res Ed)* 292(6526):983–87.

Price, T.B., D. Laurent, K.F. Petersen, D.L. Rothman, and G.I. Shulman. 2000. Glycogen Loading Alters Muscle Glycogen Resynthesis after Exercise. *J Appl Physiol* 88(2):698–704.

Qin, L.Q., J. Li, Y. Wang, J. Wang, J.Y. Xu, and T. Kaneko. 2003. The Effects of Nocturnal Life on Endocrine Circadian Patterns in Healthy Adults. *Life Sci* 73(19):2467–75.

Rabasa-Lhoret, R., J. Bourque, F. Ducros, and J.L. Chiasson. 2001. Guidelines for Premeal Insulin Dose Reduction for Postprandial Exercise of Different Intensities and Durations in Type 1 Diabetic Subjects Treated Intensively with a Basal-Bolus Insulin Regimen (Ultralente-Lispro). *Diabetes Care* 24(4):625–30.

Raben, A., T.H. Vasilaras, A.C. Moller, and A. Astrup. 2002. Sucrose Compared with Artificial Sweeteners: Different Effects on Ad Libitum Food Intake and Body Weight after 10 Wk of Supplementation in Overweight Subjects. *Am J Clin Nutr* 76(4):721–29.

Rampersaud, G.C., M.A. Pereira, B.L. Girard, J. Adams, and J.D. Metzl. 2005. Breakfast Habits, Nutritional Status, Body Weight, and Academic Performance in Children and Adolescents. *J Am Diet Assoc* 105(5):743–60.

Randle, P.J., P.B. Garland, C.N. Hales, and E.A. Newsholme. 1963. The Glucose Fatty-Acid Cycle: Its Role in Insulin Sensitivity and the Metabolic Disturbances of Diabetes Mellitus. *Lancet* 1(7285):785–89.

Rankin, J.W., L.P. Goldman, M.J. Puglisi, S.M. Nickols-Richardson, C.P. Earthman, and F.C. Gwazdauskas. 2004. Effect of Post-Exercise Supplement Consumption on Adaptations to Resistance Training. *J Am Coll Nutr* 23(4):322–30.

Rasmussen, B.B., K.D. Tipton, S.L. Miller, S.E. Wolf, and R.R. Wolfe. 2000. An Oral Essential Amino Acid-Carbohydrate Supplement Enhances Muscle Protein Anabolism after Resistance Exercise. *J Appl Physiol* 88(2):386–92.

Rauch, L.H., I. Rodger, G.R. Wilson, J.D. Belonje, S.C. Dennis, T.D. Noakes, and J.A. Hawley. 1995. The Effects of Carbohydrate Loading on Muscle Glycogen Content and Cycling Performance. *Int J Sport Nutr* 5(1):25–36.

Raue, U., D. Slivka, B. Jemiolo, C. Hollon, and S. Trappe. 2007. Proteolytic Gene Expression Differs at Rest and after Resistance Exercise between Young and Old Women. *J Gerontol* 62(12):1407–12.

Rawson, E.S., and P.M. Clarkson. 2000. Acute Creatine Supplementation in Older Men. *Int J Sports Med* 21(1):71–75.

Rawson, E.S., and J.S. Volek. 2003. Effects of Creatine Supplementation and Resistance Training on Muscle Strength and Weightlifting Performance. *J Strength Cond Res* 17(4):822–31.

Reed, M.J., J.T. Brozinick, Jr., M.C. Lee, and J.L. Ivy. 1989. Muscle Glycogen Storage Postexercise: Effect of Mode of Carbohydrate Administration. *J Appl Physiol* 66(2):720–26.

Reeds, P.J. 2000. Dispensable and Indispensable Amino Acids for Humans. *J Nutr* 130(7):1835S–40S.

Rehrer, N.J. 2001. Fluid and Electrolyte Balance in Ultra-Endurance Sport. *Sports Med* 31(10):701–15.

Rehrer, N.J., F. Brouns, E.J. Beckers, and W.H. Saris. 1994. The Effect of Beverage Composition and Gastrointestinal Function on Fluid and Nutrient Availability during Exercise. *Scand J Med Sci Sports* 4(3):159–72.

Reid, M.B. 2008. Free Radicals and Muscle Fatigue: Of Ros, Canaries, and the IOC. *Free Radic Biol Med* 44(2):169–79.

Rennie, M.J., J. Bohe, K. Smith, H. Wackerhage, and P. Greenhaff. 2006. Branched-Chain Amino Acids as Fuels and Anabolic Signals in Human Muscle. *J Nutr* 136(1 Suppl):264S–68S.

Rennie, M.J., and K.D. Tipton. 2000. Protein and Amino Acid Metabolism during and after Exercise and the Effects of Nutrition. *Annu Rev Nutr* 20:457–83.

Rennie, M.J., W.W. Winder, and J.O. Holloszy. 1976. A Sparing Effect of Increased Plasma Fatty Acids on Muscle and Liver Glycogen Content in the Exercising Rat. *Biochem J* 156(3):647–55.

Rhea, M., D. Bunker, P. Marin, and K. Lunt. 2009. Effect of Itonic Whole Body Vibration on Delayed Onset Muscle Soreness among Untrained Individuals. *J Strength Cond Res* 23(3):1677–82.

Rieu, I., M. Balage, C. Sornet, C. Giraudet, E. Pujos, J. Grizard, L. Mosoni, and D. Dardevet. 2006. Leucine Supplementation Improves Muscle Protein Synthesis in Elderly Men Independently of Hyperaminoacidaemia. *J Physiol* 575(Pt 1):305–15.

Rieu, I., C. Sornet, G. Bayle, J. Prugnaud, C. Pouyet, M. Balage, I. Papet, J. Grizard, and D. Dardevet. 2003. Leucine-Supplemented Meal Feeding for Ten Days Beneficially Affects Postprandial Muscle Protein Synthesis in Old Rats. *J Nutr* 133(4):1198–1205.

Ristow, M., K. Zarse, A. Oberbach, N. Kloting, M. Birringer, M. Kiehntopf, M. Stumvoll, C.R. Kahn, and M. Bluher. 2009. Antioxidants Prevent Health-Promoting Effects of Physical Exercise in Humans. *Proc Natl Acad Sci U S A* 106(21):8665–70.

Robergs, R.A., D.R. Pearson, D.L. Costill, W.J. Fink, D.D. Pascoe, M.A. Benedict, C.P. Lambert, and J.J. Zachweija. 1991. Muscle Glycogenolysis during Differing Intensities of Weight-Resistance Exercise. *J Appl Physiol* 70(4):1700–6.

Roberts, M.D., V.J. Dalbo, S.E. Hassell, and C.M. Kerksick. 2009. The Expression of Androgen-Regulated Genes before and after a Resistance Exercise Bout in Younger and Older Men. *J Strength Cond Res* 23(4):1060–67.

Robinson, S.M., C. Jaccard, C. Persaud, A.A. Jackson, E. Jequier, and Y. Schutz. 1990. Protein Turnover and Thermogenesis in Response to High-Protein and High-Carbohydrate Feeding in Men. *Am J Clin Nutr* 52(1):72–80.

Robinson, T.M., D.A. Sewell, E. Hultman, and P.L. Greenhaff. 1999. Role of Submaximal Exercise in Promoting Creatine and Glycogen Accumulation in Human Skeletal Muscle. *J Appl Physiol* 87(2):598–604.

Robson-Ansley, P., M. Gleeson, and L. Ansley. 2009. Fatigue Management in the Preparation of Olympic Athletes. *J Sports Sci* 27(13):1409–20.

Rockwell, J.A., J.W. Rankin, and B. Toderico. 2001. Creatine Supplementation Affects Muscle Creatine during Energy Restriction. *Med Sci Sports Exerc* 33(1):61–68.

Rodriguez, N.R., N.M. Di Marco, and S. Langley. 2009a. American College of Sports Medicine Position Stand. Nutrition and Athletic Performance. *Med Sci Sports Exerc* 41(3):709–31.

Rodriguez, N.R., N.M. Dimarco, and S. Langley. 2009b. Position of the American Dietetic Association, Dietitians of Canada, and the American College of Sports Medicine: Nutrition and Athletic Performance. *J Am Diet Assoc* 109(3):509–27.

Rokitzki, L., E. Logemann, A.N. Sagredos, M. Murphy, W. Wetzel-Roth, and J. Keul. 1994. Lipid Peroxidation and Antioxidative Vitamins under Extreme Endurance Stress. *Acta Physiol Scand* 151(2):149–58.

Rollo, I., M. Cole, R. Miller, and C. Williams. 2009. The Influence of Mouth-Rinsing a Carbohydrate Solution on 1 Hour Running Performance. *Med Sci Sports Exerc* 41(5) (Suppl. 1):21.

Rollo, I., and C. Williams. 2010. Influence of Ingesting a Carbohydrate-Electrolyte Solution before and during a 1-Hour Run in Fed Endurance-Trained Runners. *J Sports Sci* 28(6):593–601.

Rollo, I., C. Williams, N. Gant, and M. Nute. 2008. The Influence of Carbohydrate Mouth Rinse on Self-Selected Speeds during a 30-Min Treadmill Run. *Int J Sport Nutr Exerc Metab* 18(6):585–600.

Romano-Ely, B.C., M.K. Todd, M.J. Saunders, and T.S. Laurent. 2006. Effect of an Isocaloric Carbohydrate-Protein-Antioxidant Drink on Cycling Performance. *Med Sci Sports Exerc* 38(9):1608–16.

Romijn, J.A., E.F. Coyle, L.S. Sidossis, A. Gastaldelli, J.F. Horowitz, E. Endert, and R.R. Wolfe. 1993. Regulation of Endogenous Fat and Carbohydrate Metabolism in Relation to Exercise Intensity and Duration. *Am J Physiol* 265(3 Pt 1):E380–91.

Romijn, J.A., E.F. Coyle, L.S. Sidossis, J. Rosenblatt, and R.R. Wolfe. 2000. Substrate Metabolism during Different Exercise Intensities in Endurance-Trained Women. *J Appl Physiol* 88(5):1707–14.

Romijn, J.A., E.F. Coyle, L.S. Sidossis, X.J. Zhang, and R.R. Wolfe. 1995. Relationship between Fatty Acid Delivery and Fatty Acid Oxidation during Strenuous Exercise. *J Appl Physiol* 79(6):1939–45.

Rose, A.J., B. Bisiani, B. Vistisen, B. Kiens, and E.A. Richter. 2009. Skeletal Muscle eEF2 and 4EBP1 Phosphorylation during Endurance Exercise Is Dependent on Intensity and Muscle Fiber Type. *Am J Physiol Regul Integr Comp Physiol* 296(2):R326–33.

Rose, A.J., C. Broholm, K. Kiillerich, S.G. Finn, C.G. Proud, M.H. Rider, E.A. Richter, and B. Kiens. 2005. Exercise Rapidly Increases Eukaryotic Elongation Factor 2 Phosphorylation in Skeletal Muscle of Men. *J Physiol* 569(Pt 1):223–28.

Roth, S.M. 2007. *Genetics Primer for Exercise Science and Health, Primers in Exercise Science*. Champaign, IL: Human Kinetics.

Roth, S.M., G.F. Martel, F.M. Ivey, J.T. Lemmer, B.L. Tracy, E.J. Metter, B.F. Hurley, and M.A. Rogers. 2001. Skeletal Muscle Satellite Cell Characteristics in Young and Older Men and Women after Heavy Resistance Strength Training. *J Gerontol* 56(6):B240–47.

Rousset, S., P. Patureau Mirand, M. Brandolini, J.F. Martin, and Y. Boirie. 2003. Daily Protein Intakes and Eating Patterns in Young and Elderly French. *Br J Nutr* 90(6):1107–15.

Rowland, T.W., M.B. Deisroth, G.M. Green, and J.F. Kelleher. 1988. The Effect of Iron Therapy on the Exercise Capacity of Nonanemic Iron-Deficient Adolescent Runners. *Am J Dis Child (1960)* 142(2):165–69.

Rowlands, D.S., and W.G. Hopkins. 2002. Effect of High-Fat, High-Carbohydrate, and High-Protein Meals on Metabolism and Performance during Endurance Cycling. *Int J Sport Nutr Exerc Metab* 12(3):318–35.

Rowlands, D.S., K. Rossler, R.M. Thorp, D.F. Graham, B.W. Timmons, S.R. Stannard, and M.A. Tarnopolsky. 2008. Effect of Dietary Protein Content during Recovery from High-Intensity Cycling on Subsequent Performance and Markers of Stress, Inflammation, and Muscle Damage in Well-Trained Men. *Appl Physiol Nutr Metab* 33(1):39–51.

Rowlands, D.S., M.S. Thorburn, R.M. Thorp, S. Broadbent, and X. Shi. 2008. Effect of Graded Fructose Coingestion with Maltodextrin on Exogenous 14C-Fructose and 13C-Glucose Oxidation Efficiency and High-Intensity Cycling Performance. *J Appl Physiol* 104(6):1709–19.

Roy, B.D., and M.A. Tarnopolsky. 1998. Influence of Differing Macronutrient Intakes on Muscle Glycogen Resynthesis after Resistance Exercise. *J Appl Physiol* 84(3):890–96.

Roy, B.D., M.A. Tarnopolsky, J.D. MacDougall, J. Fowles, and K.E. Yarasheski. 1997. Effect of Glucose Supplement Timing on Protein Metabolism after Resistance Training. *J Appl Physiol* 82(6):1882–88.

Ruidavets, J.B., V. Bongard, V. Bataille, P. Gourdy, and J. Ferrieres. 2002. Eating Frequency and Body Fatness in Middle-Aged Men. *Int J Obes Relat Metab Disord* 26(11):1476–83.

Sallis, J.F. 2000. Age-Related Decline in Physical Activity: A Synthesis of Human and Animal Studies. *Med Sci Sports Exerc* 32(9):1598–1600.

Salmeron, J., J.E. Manson, M.J. Stampfer, G.A. Colditz, A.L. Wing, and W.C. Willett. 1997. Dietary Fiber, Glycemic Load, and Risk of Non-Insulin-Dependent Diabetes Mellitus in Women. *JAMA* 277(6):472–77.

Sandler, S. 1999. The Physiology of Soft Tissue Massage. *J Bodywork Move Ther* 3(2):117–21.

Sandri, M., C. Sandri, A. Gilbert, C. Skurk, E. Calabria, A. Picard, K. Walsh, S. Schiaffino, S.H. Lecker, and A.L. Goldberg. 2004. FOXO Transcription Factors Induce the Atrophy-Related Ubiquitin Ligase Atrogin-1 and Cause Skeletal Muscle Atrophy. *Cell* 117(3):399–412.

Satia-Abouta, J., R.E. Patterson, R.N. Schiller, and A.R. Kristal. 2002. Energy from Fat Is Associated with Obesity in U.S. Men: Results from the Prostate Cancer Prevention Trial. *Prev Med* 34(5):493–501.

Saunders, M.J., J.E. Herrick, N.D. Luden, M.K. Todd, R.J. Valentine, T.S. Laurent, and M.D. Kane. 2005. Effects of a Carbohydrate/Protein Gel on Exercise Performance in Male and Female Cyclists. *J Int Soc Sports Nutr* 2(1):1–30.

Saunders, M.J., M.D. Kane, and M.K. Todd. 2004. Effects of a Carbohydrate-Protein Beverage on Cycling Endurance and Muscle Damage. *Med Sci Sports Exerc* 36(7):1233–38.

Saunders, M.J., N.D. Luden, and J.E. Herrick. 2007. Consumption of an Oral Carbohydrate-Protein Gel Improves Cycling Endurance and Prevents Postexercise Muscle Damage. *J Strength Cond Res* 21(3):678–84.

Saunders, M.J., R.W. Moore, A.K. Kies, N.D. Luden, and C.A. Pratt. 2009. Carbohydrate and Protein Hydrolysate Coingestions Improvement of Late-Exercise Time-Trial Performance. *Int J Sport Nutr Exerc Metab* 19(2):136–49.

Saunders, M.J., M.K. Todd, R.J. Valentine, T.S. Laurent, M.D. Kane, N.D. Luden, and J.E. Herrick. 2006. Inter-Study Examination of Physiological Variables Associated with Improved Endurance Performance with Carbohydrate/Protein Administration (Abstract). *Med Sci Sports Exerc* 38(5):S113–14.

Sawka, M.N., L.M. Burke, E.R. Eichner, R.J. Maughan, S.J. Montain, and N.S. Stachenfeld. 2007. American College of Sports Medicine Position Stand. Exercise and Fluid Replacement. *Med Sci Sports Exerc* 39(2):377–90.

Schaafsma, G. 2000. The Protein Digestibility-Corrected Amino Acid Score. *J Nutr* 130(7):1865S–67S.

Schaafsma, G. 2005. The Protein Digestibility-Corrected Amino Acid Score (PDCAAS)—A Concept for Describing Protein Quality in Foods and Food Ingredients: A Critical Review. *J AOAC Int* 88(3):988–94.

Schaafsma, G. 2009. Safety of Protein Hydrolysates, Fractions Thereof and Bioactive Peptides in Human Nutrition. *Eur J Clin Nutr* 63(10):1161–68.

Schwartz, W., and J.W. Bird. 1977. Degradation of Myofibrillar Proteins by Cathepsins B and D. *Biochem J* 167(3):811–20.

Scribner, K.B., D.B. Pawlak, C.M. Aubin, J.A. Majzoub, and D.S. Ludwig. 2008. Long-Term Effects of Dietary Glycemic Index on Adiposity, Energy Metabolism, and Physical Activity in Mice. *Am J Physiol Endocrinol Metab* 295(5):E1126–31.

Secher, N.H., T. Seifert, and J.J. Van Lieshout. 2008. Cerebral Blood Flow and Metabolism during Exercise: Implications for Fatigue. *J Appl Physiol* 104(1):306–14.

Selye, Hans. 1946. The General Adaptation Syndrome and the Diseases of Adaptation. *JCEM* 6:117–230.

Selye, Hans. 1956. *The Stress of Life*. New York: McGraw-Hill, xvi, 324.

Shearer, J., and T.E. Graham. 2004. Novel Aspects of Skeletal Muscle Glycogen and Its Regulation during Rest and Exercise. *Exerc Sport Sci Rev* 32(3):120–26.

Sheffield-Moore, M., D. Paddon-Jones, A.P. Sanford, J.I. Rosenblatt, A.G. Matlock, M.G. Cree, and R.R. Wolfe. 2005. Mixed Muscle and Hepatic Derived Plasma Protein Metabolism Is Differentially Regulated in Older and Younger Men Following Resistance Exercise. *Am J Physiol Endocrinol Metab* 288(5):E922–29.

Sheffield-Moore, M., C.W. Yeckel, E. Volpi, S.E. Wolf, B. Morio, D.L. Chinkes, D. Paddon-Jones, and R.R. Wolfe. 2004. Postexercise Protein Metabolism in Older and Younger Men Following Moderate-Intensity Aerobic Exercise. *Am J Physiol Endocrinol Metab* 287(3):E513–22.

Shelmadine, B., M. Cooke, T. Buford, G. Hudson, L. Redd, B. Leutholtz, and D.S. Willoughby. 2009. Effects of 28 Days of Resistance Exercise and Consuming a Commercially Available Pre-Workout Supplement, No-Shotgun(R), on Body Composition, Muscle Strength and Mass, Markers of Satellite Cell Activation, and Clinical Safety Markers in Males. *J Int Soc Sports Nutr* 6:16.

Sherman, W.M., G. Brodowicz, D.A. Wright, W.K. Allen, J. Simonsen, and A. Dernbach. 1989. Effects of 4 h Preexercise Carbohydrate Feedings on Cycling Performance. *Med Sci Sports Exerc* 21(5):598–604.

Sherman, W.M., D.L. Costill, W.J. Fink, and J.M. Miller. 1981. Effect of Exercise-Diet Manipulation on Muscle Glycogen and Its Subsequent Utilization during Performance. *Int J Sports Med* 2(2):114–18.

Sherman, W.M., M.C. Peden, and D.A. Wright. 1991. Carbohydrate Feedings 1 h before Exercise Improves Cycling Performance. *Am J Clin Nutr* 54(5):866–70.

Shirreffs, S.M. 2009. Body Water and Its Composition. In *The Olympic Textbook of Science in Sport*, edited by R.J. Maughan. West Sussex, UK: Blackwell.

Shirreffs, S.M., L.E. Armstrong, and S.N. Cheuvront. 2004. Fluid and Electrolyte Needs for Preparation and Recovery from Training and Competition. *J Sports Sci* 22(1):57–63.

Shirreffs, S.M., and R.J. Maughan. 1998. Volume Repletion after Exercise-Induced Volume Depletion in Humans: Replacement of Water and Sodium Losses. *Am J Physiol Renal Physiol* 274(5):868.

Shirreffs, S.M., A.J. Taylor, J. Leiper, and R. Maughan. 1996. Post-Exercise Rehydration in Man: Effects of Volume Consumed and Drink Sodium Content. *Med Sci Sports Exerc* 28(10):1260–71.

Sidossis, L.S., A. Gastaldelli, S. Klein, and R.R. Wolfe. 1997. Regulation of Plasma Fatty Acid Oxidation during Low- and High-Intensity Exercise. *Am J Physiol* 272(6 Pt 1):E1065–70.

Sigal, R.J., S.J. Fisher, A. Manzon, J.A. Morais, J.B. Halter, M. Vranic, and E.B. Marliss. 2000. Glucoregulation during and after Intense Exercise: Effects of Alpha-Adrenergic Blockade. *Metabolism* 49(3):386–94.

Simon-Schnass, I., and H. Pabst. 1988. Influence of Vitamin E on Physical Performance. *Int J Vit Nutr Res* 58(1):49–54.

Sipila, I., J. Rapola, O. Simell, and A. Vannas. 1981. Supplementary Creatine as a Treatment for Gyrate Atrophy of the Choroid and Retina. *N Engl J Med* 304(15):867–70.

Slavin, J.L. 2005. Dietary Fiber and Body Weight. *Nutrition* 21(3):411–18.

Slavin, J.L. 2008. Position of the American Dietetic Association: Health Implications of Dietary Fiber. *J Am Diet Assoc* 108(10):1716–31.

Slentz, C.A., L.B. Aiken, J.A. Houmard, C.W. Bales, J.L. Johnson, C.J. Tanner, B.D. Duscha, and W.E. Kraus. 2005. Inactivity, Exercise and Visceral Fat. STRRIDE: A Randomized, Controlled Study of Exercise Intensity and Amount. *J Appl Physiol* 99(4):1613–18.

Smeets, A.J., and M.S. Westerterp-Plantenga. 2008. Acute Effects on Metabolism and Appetite Profile of One Meal Difference in the Lower Range of Meal Frequency. *Br J Nutr* 99(6):1316–21.

Smith, A.E., C.M. Lockwood, J.R. Moon, K.L. Kendall, D.H. Fukuda, S.E. Tobkin, J.T. Cramer, and J.R. Stout. 2010. Physiological Effects of Caffeine, Epigallocatechin-3-Gallate, and Exercise in Overweight and Obese Women. *Appl Physiol Nutr Metab* 35(5):607–16.

Smith, G.J., E.C. Rhodes, and R.H. Langill. 2002. The Effect of Pre-Exercise Glucose Ingestion on Performance during Prolonged Swimming. *Int J Sport Nutr Exerc Metab* 12(2):136–44.

Smith, J.A., M. Kolbuch-Braddon, I. Gillam, R.D. Telford, and M.J. Weidemann. 1995. Changes in the Susceptibility of Red Blood Cells to Oxidative and Osmotic Stress Following Submaximal Exercise. *Eur J Appl Physiol Occup Physiol* 70(5):427–36.

Smith, J.W., J.J. Zachwieja, F. Peronnet, D.H. Passe, D. Massicotte, C. Lavoie, and D.D. Pascoe. 2010. Fuel Selection and Cycling Endurance Performance with Ingestion of [13C] Glucose: Evidence for a Carbohydrate Dose Response. *J Appl Physiol* 108(6):1520–29.

Smith, K., J.M. Barua, P.W. Watt, C.M. Scrimgeour, and M.J. Rennie. 1992. Flooding with L-[1–13C]Leucine Stimulates Human Muscle Protein Incorporation of Continuously Infused L-[1–13C]Valine. *Am J Physiol* 262(3 Pt 1):E372–76.

Smith, L.L. 2000. Cytokine Hypothesis of Overtraining: A Physiological Adaptation to Excessive Stress? *Med Sci Sports Exerc* 32:317–31.

Smith, L.L. 2004. Tissue Trauma: The Underlying Cause of Overtraining Syndrome. *J Strength Cond Res* 18(1):185–93.

Smith, L.L., Keating, Madge N, D. Holbert, D. Spratt, M.R. McCammon, S. Smith, and R. Isreal. 1994. The Effects of Athletic Massage on Delayed Onset Muscle Soreness, Creating Kinase, and Neutrophil Count: A Preliminary Report. *J Orthop Sports Phys Ther* 19(2):93–99.

Solerte, S.B., C. Gazzaruso, R. Bonacasa, M. Rondanelli, M. Zamboni, C. Basso, E. Locatelli, N. Schifino, A. Giustina, and M. Fioravanti. 2008. Nutritional Supplements with Oral Amino Acid Mixtures Increases Whole-Body Lean Mass and Insulin Sensitivity in Elderly Subjects with Sarcopenia. *Am J Cardiol* 101(11A):69E–77E.

Song, W.O., O.K. Chun, S. Obayashi, S. Cho, and C.E. Chung. 2005. Is Consumption of Breakfast Associated with Body Mass Index in U.S. Adults? *J Am Diet Assoc* 105(9):1373–82.

Sparks, M.J., S.S. Selig, and M.A. Febbraio. 1998. Pre-Exercise Carbohydrate Ingestion: Effect of the Glycemic Index on Endurance Exercise Performance. *Med Sci Sports Exerc* 30(6):844–49.

Speechly, D.P., and R. Buffenstein. 1999. Greater Appetite Control Associated with an Increased Frequency of Eating in Lean Males. *Appetite* 33(3):285–97.

Speechly, D.P., G.G. Rogers, and R. Buffenstein. 1999. Acute Appetite Reduction Associated with an Increased Frequency of Eating in Obese Males. *Int J Obes Relat Metab Disord* 23(11):1151–59.

Spillane, M., R. Schoch, M. Cooke, T. Harvey, M. Greenwood, R. Kreider, and D.S. Willoughby. 2009. The Effects of Creatine Ethyl Ester Supplementation Combined with Heavy Resistance Training on Body Composition, Muscle Performance, and Serum and Muscle Creatine Levels. *J Int Soc Sports Nutr* 6:6.

Spiller, G.A., C.D. Jensen, T.S. Pattison, C.S. Chuck, J.H. Whittam, and J. Scala. 1987. Effect of Protein Dose on Serum Glucose and Insulin Response to Sugars. *Am J Clin Nutr* 46(3):474–80.

Sport Nutrition and Weight Loss Report. 2011. *Nutrition Business Journal.*

Spriet, L.L., M.I. Lindinger, R.S. McKelvie, G.J. Heigenhauser, and N.L. Jones. 1989. Muscle Glycogenolysis and H$^+$ Concentration during Maximal Intermittent Cycling. *J Appl Physiol* 66(1):8–13.

Srinivasan, K. 2007. Black Pepper and Its Pungent Principle-Piperine: A Review of Diverse Physiological Effects. *Crit Rev Food Sci Nutr* 47(8):735–48.

Stanton, J.L., Jr., and D.R. Keast. 1989. Serum Cholesterol, Fat Intake, and Breakfast Consumption in the United States Adult Population. *J Am Coll Nutr* 8(6):567–72.

Staples, A.W., N.A. Burd, D.W. West, K.D. Currie, P.J. Atherton, D.R. Moore, M.J. Rennie, M.J. Macdonald, S.K. Baker, and S.M. Phillips. 2011. Carbohydrate Does Not Augment Exercise-Induced Protein Accretion versus Protein Alone. *Med Sci Sports Exerc* 43(7):1154–61.

Stear, S.J., L.M. Burke, and L.M. Castell. 2009. BJSM Reviews: A–Z of Nutritional Supplements: Dietary Supplements, Sports Nutrition Foods and Ergogenic Aids for Health and Performance Part 3. *Br J Sports Med* 43(12):890–92.

Stellingwerff, T., M.K. Boit, and P.T. Res. 2007. Nutritional Strategies to Optimize Training and Racing in Middle-Distance Athletes. *J Sports Sci* 25(Suppl 1):S17–28.

Stellingwerff, T., H. Boon, A.P. Gijsen, J.H. Stegen, H. Kuipers, and L.J. Van Loon. 2007. Carbohydrate Supplementation during Prolonged Cycling Exercise Spares Muscle Glycogen but Does Not Affect Intramyocellular Lipid Use. *Pflugers Arch* 454(4):635–47.

Stellingwerff, T., L.L. Spriet, M.J. Watt, N.E. Kimber, M. Hargreaves, J.A. Hawley, and L.M. Burke. 2006. Decreased PDH Activation and Glycogenolysis during Exercise Following Fat Adaptation with Carbohydrate Restoration. *Am J Physiol Endocrinol Metab* 290(2):E380–88.

Stephens, F.B., M. Roig, G. Armstrong, and P.L. Greenhaff. 2008. Post-Exercise Ingestion of a Unique, High Molecular Weight Glucose Polymer Solution Improves Performance during a Subsequent Bout of Cycling Exercise. *J Sports Sci* 26(2):149–54.

Stevenson, E.J., C. Williams, L.E. Mash, B. Phillips, and M.L. Nute. 2006. Influence of High-Carbohydrate Mixed Meals with Different Glycemic Indexes on Substrate Utilization during Subsequent Exercise in Women. *Am J Clin Nutr* 84(2):354–60.

Stewart, J.G., D.A. Ahlquist, D.B. McGill, D.M. Ilstrup, S. Schwartz, and R.A. Owen. 1984. Gastrointestinal Blood Loss and Anemia in Runners. *Ann Intern Med* 100(6):843–45.

Stipanuk, M.H. 2007. Leucine and Protein Synthesis: mTOR and Beyond. *Nutr Rev* 65(3):122–29.

Stout, J.R., B.S. Graves, J.T. Cramer, E.R. Goldstein, P.B. Costa, A.E. Smith, and A.A. Walter. 2007. Effects of Creatine Supplementation on the Onset of Neuromuscular Fatigue Threshold and Muscle Strength in Elderly Men and Women (64–86 Years). *J Nutr Health Aging* 11(6):459–64.

Stover, E.A., H.J. Petrie, D. Passe, C.A. Horswill, B. Murray, and R. Wildman. 2006. Urine Specific Gravity in Exercisers Prior to Physical Training. *Appl Physiol Nutr Metab* 31(3):320–27.

Summerbell, C.D., R.C. Moody, J. Shanks, M.J. Stock, and C. Geissler. 1996. Relationship between Feeding Pattern and Body Mass Index in 220 Free-Living People in Four Age Groups. *Eur J Clin Nutr* 50(8):513–19.

Surwit, R.S., M.N. Feinglos, C.C. McCaskill, S.L. Clay, M.A. Babyak, B.S. Brownlow, C.S. Plaisted, and P.H. Lin. 1997. Metabolic and Behavioral Effects of a High-Sucrose Diet during Weight Loss. *Am J Clin Nutr* 65(4):908–15.

Swenson, C., L. Sward, and J. Karlsson. 1996. Cryotherapy in Sports Medicine. *Scand J Med Sci Sports* 6(4):193–200.

Symons, T.B., S.E. Schutzler, T.L. Cocke, D.L. Chinkes, R.R. Wolfe, and D. Paddon-Jones. 2007. Aging Does Not Impair the Anabolic Response to a Protein-Rich Meal. *Am J Clin Nutr* 86(2):451–56.

Takeuchi, L., G.M. Davis, M. Plyley, R. Goode, and R.J. Shephard. 1985. Sleep Deprivation, Chronic Exercise and Muscular Performance. *Ergonomics* 28(3):591–601.

Tang, J.E., D.R. Moore, G.W. Kujbida, M.A. Tarnopolsky, and S.M. Phillips. 2009. Ingestion of Whey Hydrolysate, Casein, or Soy Protein Isolate: Effects on Mixed Muscle Protein Synthesis at Rest and Following Resistance Exercise in Young Men. *J Appl Physiol* 107(3):987–92.

Tang, J.E., J.G. Perco, D.R. Moore, S.B. Wilkinson, and S.M. Phillips. 2008. Resistance Training Alters the Response of Fed State Mixed Muscle Protein Synthesis in Young Men. *Am J Physiol Regul Integr Comp Physiol* 294(1):R172–78.

Tarnopolsky, M.A., M. Bosman, J.R. Macdonald, D. Vandeputte, J. Martin, and B.D. Roy. 1997. Postexercise Protein-Carbohydrate and Carbohydrate Supplements Increase Muscle Glycogen in Men and Women. *J Appl Physiol* 83(6):1877–83.

Tarpenning, K.M., R.A. Wiswell, S.A. Hawkins, and T.J. Marcell. 2001. Influence of Weight Training Exercise and Modification of Hormonal Response on Skeletal Muscle Growth. *J Sci Med Sport* 4(4):431–46.

Taylor, J., G. Allen, J. Butler, and S. Gandevia. 2000. Supraspinal Fatigue during Intermittent Maximal Voluntary Contractions of the Human Elbow. *J Appl Physiol* 89:305–13.

Taylor, M.A., and J.S. Garrow. 2001. Compared with Nibbling, Neither Gorging nor a Morning Fast Affect Short-Term Energy Balance in Obese Patients in a Chamber Calorimeter. *Int J Obes Relat Metab Disord* 25(4):519–28.

Telford, R.D., E.A. Catchpole, V. Deakin, A.G. Hahn, and A.W. Plank. 1992. The Effect of 7 to 8 Months of Vitamin/Mineral Supplementation on Athletic Performance. *Int J Sport Nutr* 2(2):135–53.

Tharion, W.J., B. Shukitt-Hale, and H.R. Lieberman. 2003. Caffeine Effects on Marksmanship during High-Stress Military Training with 72 Hour Sleep Deprivation. *Aviat Space Environ Med* 74(4):309–14.

Thomas, D.E., J.R. Brotherhood, and J.C. Brand. 1991. Carbohydrate Feeding before Exercise: Effect of Glycemic Index. *Int J Sports Med* 12(2):180–86.

Thomas, D.E., J.R. Brotherhood, and J.B. Miller. 1994. Plasma Glucose Levels after Prolonged Strenuous Exercise Correlate Inversely with Glycemic Response to Food Consumed before Exercise. *Int J Sport Nutr* 4(4):361–73.

Thompson, H.S., and S.P. Scordilis. 1994. Ubiquitin Changes in Human Biceps Muscle Following Exercise-Induced Damage. *Biochem Biophys Res Commun* 204(3):1193–98.

Thorburn, M.S., B. Vistisen, R.M. Thorp, M.J. Rockell, A.E. Jeukendrup, X. Xu, and D.S. Rowlands. 2006. Attenuated Gastric Distress but No Benefit to Performance with Adaptation to Octanoate-Rich Esterified Oils in Well-Trained Male Cyclists. *J Appl Physiol* 101(6):1733–43.

Thorburn, M.S., Vistisen, B., Thorp, R.M., Rockell, M.J., Jeukendrup, A.E., Xu, X., Rowlands, D.S. 2007. No Attenuation of Gastric Distress or Benefit to Performance with Adaptation to Octanoate-Rich Esterified Oils in Female Cyclists. *Eur J Sport Sci* 7(4):179–92.

Timlin, M.T., and M.A. Pereira. 2007. Breakfast Frequency and Quality in the Etiology of Adult Obesity and Chronic Diseases. *Nutr Rev* 65(6 Pt 1):268–81.

Tipton, K.D., E. Borsheim, S.E. Wolf, A.P. Sanford, and R.R. Wolfe. 2003. Acute Response of Net Muscle Protein Balance Reflects 24-h Balance after Exercise and Amino Acid Ingestion. *Am J Physiol Endocrinol Metab* 284(1):E76–E89.

Tipton, K.D., T.A. Elliott, M.G. Cree, A.A. Aarsland, A.P. Sanford, and R.R. Wolfe. 2007. Stimulation of Net Muscle Protein Synthesis by Whey Protein Ingestion before and after Exercise. *Am J Physiol Endocrinol Metab* 292(1):E71–E76.

Tipton, K.D., T.A. Elliott, M.G. Cree, S.E. Wolf, A.P. Sanford, and R.R. Wolfe. 2004. Ingestion of Casein and Whey Proteins Result in Muscle Anabolism after Resistance Exercise. *Med Sci Sports Exerc* 36(12):2073–81.

Tipton, K.D., and A.A. Ferrando. 2008. Improving Muscle Mass: Response of Muscle Metabolism to Exercise, Nutrition and Anabolic Agents. *Essays Biochem.* 44:85–98.

Tipton, K.D., A.A. Ferrando, S.M. Phillips, D. Doyle, Jr., and R.R. Wolfe. 1999. Postexercise Net Protein Synthesis in Human Muscle from Orally Administered Amino Acids. *Am J Physiol* 276(4 Pt 1):E628–34.

Tipton, K.D., B.E. Gurkin, S. Matin, and R.R. Wolfe. 1999. Nonessential Amino Acids Are Not Necessary to Stimulate Net Muscle Protein Synthesis in Healthy Volunteers. *J Nutr Biochem* 10(2):89–95.

Tipton, K.D., B.B. Rasmussen, S.L. Miller, S.E. Wolf, S.K. Owens-Stovall, B.E. Petrini, and R.R. Wolfe. 2001. Timing of Amino Acid-Carbohydrate Ingestion Alters Anabolic Response of Muscle to Resistance Exercise. *Am J Physiol Endocrinol Metab* 281(2):E197–E206.

Tipton, K.D., and O.C. Witard. 2007. Protein Requirements and Recommendations for Athletes: Relevance of Ivory Tower Arguments for Practical Recommendations. *Clin Sports Med* 26(1):17–36.

Toone, R.J., and J.A. Betts. 2010. Isocaloric Carbohydrate Versus Carbohydrate-Protein Ingestion and Cycling Time-Trial Performance. *Int J Sport Nutr Exerc Metab* 20(1):34–43.

Tordoff, M.G., and A.M. Alleva. 1990. Effect of Drinking Soda Sweetened with Aspartame or High-Fructose Corn Syrup on Food Intake and Body Weight. *Am J Clin Nutr* 51(6):963–69.

Tran, H., A. Brunet, E.C. Griffith, and M.E. Greenberg. 2003. The Many Forks in FOXO's Road. *Sci STKE* 2003(172):RE5.

Trappe, T.A., U. Raue, and P.A. Tesch. 2004. Human Soleus Muscle Protein Synthesis Following Resistance Exercise. *Acta Physiol Scand* 182(2):189–96.

Tsintzas, K., and C. Williams. 1998. Human Muscle Glycogen Metabolism during Exercise. Effect of Carbohydrate Supplementation. *Sports Med* 25(1):7–23.

Tsintzas, O.K., C. Williams, L. Boobis, and P. Greenhaff. 1995. Carbohydrate Ingestion and Glycogen Utilization in Different Muscle Fibre Types in Man. *J Physiol* 489(Pt 1):243–50.

Tsintzas, O.K., C. Williams, L. Boobis, and P. Greenhaff. 1996. Carbohydrate Ingestion and Single Muscle Fiber Glycogen Metabolism during Prolonged Running in Men. *J Appl Physiol* 81(2):801–9.

Tsintzas, O.K., C. Williams, W. Wilson, and J. Burrin. 1996. Influence of Carbohydrate Supplementation Early in Exercise on Endurance Running Capacity. *Med Sci Sports Exerc* 28(11):1373–79.

Vaile, J., S. Halson, N. Gill, and B. Dawson. 2008. Effect of Hydrotherapy on Recovery from Fatigue. *Int J Sports Med* 29:539–44.

Valentine, R.J., T.S. Laurent, M.J. Saunders, M.K. Todd, and J.A. Flohr. 2006. Comparison of Responses to Exercise When Consuming Carbohydrate and Carbohydrate/Protein Beverages (Abstract). *Med Sci Sports Exerc* 38(5):S341.

Valentine, R.J., M.J. Saunders, M.K. Todd, and T.G. St. Laurent. 2008. Influence of Carbohydrate-Protein Beverage on Cycling Endurance and Indices of Muscle Disruption. *Int J Sport Nutr Exerc Metab* 18(4):363–78.

Van Essen, M., and M.J. Gibala. 2006. Failure of Protein to Improve Time Trial Performance When Added to a Sports Drink. *Med Sci Sports Exerc* 38(8):1476–83.

Van Hall, G., J.S. Raaymakers, W.H. Saris, and A.J. Wagenmakers. 1995. Ingestion of Branched-Chain Amino Acids and Tryptophan during Sustained Exercise in Man: Failure to Affect Performance. *J Physiol* 486(Pt 3):789–94.

Van Hall, G., S.M. Shirreffs, and J.A. Calbet. 2000. Muscle Glycogen Resynthesis during Recovery from Cycle Exercise: No Effect of Additional Protein Ingestion. *J Appl Physiol* 88(5):1631–36.

Van Loon, L.J., P.L. Greenhaff, D. Constantin Teodosiu, W.H. Saris, and A.J. Wagenmakers. 2001. The Effects of Increasing Exercise Intensity on Muscle Fuel Utilisation in Humans. *J Physiol* 536(Pt 1):295–304.

Van Loon, L.J., W.H. Saris, M. Kruijshoop, and A.J. Wagenmakers. 2000. Maximizing Postexercise Muscle Glycogen Synthesis: Carbohydrate Supplementation and the Application of Amino Acid or Protein Hydrolysate Mixtures. *Am J Clin Nutr* 72(1):106–11.

Van Loon, L.J., W.H. Saris, H. Verhagen, and A.J. Wagenmakers. 2000. Plasma Insulin Responses after Ingestion of Different Amino Acid or Protein Mixtures with Carbohydrate. *Am J Clin Nutr* 72(1):96–105.

Van Zyl, C.G., E.V. Lambert, J.A. Hawley, T.D. Noakes, and S.C. Dennis. 1996. Effects of Medium-Chain Triglyceride Ingestion on Fuel Metabolism and Cycling Performance. *J Appl Physiol* 80(6):2217–25.

Vary, T.C., L.S. Jefferson, and S.R. Kimball. 2001. Insulin Fails to Stimulate Muscle Protein Synthesis in Sepsis Despite Unimpaired Signaling to 4E-BP1 and S6K1. *Am J Physiol Endocrinol Metab* 281(5):E1045–53.

Vary, T.C., and C.J. Lynch. 2006. Meal Feeding Stimulates Phosphorylation of Multiple Effector Proteins Regulating Protein Synthetic Processes in Rat Hearts. *J Nutr* 136(9):2284–90.

Vaschillo, E., P. Lehrer, N. Rishe, and M. Konstantinov. 2002. Heart Rate Variability Biofeedback as a Method for Assessing Baroreflex Function: A Preliminary Study of Resonance in the Cardiovascular System. *Appl Psychophysiol Biofeedback* 27:1–27.

Vaschillo, E., B. Vaschillo, and P. Lehrer. 2004. Heart Rate Variability Biofeedback Increases Baroreflex Gain and Peak Expiratory Flow. *Psychosom Med* 2003(5):796–805.

Verboeket-Van De Venne, W.P., and K.R. Westerterp. 1993. Frequency of Feeding, Weight Reduction and Energy Metabolism. *Int J Obes Relat Metab Disord* 17(1):31–36.

Verdijk, L.B., B.G. Gleeson, R.A. Jonkers, K. Meijer, H.H. Savelberg, P. Dendale, and L.J. Van Loon. 2009. Skeletal Muscle Hypertrophy Following Resistance Training Is Accompanied by a Fiber Type-Specific Increase in Satellite Cell Content in Elderly Men. *J Gerontol* 64(3):332–39.

Verdijk, L.B., R.A. Jonkers, B.G. Gleeson, M. Beelen, K. Meijer, H.H. Savelberg, W.K. Wodzig, P. Dendale, and L.J. Van Loon. 2009. Protein Supplementation before and after Exercise Does Not Further Augment Skeletal Muscle Hypertrophy after Resistance Training in Elderly Men. *Am J Clin Nutr* 89(2):608–16.

Verdijk, L.B., R. Koopman, G. Schaart, K. Meijer, H.H. Savelberg, and L.J. Van Loon. 2007. Satellite Cell Content Is Specifically Reduced in Type II Skeletal Muscle Fibers in the Elderly. *Am J Physiol Endocrinol Metab* 292(1):E151–17.

Vergauwen, L., F. Brouns, and P. Hespel. 1998. Carbohydrate Supplementation Improves Stroke Performance in Tennis. *Med Sci Sports Exerc* 30(8):1289–95.

Verhoeven, S., K. Vanschoonbeek, L.B. Verdijk, R. Koopman, W.K. Wodzig, P. Dendale, and L.J. Van Loon. 2009. Long-Term Leucine Supplementation Does Not Increase Muscle Mass or Strength in Healthy Elderly Men. *Am J Clin Nutr* 89(5):1468–75.

Veves, A., R. Saouaf, V.M. Donaghue, C.A. Mullooly, J.A. Kistler, J.M. Giurini, E.S. Horton, and R.A. Fielding. 1997. Aerobic Exercise Capacity Remains Normal Despite Impaired Endothelial Function in the Micro- and Macrocirculation of Physically Active IDDM Patients. *Diabetes* 46(11):1846–52.

Vist, G.E., and R.J. Maughan. 1995. The Effect of Osmolality and Carbohydrate Content on the Rate of Gastric Emptying of Liquids in Man. *J Physiol* 486(Pt 2):523–31.

Vistisen, B., L. Nybo, X. Xu, C.E. Hoy, and B. Kiens. 2003. Minor Amounts of Plasma Medium-Chain Fatty Acids and No Improved Time Trial Performance after Consuming Lipids. *J Appl Physiol* 95(6):2434–43.

Volek, J.S. 2004. Influence of Nutrition on Responses to Resistance Training. *Med Sci Sports Exerc* 36(4):689–96.

Volek, J.S., A.L. Gomez, T.P. Scheett, M.J. Sharman, D.N. French, M.R. Rubin, N.A. Ratamess, M.M. McGuigan, and W.J. Kraemer. 2003. Increasing Fluid Milk Favorably Affects Bone Mineral Density Responses to Resistance Training in Adolescent Boys. *J Am Diet Assoc* 103(10):1353–56.

Volpi, E., H. Kobayashi, M. Sheffield-Moore, B. Mittendorfer, and R.R. Wolfe. 2003. Essential Amino Acids Are Primarily Responsible for the Amino Acid Stimulation of Muscle Protein Anabolism in Healthy Elderly Adults. *Am J Clin Nutr* 78(2):250–58.

Von Liebig, J. 1840. *Animal Chemistry or Organic Chemistry in Its Application to Physiology and Pathology*. W. Gregory, Trans. Cambridge, MA: Owen.

Vukovich, M.D., D.L. Costill, M.S. Hickey, S.W. Trappe, K.J. Cole, and W.J. Fink. 1993. Effect of Fat Emulsion Infusion and Fat Feeding on Muscle Glycogen Utilization during Cycle Exercise. *J Appl Physiol* 75(4):1513–18.

Wagenmakers, A.J., J.H. Coakley, and R.H. Edwards. 1990. Metabolism of Branched-Chain Amino Acids and Ammonia during Exercise: Clues from McArdle's Disease. *Int J Sports Med* 11(Suppl 2):S101–13.

Walberg-Rankin, J. 1997. Glycemic Index and Exercise Metabolism. *Sports Sci Exch* 10(1):1–7.

Wallis, G.A., D.S. Rowlands, C. Shaw, R.L. Jentjens, and A.E. Jeukendrup. 2005. Oxidation of Combined Ingestion of Maltodextrins and Fructose during Exercise. *Med Sci Sports Exerc* 37(3):426–32.

Walrand, S., and Y. Boirie. 2005. Optimizing Protein Intake in Aging. *Curr Opin Clin Nutr Metab Care* 8(1):89–94.

Wang, Y., C. Monteiro, and B.M. Popkin. 2002. Trends of Obesity and Underweight in Older Children and Adolescents in the United States, Brazil, China, and Russia. *Am J Clin Nutr* 75(6):971–77.

Wanke, T., D. Formanek, M. Auinger, H. Zwick, and K. Irsigler. 1992. Pulmonary Gas Exchange and Oxygen Uptake during Exercise in Patients with Type 1 Diabetes Mellitus. *Diabet Med* 9(3):252–57.

Wasserman, D.H. 2009. Four Grams of Glucose. *Am J Physiol Endocrinol Metab* 296(1):E11–E21.

Watson, P., S.M. Shirreffs, and R.J. Maughan. 2004. The Effect of Acute Branched-Chain Amino Acid Supplementation on Prolonged Exercise Capacity in a Warm Environment. *Eur J Appl Physiol* 93(3):306–14.

Weigle, D.S., P.A. Breen, C.C. Matthys, H.S. Callahan, K.E. Meeuws, V.R. Burden, and J.Q. Purnell. 2005. A High-Protein Diet Induces Sustained Reductions in Appetite, Ad Libitum Caloric Intake, and Body Weight Despite Compensatory Changes in Diurnal Plasma Leptin and Ghrelin Concentrations. *Am J Clin Nutr* 82(1):41–48.

Welle, S., C. Thornton, and M. Statt. 1995. Myofibrillar Protein Synthesis in Young and Old Human Subjects after Three Months of Resistance Training. *Am J Physiol* 268(3 Pt 1):E422–27.

Welle, S., S. Totterman, and C. Thornton. 1996. Effect of Age on Muscle Hypertrophy Induced by Resistance Training. *J Gerontol A Biol Sci Med Sci* 51(6):M270–75.

Wendt, D., L.J. Van Loon, and W.D. Lichtenbelt. 2007. Thermoregulation during Exercise in the Heat: Strategies for Maintaining Health and Performance. *Sports Med* 37(8):669–82.

West, D.W., N.A. Burd, J.E. Tang, D.R. Moore, A.W. Staples, A.M. Holwerda, S.K. Baker, and S.M. Phillips. 2010. Elevations in Ostensibly Anabolic Hormones with Resistance Exercise Enhance Neither Training-Induced Muscle Hypertrophy nor Strength of the Elbow Flexors. *J Appl Physiol* 108(1):60–67.

West, D.W., G.W. Kujbida, D.R. Moore, P. Atherton, N.A. Burd, J.P. Padzik, M. De Lisio, J.E. Tang, G. Parise, M.J. Rennie, S.K. Baker, and S.M. Phillips. 2009. Resistance Exercise-Induced Increases in Putative Anabolic Hormones Do Not Enhance Muscle Protein Synthesis or Intracellular Signalling in Young Men. *J Physiol* 587(Pt 21):5239–47.

Westerterp, K.R., W.H. Saris, M. Van Es, and F. Ten Hoor. 1986. Use of the Doubly Labeled Water Technique in Humans during Heavy Sustained Exercise. *J Appl Physiol* 61(6):2162–67.

Westerterp-Plantenga, M.S., E.M. Kovacs, and K.J. Melanson. 2002. Habitual Meal Frequency and Energy Intake Regulation in Partially Temporally Isolated Men. *Int J Obes Relat Metab Disord* 26(1):102–10.

White, J.P., J.M. Wilson, K.G. Austin, B.K. Greer, N. St. John, and L.B. Panton. 2008. Effect of Carbohydrate-Protein Supplement Timing on Acute Exercise-Induced Muscle Damage. *J Int Soc Sports Nutr* 5:5.

Whitham, M., and J. McKinney. 2007. Effect of a Carbohydrate Mouthwash on Running Time-Trial Performance. *J Sports Sci* 25(12):1385–92.

Whitley, H.A., S.M. Humphreys, I.T. Campbell, M.A. Keegan, T.D. Jayanetti, D.A. Sperry, D.P. MaClaren, T. Reilly, and K.N. Frayn. 1998. Metabolic and Performance Responses during Endurance Exercise after High-Fat and High-Carbohydrate Meals. *J Appl Physiol* 85(2):418–24.

Wilborn, C.D., C.M. Kerksick, B.I. Campbell, L.W. Taylor, B.M. Marcello, C.J. Rasmussen, M.C. Greenwood, A. Almada, and R.B. Kreider. 2004. Effects of Zinc Magnesium Aspartate (ZMA) Supplementation on Training Adaptations and Markers of Anabolism and Catabolism. *J Int Soc Sports Nutr* 1(2):12–20.

Wildman, R.E.C., B. Campbell, and C.M. Kerksick. 2010. Carbohydrate, Exercise and Sport Performance. *Strength and Cond J* 32(1):21–29.

Wilkinson, S.B., S.M. Phillips, P.J. Atherton, R. Patel, K.E. Yarasheski, M.A. Tarnopolsky, and M.J. Rennie. 2008. Differential Effects of Resistance and Endurance Exercise in the Fed State on Signalling Molecule Phosphorylation and Protein Synthesis in Human Muscle. *J Physiol* 586(Pt 15):3701–17.

Wilkinson, S.B., M.A. Tarnopolsky, M.J. Macdonald, J.R. MacDonald, D. Armstrong, and S.M. Phillips. 2007. Consumption of Fluid Skim Milk Promotes Greater Muscle Protein Accretion after Resistance Exercise Than Does Consumption of an Isonitrogenous and Isoenergetic Soy-Protein Beverage. *Am J Clin Nutr* 85(4):1031–40.

Williams, A.B., G.M. Decourten-Myers, J.E. Fischer, G. Luo, X. Sun, and P.O. Hasselgren. 1999. Sepsis Stimulates Release of Myofilaments in Skeletal Muscle by a Calcium-Dependent Mechanism. *FASEB J* 13(11):1435–43.

Williams, C., M.G. Nute, L. Broadbank, and S. Vinall. 1990. Influence of Fluid Intake on Endurance Running Performance. A Comparison between Water, Glucose and Fructose Solutions. *Eur J Appl Physiol Occup Physiol* 60(2):112–19.

Williams, M.H. 2004. Dietary Supplements and Sports Performance: Introduction and Vitamins. *J Int Soc Sports Nutr* 1:1–6.

Willis, K.S., N.J. Peterson, and D.E. Larson-Meyer. 2008. Should We Be Concerned About the Vitamin D Status of Athletes? *Int J Sport Nutr Exerc Metab* 18(2):204–24.

Willoughby, D.S., and J. Rosene. 2001. Effects of Oral Creatine and Resistance Training on Myosin Heavy Chain Expression. *Med Sci Sports Exerc* 33(10):1674–81.

Willoughby, D.S., J.R. Stout, and C.D. Wilborn. 2007. Effects of Resistance Training and Protein Plus Amino Acid Supplementation on Muscle Anabolism, Mass, and Strength. *Amino Acids* 32(4):467–77.

Wilson, J.M., J.S. Kim, S.R. Lee, J.A. Rathmacher, B. Dalmau, J.D. Kingsley, H. Koch, A.H. Manninen, R. Saadat, and L.B. Panton. 2009. Acute and Timing Effects of Beta-Hydroxy-Beta-Methylbutyrate (HMB) on Indirect Markers of Skeletal Muscle Damage. *Nutr Metab (Lond)* 6:6.

Winnick, J.J., J.M. Davis, R.S. Welsh, M.D. Carmichael, E.A. Murphy, and J.A. Blackmon. 2005. Carbohydrate Feedings during Team Sport Exercise Preserve Physical and CNS Function. *Med Sci Sports Exerc* 37(2):306–15.

Witard, O.C., M. Tieland, M. Beelen, K.D. Tipton, L.J. Van Loon, and R. Koopman. 2009. Resistance Exercise Increases Postprandial Muscle Protein Synthesis in Humans. *Med Sci Sports Exerc* 41(1):144–54.

Wolever, T.M., and C. Bolognesi. 1996. Source and Amount of Carbohydrate Affect Postprandial Glucose and Insulin in Normal Subjects. *J Nutr* 126(11):2798–806.

Wolever, T.M., D.J. Jenkins, A.L. Jenkins, and R.G. Josse. 1991. The Glycemic Index: Methodology and Clinical Implications. *Am J Clin Nutr* 54(5):846–54.

Wolf, D.H., and W. Hilt. 2004. The Proteasome: A Proteolytic Nanomachine of Cell Regulation and Waste Disposal. *Biochim Biophys Acta* 1695(1–3):19–31.

Wolfe, R.R. 2005. Regulation of Skeletal Muscle Protein Metabolism in Catabolic States. *Curr Opin Clin Nutr Metab Care* 8(1):61–65.

Wolfe, R.R. 2006. The Underappreciated Role of Muscle in Health and Disease. *Am J Clin Nutr* 84(3):475–82.

Wolfe, R.R., D.L. Chinkes, and R.R. Wolfe. 2005. *Isotope Tracers in Metabolic Research: Principles and Practice of Kinetic Analysis.* 2nd ed. Hoboken, NJ: Wiley-Liss.

Wolfe, R.R., and S.L. Miller. 2008. The Recommended Dietary Allowance of Protein: A Misunderstood Concept. *JAMA* 299(24):2891–93.

Wolfram, G., M. Kirchgessner, H.L. Muller, and S. Hollomey. 1987. Thermogenesis in Humans after Varying Meal Time Frequency. *Ann Nutr Metab* 31(2):88–97.

Wu, C.L., C. Nicholas, C. Williams, A. Took, and L. Hardy. 2003. The Influence of High-Carbohydrate Meals with Different Glycaemic Indices on Substrate Utilisation during Subsequent Exercise. *Br J Nutr* 90(6):1049–56.

Wyatt, H.R., G.K. Grunwald, C.L. Mosca, M.L. Klem, R.R. Wing, and J.O. Hill. 2002. Long-Term Weight Loss and Breakfast in Subjects in the National Weight Control Registry. *Obes Res* 10(2):78–82.

Yang, Y., B. Jemiolo, and S. Trappe. 2006. Proteolytic mRNA Expression in Response to Acute Resistance Exercise in Human Single Skeletal Muscle Fibers. *J Appl Physiol* 101(5):1442–50.

Yannakoulia, M., L. Melistas, E. Solomou, and N. Yiannakouris. 2007. Association of Eating Frequency with Body Fatness in Pre- and Postmenopausal Women. *Obesity (Silver Spring)* 15(1):100–6.

Yaspelkis, B.B., 3rd, J.G. Patterson, P.A. Anderla, Z. Ding, and J.L. Ivy. 1993. Carbohydrate Supplementation Spares Muscle Glycogen during Variable-Intensity Exercise. *J Appl Physiol* 75(4):1477–85.

Yeo, W.K., S.L. McGee, A.L. Carey, C.D. Paton, A.P. Garnham, M. Hargreaves, and J.A. Hawley. 2010. Acute Signalling Responses to Intense Endurance Training Commenced with Low or Normal Muscle Glycogen. *Exp Physiol* 95(2):351–58.

Young, R.B., and R.M. Denome. 1984. Effect of Creatine on Contents of Myosin Heavy Chain and Myosin-Heavy-Chain mRNA in Steady-State Chicken Muscle-Cell Cultures. *Biochem J* 218(3):871–76.

Young, S. 1986. The Clinical Psychopharmacology of Trytophan. In *Nutrition and the Brain*, edited by R. Wurtman and J.J. Wurtman. New York: Raven Press.

Zanchi, N.E., F. Gerlinger-Romero, L. Guimaraes-Ferreira, M.A. De Siqueira Filho, V. Felitti, F.S. Lira, M. Seelaender, and A.H. Lancha, Jr. 2011. HMB Supplementation: Clinical and Athletic Performance-Related Effects and Mechanisms of Action. *Amino Acids* 40(4):1015–25.

Zanni, E., D.H. Calloway, and A.Y. Zezulka. 1979. Protein Requirements of Elderly Men. *J Nutr* 109(3):513–24.

Zavorsky, G.S., S. Kubow, V. Grey, V. Riverin, and L.C. Lands. 2007. An Open-Label Dose-Response Study of Lymphocyte Glutathione Levels in Healthy Men and Women Receiving Pressurized Whey Protein Isolate Supplements. *Int J Food Sci Nutr* 58(6):429–36.

Zawadzki, K.M., B.B. Yaspelkis, III, and J.L. Ivy. 1992. Carbohydrate-Protein Complex Increases the Rate of Muscle Glycogen Storage after Exercise. *J Appl Physiol* 72(5):1854–59.

Zerguini, Y., J. Dvorak, R.J. Maughan, J.B. Leiper, Z. Bartagi, D.T. Kirkendall, M. Al-Riyami, and A. Junge. 2008. Influence of Ramadan Fasting on Physiological and Performance Variables in Football Players: Summary of the F-MARC 2006 Ramadan Fasting Study. *J Sports Sci* 26(Suppl 3):S3–S6.

Zhang, Y., K. Guo, R.E. Leblanc, D. Loh, G.J. Schwartz, and Y.H. Yu. 2007. Increasing Dietary Leucine Intake Reduces Diet-Induced Obesity and Improves Glucose and Cholesterol Metabolism in Mice via Multimechanisms. *Diabetes* 56(6):1647–54.

Zinman, B., N. Ruderman, B.N. Campaigne, J.T. Devlin, and S.H. Schneider. 2004. Physical Activity/Exercise and Diabetes. *Diabetes Care* 27(Suppl 1):S58–S62.

Zotova, E.V., K.V. Savost'ianov, D.A. Chistiakov, T.R. Bursa, I.V. Galeev, I.A. Strokov, and V.V. Nosikov. 2004. Search for the Association of Polymorphic Markers for Genes Coding for Antioxidant Defense Enzymes, with Development of Diabetic Polyneuropathies in Patients with Type 1 Diabetes Mellitus. *Molekuliarnaia Biologiia* 38(2):244–49.

Zuluaga, M., C. Briggs, J. Carlisle, V. McDonald, J. McMeeken, W. Nickson, P. Oddy, and D. Wilson, eds. 1995. *Sports Physiotherapy: Applied Science and Practice*. Melbourne: Churchill Livingstone.

Zuntz, N., and W. Loeb. 1894. Über Die Bedeutung Der Verschiedene Nährstoff Als Energiequelle Der Muskelkraft. *Archiv Anat Physiol* 18:541–43.

Index